Self-Assessment C

Small Animal
Cardiopulmonary
Medicine

Wendy A Ware
DVM, MS, DipACVIM(Cardiology)
Professor, Departments of Veterinary Clinical Sciences
and Biomedical Sciences
College of Veterinary Medicine
Iowa State University
Ames, Iowa, USA

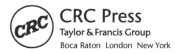
CRC Press
Taylor & Francis Group
Boca Raton London New York

CRC Press is an imprint of the
Taylor & Francis Group, an **informa** business

Self-Assessment Color Review

Small Animal Cardiopulmonary Medicine

Wendy A Warc
DVM, MS, DipACVIM(Cardiology)
Professor, Departments of Veterinary Clinical Sciences
and Biomedical Sciences
College of Veterinary Medicine
Iowa State University
Ames, Iowa, USA

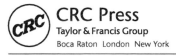

CRC Press
Taylor & Francis Group
Boca Raton London New York

CRC Press is an imprint of the
Taylor & Francis Group, an **informa** business

CRC Press
Taylor & Francis Group
6000 Broken Sound Parkway NW, Suite 300
Boca Raton, FL 33487-2742

© 2012 by Taylor & Francis Group, LLC
CRC Press is an imprint of Taylor & Francis Group, an Informa business

No claim to original U.S. Government works

ISBN-13: 9781840761641

Visit the Taylor & Francis Web site at
http://www.taylorandfrancis.com

and the CRC Press Web site at
http://www.crcpress.com

Acknowledgements

I am grateful to my colleagues who contributed cases and images to this book and to Lori Moran for technical support, as well as to commissioning editor Jill Northcott, Michael Manson, and the staff at Manson Publishing. All your help in developing and creating this publication is truly appreciated. Also, and very importantly, I am indebted to many others who, in various ways, contributed to this book, especially the pets and their owners, referring veterinarians, and hospital staff with whom my contributors and I worked and who made this collection of cases possible. Finally, but certainly not least, I owe many thanks to my family – for your continuing love, support, and patience.

Disclaimer: Every effort has been made to eliminate inaccuracies but readers are advised to confirm recommended doses in the drug data sheets before prescribing regimens. The advice and information given in this book are believed to be true and accurate at the time of going to press, but neither the editor nor the publisher can accept any legal responsibility or liability for any errors or omissions that have been made.

Preface

This book brings together a wide variety of cases involving cardiac and pulmonary diseases, or related clinical signs, that are relevant to the practicing veterinarian. The collection is appropriate not only for general practitioners looking for a quick review or reference for cardiac, respiratory, and other intrathoracic disorders, but additionally for those studying towards a higher professional qualification. Veterinary students should also find these cases useful when preparing for professional examinations. The book is also appropriate for veterinary technicians and nurses studying towards further qualifications. In addition, this collection is intended to provide an enjoyable way for practicing veterinarians to 'test' and expand their knowledge of canine and feline cardiothoracic problems.

The cases presented here largely focus on causes of respiratory distress, cough, or other signs that mainly relate to lower respiratory, cardiac, and intrathoracic disorders. The decision to emphasize diseases of intrathoracic structures was intentional. While upper respiratory conditions such as nasal and nasopharyngeal disorders clearly are important, their presenting clinical signs (e.g. nasal discharge, stridor) are often different and tend to be more easily localizable. Many cases in this book involve common diseases, with a focus on important principles of diagnosis and management. Others are more challenging or unusual. Some cases contained in this book reflect diseases (e.g. parasitic) that are common in some geographical regions, but occur with low prevalence, or not at all, in others. Because of their importance in areas where they do occur and the fact that the worldwide distribution of some diseases (e.g. heartworm disease and angiostrongylosis) appears to be increasing, it is hoped that readers living in unaffected regions will forgive their inclusion.

The cases are ordered randomly throughout the book, as they are likely to occur in clinical practice. The format is similar to other books in the 'Self-Assessment' series. The cases and related questions are presented on one page, so the reader is encouraged to think about specific answers or management strategies before turning the page to see the written explanations/answers (unless you peek!). A Classification of cases, a Further reading list arranged by topic, an Appendix listing Drugs used for cardiac and respiratory diseases, and an Index are included for reference and to facilitate a review of specific problems and their management. It is my hope that you, the reader, will find this book interesting and enjoyable, as well as useful in your practice.

Wendy A Ware

Contributors

Luca Ferasin DVM, PhD, CertVC,
DipECVIM-CA(Cardiology),
MRCVS
Specialist Veterinary Cardiology
Consultancy Ltd
Newbury, Berkshire, UK

Shannon Jones Hostetter DVM, PhD,
DipACVP(Clinical Pathology)
Assistant Professor, Department of
Veterinary Pathology
Staff Clinical Pathologist, Lloyd
Veterinary Medical Center
College of Veterinary Medicine
Iowa State University
Ames, Iowa, USA

FA (Tony) Mann DVM, MS,
DipACVS, DipACVECC
Professor, Department of Veterinary
Medicine and Surgery
Director, Small Animal Emergency and
Critical Care Services
Small Animal Soft Tissue Surgery
Service Chief
Small Animal Surgery/Neurology
Instructional Leader
Veterinary Medical Teaching Hospital
University of Missouri
Columbia, Missouri, USA

O Lynne Nelson DVM, MS,
DipACVIM(Internal Medicine and
Cardiology)
Associate Professor of Cardiology
Staff Cardiologist, Veterinary Teaching
Hospital
College of Veterinary Medicine
Washington State University
Pullman, Washington, USA

Elizabeth Riedesel DVM, DipACVR
Associate Professor, Department of
Veterinary Clinical Sciences
Staff Radiologist, Lloyd Veterinary
Medical Center
College of Veterinary Medicine
Iowa State University
Ames, Iowa, USA

Wendy A Ware DVM, MS,
DipACVIM(Cardiology)
Professor, Departments of Veterinary
Clinical Sciences and
Biomedical Sciences
Staff Cardiologist, Lloyd Veterinary
Medical Center
Iowa State University
Ames, Iowa, USA

Additional image acknowledgements

162a, c, 218a, b, c   Courtesy Dr. Oliver Garrdod
79a, b   Courtesy Dr. Phyllis Frost
103a, b, c   Courtesy Drs. Jessica Clemans and Krysta Deitz
151a, b, 195a, b   Courtesy Dr. JoAnn Morrison
8a, b   Courtesy Dr. Leslie Fox
2a, b, 116a, b   Courtesy Dr. Krysta Deitz

Abbreviations

A/Ao	aorta/aortic root	PaCO$_2$	partial pressure of carbon dioxde in arterial blood
AV	atrioventricular		
BAL	bronchoalveolar lavage	PAO$_2$	partial pressure of O$_2$ in the alveolus
BP	blood pressure		
bpm	beats per minute	PaO$_2$	partial pressure of O$_2$ in arterial blood
CBC	complete blood count		
CO$_2$	carbon dioxide	PCO$_2$	carbon dioxide partial pressure or tension
CRI	constant rate infusion		
CT	computed tomography	PCR	polymerase chain reaction
DLH	domestic longhair (cat)	PCV	packed cell volume
DSH	domestic shorthair (cat)	PO	per os
DV	dorsoventral	PRN	pro re nate (according to circumstances)
ECG	electrocardiogram		
FS	fractional shortening	PT	prothrombin time
HCO$_3$	bicarbonate	aPTT	activated partial thromboplastin time
HR	heart rate		
IM	intramuscular	RA	right atrium/atrial
IV	intravenous	RNA	ribonucleic acid
IVS	interventricular septum	RV	right ventricle/ventricular
LA	left atrium/atrial	SC	subcutaneous
LV	left ventricle/ventricular	SG	specific gravity
MRI	magnetic resonance imaging	VD	ventrodorsal
O$_2$	oxygen	VHS	vertebral heart size
PA	pulmonary artery/arterial		

Classification of cases

Airway diseases: 5, 9, 10, 15, 16, 21, 28, 39, 40, 57, 58, 72, 96, 99, 133, 151, 164, 176, 195, 200

Cardiac arrhythmias: 4, 18, 36, 37, 38, 49, 53, 54, 67, 77, 87, 91, 113, 114, 115, 130, 135, 143, 145, 173, 181, 183, 204, 217

Cardiac valvular disease, acquired: 48, 85, 86, 127, 128, 189, 211, 214, 216

Cardiomyopathies: 18, 32, 35, 36, 47, 67, 90, 110, 117, 148, 165, 170, 171, 207, 208

Cardiopulmonary tests: 20, 24, 29, 33, 44, 53, 54, 68, 75, 102, 152, 159

Collapse or weakness: 112

Congenital malformations: 13, 26, 31, 45, 50, 63, 79, 80, 88, 92, 118, 119, 120, 121, 125, 131, 139, 146, 149, 156, 163, 174, 175, 186, 188, 203, 205, 206

Congestive heart failure: 73, 117, 124, 157, 171, 187, 189, 190, 205

Diagphragmatic hernia: 3, 74, 84, 98, 140

Esophageal abnormalities: 139, 191, 200

Foreign body: 103, 167, 179

Hypertension, systemic or pulmonary: 83, 129, 131, 132, 156, 201, 211

Mediastinal diseases: 52, 93, 122, 213

Miscellaneous: 14, 56, 66, 92, 101, 142

Neoplasia: 2, 6, 8, 17, 70, 71, 76, 82, 93, 94, 109, 111, 116, 122, 123, 134, 141, 142, 158, 168, 172, 192, 209, 212, 213, 219

Parasitic diseases: 27, 55, 64, 108, 136, 137, 154, 162, 185, 199, 210, 218

Pericardial diseases: 46, 69, 140, 144, 160, 161, 209, 219

Physical examination abnormalities: 7, 12, 23, 26, 41, 51, 109, 120, 198

Pleural space abnormalities (effusion or pneumothorax): 19, 25, 30, 59, 60, 61, 78, 123, 134, 155, 193

Pneumonias and other pulmonary diseases: 11, 22, 56, 62, 65, 81, 89, 101, 105, 106, 126, 134, 150, 153, 166, 169, 177, 184, 191, 196, 197

Respiratory signs: 1, 104, 137

Respiratory therapy: 42, 43, 100, 215

Thromboembolic disease: 34, 97, 107, 129, 180

Toxicity: 65, 104, 138, 143

Trauma: 30, 81, 147, 178, 182, 194, 202

Contributed cases

LF: 19, 36, 47, 50, 53, 54, 59, 60, 72, 90, 95, 99, 123, 162, 165, 166, 177, 198, 200, 211, 218

SH: 6, 10, 25, 61, 71, 78, 141, 169, 197

TM: 42, 43, 57, 58, 66, 69, 70, 84, 118, 119, 134, 182, 213, 215

LN: 5, 13, 14, 15, 21, 34, 45, 77, 105, 106, 111, 114, 115, 126, 129, 138, 159, 163, 184, 204

ER: 3, 9, 11, 16, 17, 22, 28, 30, 39, 40, 56, 62, 65, 74, 81, 89, 93, 94, 98, 101, 108, 122, 142, 147, 155, 164, 167, 176, 178, 179, 191, 192, 193, 196, 202, 212

1 A 4-year-old male Rottweiler (1) is presented with a history of a chronic dry cough. Lately he has become anorexic and he now is having trouble breathing. You observe increased respiratory rate and effort. On auscultation you hear no cardiac murmur, but notice increased breath sounds and pulmonary crackles.

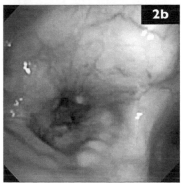

i. Describe characteristics of the dog's appearance that indicate respiratory distress.

ii. How can respiratory pattern help suggest the location of disease in patients with respiratory distress?

2 A 13-year-old neutered male Shih Tzu has been coughing for the past 3 weeks, after he was at a boarding facility for several weeks. Decreased appetite and weight loss were noted recently. Amoxicillin with clavulanate and hydrocodone were prescribed elsewhere for suspected bronchitis, but the owner has had trouble administering the medication. The dog is quiet, but alert and responsive. Body temperature, HR, and respiratory rate are normal. Soft pulmonary crackles are heard over the left hemithorax. Tracheal palpation elicits a non-productive cough. The rest of the physical examination is normal. Chest radiographs show a moderate to severe bronchointerstitial pattern in the caudal lung with alveolar infiltrates in the right cranial lobe. Cardiac size and pulmonary vasculature are normal. A hemogram shows mild thrombocytosis, but is otherwise normal; serum chemistries and urinalysis are unremarkable. Bronchoscopy (2a, b) and BAL are performed.

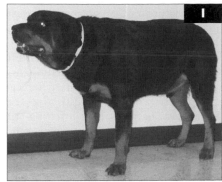

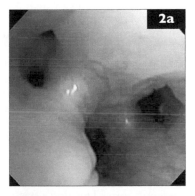

i. What findings are shown in the bronchoscopic images?

ii. What differential diagnoses should be considered?

iii. How would you proceed with this case?

1 i. His posture suggests severe respiratory distress ('orthopnea'). Dogs with orthopnea stand or sit with their elbows abducted (allowing full rib expansion) and neck extended, resist lateral or dorsally recumbent positions, and are reluctant to eat and drink or even swallow saliva (note saliva hanging from this dog's mouth). Dilated pupils also suggest anxiety (note tapetal reflection in photograph).

ii. Respiratory rate and character can provide diagnostic clues. Reduced lung compliance produces a 'restrictive' (rapid and shallow) breathing pattern, which minimizes the work of ventilating stiffer lungs. Exhalation or both phases may appear labored. Pulmonary edema, other interstitial infiltrative disease (e.g. bacterial pneumonia, as in this dog), and pulmonary fibrosis produce this pattern; inspiratory pulmonary crackles are common. Partial lung collapse from pleural effusion or other pleural space disease also decreases lung compliance, although large-volume effusion can cause slow, labored inspiration with pronounced abdominal effort.

Airway narrowing causes an 'obstructive' breathing pattern. Slower, deeper breaths reduce frictional resistance and respiratory work, although respiratory rate can be normal or increased with peripheral airway disease. The location of the narrowing determines which phase is more labored and (often) prolonged. Lower airway obstruction causes expiratory difficulty, sometimes with wheezing. Upper airway obstruction produces slow or labored inspiration, with or without stridor.

2 i. The airways appear diffusely edematous with mild erythema consistent with generalized bronchial inflammation. Small yellowish tan nodules are seen on some surfaces (**2b**, from right cranial bronchus).

ii. The radiographic pattern suggests pneumonia or an infiltrative inflammatory or neoplastic disease. Given the history of boarding, infectious tracheobronchitis with secondary pneumonia is a consideration. Small nodules within the airways most often result from chronic inflammation and mucosal proliferation secondary to chronic bronchitis, but neoplastic infiltration is another consideration. Nodules found only near the carina may signal infection with the parasite *Oslerus osleri* in endemic areas. This dog's systemic signs, along with the relatively recent onset of coughing, are not typical for chronic bronchitis.

iii. In addition to BAL cytologic analysis and culture, airway brushings and pinch biopsy of a nodule should be obtained during the bronchoscopic procedure. If evaluation of these samples does not yield a definitive diagnosis, lung biopsy is recommended. In this dog, cytologic evaluation revealed mild purulent inflammation, mild chronic hemorrhage, and variably-sized cohesive clusters of highly vacuolated cells thought to be carcinoma cells. BAL cultures yielded no aerobic or anaerobic growth.

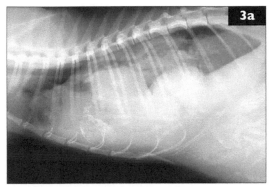

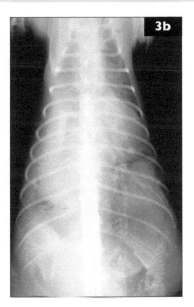

3 A 3-year-old female DSH cat is presented for 1 week of lethargy and increased respiratory effort. She is at 56 days of gestation. A similar episode occurred with the previous pregnancy and responded favorably to antibiotic therapy. This episode seems to be worse. Right lateral (3a) and DV (3b) thoracic radiographs are made.
i. What radiographic abnormalities are evident?
ii. What is the radiographic diagnosis?

4 A 9-year-old female Dalmation is presented because of a collapse episode earlier in the day. She has been less active lately and becomes winded easily when on walks. The dog appears anxious and slightly tachypneic. Mucous membranes are pink, femoral pulses are weak and of variable intensity, and the HR is rapid and irregular. There is a soft systolic murmur heard best at the right apex,

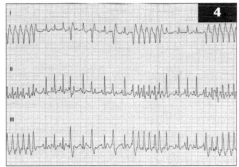

but also heard at the left apex. Lung sounds are increased. You record an ECG. Simultaneous leads I, II, and III at 25 mm/s, 1 cm = 1 mV are shown (4).
i. What is the ECG diagnosis?
ii. How would you initially manage this case?
iii. What do you recommend next?

3 i. There is increased opacity in the ventral and right halves of the thoracic cavity. Only a short dorsal segment of the left crus of the diaphragm is distinct; the remainder is effaced by the increased thoracic opacity. The trachea is displaced dorsally, but remains mid-line in the DV view. The heart is shifted dorsally and to the left. Only the left lung lobes are well inflated with well-defined vessels. The increased thoracic opacity is a mix of solid soft tissue or fluid and mineralized opacity of fetal skeletal structures. A fetal skull is evident ventrally at the 5th intercostal space and a different fetal lumbar spine crosses the pleura-peritoneal junction ventrally.
ii. Right-sided diaphragmatic hernia with thoracic displacement of gravid uterus and probably liver. The degree of fetal skeletal mineralization is consistent with late-term gestation. No signs of fetal death are evident. Ultrasound would be valuable to determine fetal viability. In several reports, the most common organs to be herniated through a tear in the diaphragm are liver, stomach, and small intestine. Several case reports of diaphragmatic herniation of gravid uterus in dogs appear in the literature.

4 i. Paroxysmal ventricular tachycardia (at 300 bpm) is seen at the beginning of the strip, just after the middle, and at the right edge. Sinus tachycardia (at 180 bpm) is evident intermittently. Single ventricular premature complexes also occur, and are easier to distinguish in leads I and III. The sinus complexes indicate a normal mean electrical axis. P waves are slightly wide (0.05 second) consistent with LA enlargement; sinus QRS complexes are also wide (~0.08 second), suggesting myocardial disease and abnormal intraventricular conduction. Other complex measurements are normal. Each 1 mm box = 0.04 second at 25 mm/s.
ii. IV lidocaine is the initial drug of choice for acute treatment of ventricular tachyarrhythmias. An IV catheter is placed as soon as possible. Supplemental O_2 may be helpful. The dog should be carried/carted if it must be moved; stress should be minimized.
iii. Identify underlying abnormalities as soon as possible; screen for electrolyte or other metabolic or hematologic abnormalities, obtain thoracic (and possibly abdominal) radiographs, as well as an echocardiogram to assess cardiac structure and function. Additional antiarrhythmic strategies are used if lidocaine is ineffective and for long-term therapy (see Further reading). Additional therapy depends on test results. This dog had dilated cardiomyopathy.

5 The owner of a 12-week-old kitten complains of 'noisy breathing'. The kitten was adopted 4 weeks ago from the animal shelter and has always made a lot of noise with normal breathing. However, the sound has become more pronounced as the kitten has grown. Breathing is especially noisy when the kitten plays or is excited. Occasionally the kitten gags when eating, but otherwise has been normal. High-pitched inspiratory stridor and exaggerated inspiratory effort are the most obvious physical findings. The image was obtained with a bronchoscope

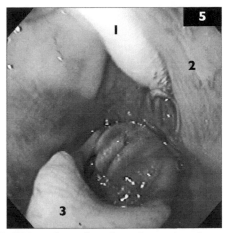

camera after heavy sedation (5; 1 – swab lifting the soft palate, 2 – soft palate, 3 – epiglottis).
i. What abnormality is shown?
ii. What conditions could cause this?
iii. How would you manage this case?

6 A 12-year-old spayed female Springer Spaniel develops lethargy and respiratory distress. Physical examination findings include weakness, labored respiration, muffled heart sounds, jugular vein distension, and abdominal distension with a pronounced fluid wave. Peri-cardial effusion with cardiac tamponade is suspected based on radiographic findings and the electrical alternans evident on an ECG. Echocardiographic

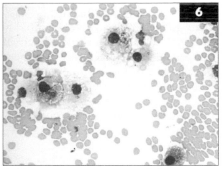

examination is desired, but not readily available at present. In view of the patient's urgent status, pericardiocentesis is done to relieve the tamponade. Approximately 300 ml of red, turbid pericardial effusion is removed. The fluid is grossly bloody, with a cell count of 6110/µl, pH of 6.4, protein content of 57 g/l (5.7 g/dl), and PCV of 0.73 l/l (73%). A cytospin preparation of the effusion is shown (6, Wright's stain, 50× oil).
i. What cytologic features reveal this to be pathologic rather than iatrogenic hemorrhage?
ii. What etiologies are most likely for the hemorrhagic pericardial effusion in this dog?

5 i. This image of the larynx was taken during inspiration. It shows failure of the laryngeal arytenoid cartilages and vocal folds to abduct. This finding is the hallmark of laryngeal paralysis.

ii. Laryngeal paralysis was suspected to be congenital in this case. Congenital laryngeal paralysis has been most commonly reported in dogs, especially Siberian Huskies, Bouvier des Flandres, and Bull Terriers. Paralysis could occur as a result of trauma to the cervical region; the earlier history in this kitten was unknown. Acquired laryngeal paralysis usually occurs in older animals and may be idiopathic (such as with the Labrador Retriever) or secondary to a polyneuropathy (e.g. myasthenia gravis, hypothyroidism), anterior thoracic neoplasia, or other mass lesion. (**Note:** Other potential causes for upper airway obstruction in cats include nasopharyngeal polyp, laryngeal lymphoma, or other mass lesions.)

iii. A unilateral arytenoid lateralization surgical procedure is the best method to alleviate the upper airway obstruction. Good results are usually obtained. Aspiration pneumonia can sometimes be a complicating factor after repair.

6 i. The presence of phagocytized erythrocytes within the cytoplasm of macrophages (erythrophagia) and lack of platelets in this sample are indicators of pathologic hemorrhage. Hemosiderin (seen in the image as deep blue-black pigment within the cytoplasm of macrophages) is an additional indicator of pathologic hemorrhage. Hemosiderin is an intracellular iron storage complex resulting from erythrocyte breakdown. Hematoidin, a yellow crystal that forms secondary to hemoglobin degradation, is another indicator of pathologic hemorrhage.

With iatrogenic hemorrhage, platelets are present and erythrophagia is not evident unless a prolonged time has occurred between sample acquisition and analysis. Hemosiderin and hematoidin are not seen with iatrogenic hemorrhage.

ii. Neoplastic effusion is most likely in a dog of this age. Hemangiosarcoma and, less often, chemodectoma are the tumors most commonly associated with pericardial effusion in the dog. A thorough echocardiographic examination often reveals the mass lesion in such cases. Mesothelioma and occasionally other neoplasms are other potential causes of pericardial effusion. Although idiopathic pericardial effusion also occurs frequently in dogs, it usually affects younger individuals. In this case, hemangiosarcoma involving the right auricle was found at necropsy.

7 A dog of unknown age is presented because the owner thinks its exercise tolerance has decreased. Physical examination is unremarkable except for a murmur, which is loudest on the left side.

i. When a murmur is auscultated, what characteristics are the most important to identify?

ii. What are the main causes of a systolic murmur heard best over the left chest wall?

8 An 11-year-old spayed female Cocker Spaniel is presented for coughing episodes that began a week ago, after a hiking trip to the mountains. The cough is becoming more severe and is worse in the morning and after periods of rest. The dog was referred for suspected congestive heart failure, but initial furosemide treatment has not improved the cough. Prior medical history includes a patent ductus arteriosus (closed at 3 months of age), pyometra (resolved after spay 2 years ago), mammary gland adenocarcinoma and mammary mixed-cell fibrosarcoma (removed 1.5 years ago, with no evidence of metastasis), early degenerative AV valve disease, hypertension, and occasional second degree AV block. She is being treated with oral cyclo phosphamide, piroxicam, and enalapril. A grade 1/6 systolic murmur is heard over the tricuspid region and a clicking sound is noted on inspiration; otherwise, the physical examination is unremarkable. Thoracic radiographs reveal a singular pulmonary nodule in the periphery of the right caudal lung lobe. The nodule appears distant to the major lobar bronchus. No other radiographic abnormalities are evident. Bron-

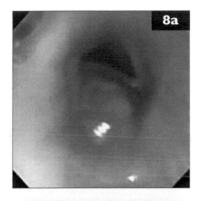

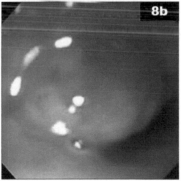

choscopy is performed to evaluate the airways and collect samples for cytology and culture. Images are from the right caudal bronchus (8a, b).

i. Would a single peripheral lung mass be expected to cause severe paroxysmal coughing?

ii. What other problems should be considered?

iii. What does bronchoscopy reveal?

7 i. Timing (e.g. systolic, diastolic, continuous), point of maximal intensity (PMI), and intensity (loudness) at the PMI. A murmur's timing within the cardiac cycle helps identify its origin. Knowing what events generate normal heart sounds (S_1 and S_2), and understanding the timing of systole (between S_1 and S_2) and diastole (after S_2 until the next S_1) in each patient is important. PMI is described by the hemithorax and valve area (or terms 'apex' or 'base') where the murmur is loudest. Murmur intensity is usually graded on a 1–6 scale.

Grade	Murmur
1	Very soft murmur; heard only in quiet surroundings.
2	Soft murmur, but easily heard.
3	Moderate intensity murmur.
4	Loud murmur, but no precordial thrill.
5	Loud murmur with palpable precordial thrill.
6	Very loud murmur with precordial thrill; also heard when stethoscope lifted slightly away from chest wall.

The murmur's 'shape', radiation, quality, and pitch are other characteristics.

ii. Left basilar systolic murmurs usually are ejection-type (crescendo–decrescendo) murmurs, often caused by ventricular outflow obstruction. Physiologic murmurs (as with fever, exercise, hyperthyroidism, anemia) occur from increased ejection velocity or turbulence. Increased flow volume can cause a murmur of 'relative' valve stenosis. A soft (innocent or functional) murmur sometimes occurs in structurally normal hearts. Mitral regurgitation produces a holosystolic (or decrescendo) murmur loudest near the left apex. Causes include mitral degeneration, infection, congenital malformation, and LV dilation.

8 i. Given the peripheral location of this nodule, and its apparent distance from a major airway, the dog's violent coughing episodes seemed unusual. Primary disease involving a large airway was thought more likely. Therefore, bronchoscopic examination with BAL was done prior to surgical mass removal (right caudal lobectomy).

ii. Major airway collapse, infectious or allergic bronchitis, airway foreign body (such as inhaled plant material), as well as neoplastic invasion of the airways.

iii. A smooth fleshy bump is seen on the approach to the right caudal bronchus (8a). The pale mass is seen more clearly within this bronchus (8b). Although not evident radiographically, the pulmonary nodule had invaded the right caudal bronchus, triggering the cough. The remaining airways were normal. Histopathology of the surgically-excised mass revealed a poorly differentiated pulmonary sarcoma. Late metastasis from the dog's previous mammary mixed-cell fibrosarcoma was suspected, although a primary lung tumor could not be ruled out.

9 A 16-year-old male Poodle is referred for evaluation of a long-term intermittent cough with excitement that has been more persistent in the last month. Over the last several days the dog has developed trouble breathing, and on presentation has dyspnea with marked inspiratory effort and cyanosis. An emergency lateral radiograph is taken (9a).

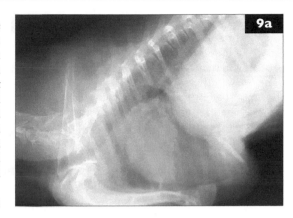

i. Is a cause for the dyspnea evident?

ii. What are the etiologic differential diagnoses?

iii. What is the explanation for the shape of the ventral thoracic-to-abdominal body wall contour?

10 An 8-year-old intact male Basenji is presented for chronic coughing. A dry, non-productive cough is observed during the physical examination and is easily elicited with tracheal palpation. Thoracic auscultation reveals normal heart sounds and increased breath sounds, with pulmonary crackles heard ventrally. A diffuse bronchointerstitial pattern is seen on thoracic radiographs. BAL is performed. A cytospin preparation of bronchoalveolar fluid (10a, Wright's stain, 100× oil) and a direct smear from BAL fluid (10b, Wright's stain, 20×) are shown.

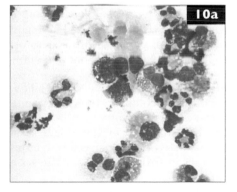

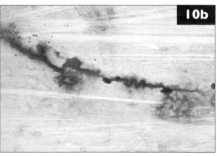

i. Describe the findings in 10a.

ii. Identify the structure visible in 10b and describe its significance in a BAL sample.

iii. Are additional diagnostic tests indicated? If so, what would you recommend?

9 i. Yes. A soft tissue/fluid intratracheal opacity (mass effect), at the 1st intercostal space, obliterates the dorsal tracheal border and markedly narrows the lumen. The 'mass' tapers at the dorsal tracheal border, suggesting either a mural or broad-based luminal lesion. Lung inflation is poor despite a wide tracheal diameter caudal to the lesion. Because of the diaphragmatic cupola's marked cranio-dorsal shift and vertical xiphoid orien-

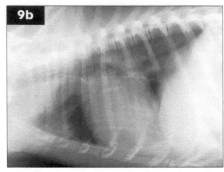

tation, the cranioventral abdominal wall appears to be pulled into the thoracic cavity.
ii. Obstructive tracheal lesions include: mural mass (inflammatory [e.g. polyp, granuloma] or neoplastic); intraluminal lesion (e.g. abscess, granuloma, tracheal parasites, foreign body); extratracheal lesion (e.g. peritracheal hemorrhage, neoplasia, abscess, granuloma). In this dog, a thin-walled, fluid-filled tracheal cyst was excised during emergency surgery. Postoperatively, thoracic contour is normal (**9b**).
iii. The diaphragm's position and 'sucked-in' appearance of the xiphoid and abdominal wall during inspiration are consistent with severe upper airway obstruction. As external intercostal muscle contraction pulls the ribs outward, strong negative intrapleural pressure sucks the ventral diaphragm and xiphoid craniodorsally and mimics pectus excavatum. Such paradoxical inspiratory movement has been reported in English Bulldogs with sleep apnea. Dorsal sternal deflection in patients with respiratory distress should prompt investigation for upper airway (including nasopharynx) obstruction.

10 i. This sample shows eosinophilic and neutrophilic inflammation. Additionally, two ciliated columnar respiratory epithelial cells, two alveolar macrophages, and a mast cell are present.
ii. The structure in this image is a Curschmann's spiral. These form when bronchioles become plugged with inspissated mucus. The presence of Curschmann's spirals in BAL samples indicates small airway disease with increased mucus production.
iii. Yes. Microbiological culture of the BAL sample is warranted to rule out infectious causes of bronchitis. Heartworm and lungworm testing is also indicated to rule out a parasitic disease, especially because eosinophilic inflammation is present. ECG and echocardiography are useful to rule out cardiac disease (none seen in this case). A CBC, serum biochemistry panel, and urinalysis may also provide helpful information. In this particular case, an underlying cause was not determined and the patient was treated for chronic bronchitis.

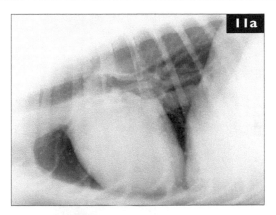

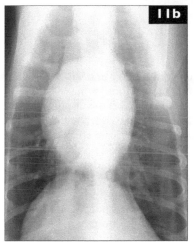
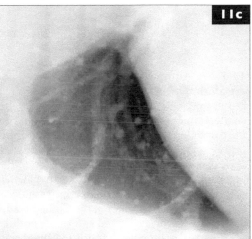

11 An 11-year-old male Collie is presented for evaluation of a lump on the nose. Over the course of a month the lump has gone from soft to firm. Due to the older age of the patient, right lateral (**11a, c**) and DV (**11b**) thoracic radiographs are taken for evaluation of potential metastasis.

i. Are there findings consistent with pulmonary metastasis?

ii. How will you differentiate benign from malignant pulmonary nodules?

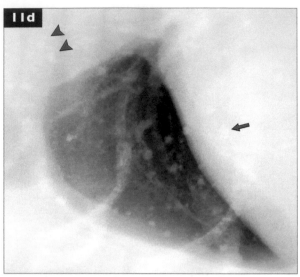

11 i. No. Although there is a diffuse small nodular pulmonary pattern, the nodules are all similar in size and strikingly opaque, similar to regional bone opacity. The red arrow heads in **11d** (enlargement of the cranioventral thorax) point to two small nodules that appear summated (superimposed) with the overlying rib opacity. One nodule (small red arrow) has a peripheral mineral opaque ring. Also, some nodules are not spherical, but mildly irregular in shape. This is the typical appearance of mineralized pulmonary nodules, also known as pulmonary osteoma, heterotopic bone formation (abnormal formation of true bone within extraskeletal soft tissues), or mineralized inactive granulomas. Although this can be seen in many dogs, it is not uncommon in the Collie breed. It is considered an incidental finding. There are no variably sized soft tissue nodules typical of pulmonary metastases.

ii. Without a biopsy, definitive differentiation between benign and malignant pulmonary nodules is not possible. Repeat radiographs can be used to assess changes in number or size of the nodules; generally, an increase in number and/or size indicates biological activity. Malignant nodules are likely to progress more rapidly than a benign process. Nodules static in size and number over several months are likely inactive and benign. Untreated infectious granulomas are likely to continue to progress. Ultimately, biopsy may be needed to make the differentiation.

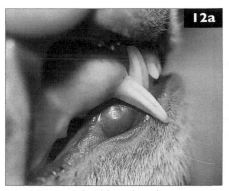
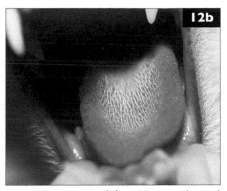

12 A 6-month-old male Lilac Point Siamese cat is presented for tiring easily and increased breathing effort. The kitten appears alert and anxious. HR is 200 bpm, with a regular rhythm. On auscultation, a grade 3–4/6 systolic murmur is heard, loudest at the right sternal border; breath sounds are fairly loud. The precordial impulse is strong bilaterally. Femoral pulses are normal. Jugular veins appear normal. Oral examination is shown (**12a, b**).

i. What abnormality is evident on the oral examination?

ii. What are the potential causes of this?

iii. What tests would you do next in this case?

13 A routine physical examination is performed on a 1-year-old male DSH cat that was recently adopted from the animal shelter. The examination is normal except for a loud holosystolic murmur heard best at the left cardiac apex. This ECG is obtained (**13**; leads I, II, and III at 50 mm/s, 1 cm = 1 mV).

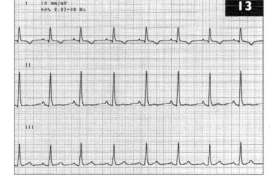

i. Identify the HR and rhythm.

ii. Are abnormalities of ECG complex size or configuration present? If so, what do they suggest?

iii. What are some potential differential diagnoses for the murmur, based on the information available?

12 i. Cyanosis. The oral mucous membranes and tongue appear bluish/grayish ('muddy').

ii. 'Central' cyanosis is associated with generalized hypoxemia; 'peripheral' cyanosis refers to local hemoglobin desaturation caused by poor peripheral circulation (as with arterial thromboembolism or cold exposure). Hypoxemia causes visible cyanosis when desaturated hemoglobin exceeds 50 g/l (5 g/dl). Chronic arterial hypoxemia stimulates erythropoiesis and erythrocytosis (polycythemia), which increases blood O_2 carrying capacity. In animals with normal PCV, visible cyanosis usually indicates severe hypoxemia (PaO_2 <45–50 mmHg). Polycythemic animals can appear cyanotic with milder hypoxemia because of greater hemoglobin content. Anemic animals may be severely hypoxemic without cyanosis. Hypoxemia and cyanosis are difficult to detect with carbon monoxide toxicity or methemoglobinemia because mucous membrane color is altered; even with a normal PaO_2, total blood O_2 content is reduced.

Common causes of central cyanosis include severe pulmonary or pleural space disease, airway obstruction, pulmonary edema, hypoventilation, and right-to-left shunting congenital cardiac defects. Exercise increases right-to-left shunting and cyanosis because peripheral vascular resistance decreases as skeletal muscle blood flow increases.

iii. Thoracic radiographs are indicated next. If a primary respiratory cause is not evident, echocardiography with Doppler is indicated to evaluate for congenital malformations. A PCV will detect erythrocytosis.

13 i. The HR is approximately 160 bpm and the rhythm is normal sinus rhythm.
ii. The P waves appear normal in size (0.03 s × 0.2 mV) and the PR interval is normal (0.08 seconds). The QRS is both prolonged (0.06 seconds) and tall (2.2 mV, lead II), which suggests LV enlargement. The QT interval is normal (~0.18 seconds).
iii. Congenital mitral valve dysplasia is a leading differential considering the signalment, murmur location, and criteria for LV enlargement. Early onset hypertrophic or dilated cardiomyopathy with secondary mitral regurgitation also is possible, but is fairly uncommon at such a young age. Ventricular septal defect (VSD) is a common congenital anomaly in the cat and usually causes LV enlargement, but the VSD murmur typically is heard best at the right sternal border. This cat was ultimately diagnosed with severe mitral valve dysplasia.

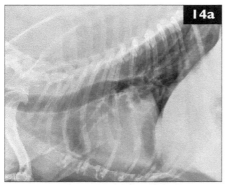
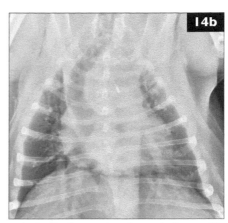

14 The owner of a 14-year-old Scottish Terrier requests removal of a small eyelid growth on her dog. During the general physical examination a holosystolic murmur is ausculted at the left cardiac apex consistent with mitral valve regurgitation. Radiographs (**14a, b**) are taken to estimate the severity of mitral regurgitation prior to anesthesia for eyelid growth removal. No cardiopulmonary clinical signs have been noted.

i. What is your assessment in this case, and is there evidence for a mass lesion?
ii. How would you clarify this?

15 The owner of a 9-year old male Pomeranian-cross complains that his dog has been coughing chronically, especially with activity. The owner reports that the dog is active and behaves normally. The cough is described as a loud, hacking sound. A grade 2/6 holosystolic murmur is heard at the left apex, consistent with mitral valve regurgitation. Thoracic radiographs reveal mild LA enlargement and no evidence of congestive heart failure. Bronchoscopy is done; the tracheal bifurcation region is shown in the image (**15**).

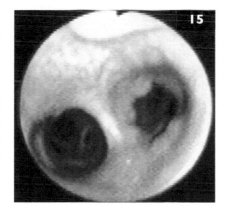

i. Describe the bronchoscopic findings.
ii. What can cause this?
iii. How should this case be managed?

14 i. There is equivocal evidence of LA enlargement on these films. The cardiac silhouette is primarily affected by the chest conformation in this dog (short and wide thoracic cavity) leading to an overall initial appearance of a larger cardiac silhouette. The VHS is only mildly increased (VHS 10.7 v). The pulmonary vessels appear normal in size. There is a mild increase in bronchointerstitial markings that is often identified in older dogs. The mitral regurgitation ausculted in this case would be assessed as hemodynamically mild at this time. There is a curious rightward bowing of the distal trachea before the main bronchial

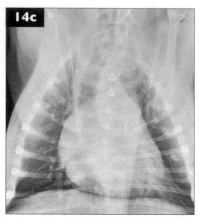

branches on the DV projection. The cranial mediastinum is slightly wide on this view, which could be suspicious for a mass lesion. However, the lateral view does not suggest tracheal deviation or an obvious increase in soft tissue opacity in this region.

ii. The trachea is a dynamic structure and its position will often shift rightward with cervical ventroflexion in the dog. Repositioning the dog with the neck extended while repeating the radiographs will often clarify 'dynamic trachea versus mass lesion' (14c).

15 i. The lumen of the left main bronchus appears narrower than the right. The tissue appears undulating and redundant and it 'sags' into the bronchial lumen.

ii. Bronchial ring weakening with mucosal membrane redundancy can occur as a part of the tracheal collapse complex. Classically, the cervical and/or thoracic trachea are affected; redundant membranes may be obvious on radiographs as the dorsal trachealis membrane sags into the tracheal lumen. When bronchial airways are affected (alone or with tracheal collapse), their radiographic appearance may be normal. Bronchoscopy or fluoroscopy may be needed to diagnose bronchial collapse. In some cases, airway collapse is caused by external compression from a mass lesion or severe LA enlargement. The LA was not considered large enough to cause compression in this dog.

iii. Airway collapse is usually managed medically. This often consists of a cough suppressant to reduce coughing 'fits' (which stimulate local inflammation), exercise restriction, and weight reduction in obese patients (to reduce intrathoracic pressure and compression). Bronchodilators, sometimes with short-term corticosteroid use, can help, especially if small airway disease is concurrent. In severe cases, where complete airway collapse leads to life-threatening hypoxia, stents may be implanted to maintain airway patency.

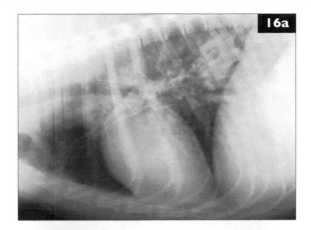

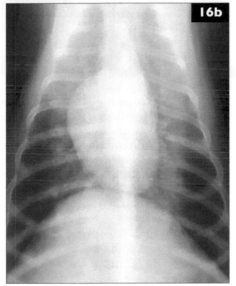

16 A 2-year-old neutered male Brittany is presented after 4 weeks of productive coughing. A 2-week course of antibiotic therapy for suspected pneumonia has had no effect. CBC reveals 38,800/μl WBCs, with 24,900/μl neutrophils, 1,880/μl lymphocytes, 287/μl monocytes, and 11,800/μl eosinophils. Thoracic radiographs are made (**16a, b**).

i. What pulmonary pattern is present?

ii. What are the etiologic differentials for this pattern in the dog?

iii. What additional diagnostic tests should be done?

23

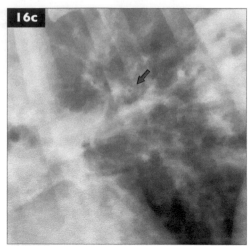

16 i. Mild diffuse bronchial pattern with a focal mass in the right dorsomedial caudal lung lobe.

ii. Evaluation of bronchial wall features is important when bronchial shadows are prominent. In dogs, thin and well-defined walls are most likely related to calcification, considered to be an aging change without clinical significance. If the walls are thickened, with both inner and outer surfaces reasonably well defined, chronic inflammation is most likely; etiologic differentials should include allergic response, inhaled irritants (smoke), parasitic inflammation, and eosinophilic infiltrates. Thickened bronchial walls with a well-defined internal border and a hazy loss of the external border has been referred to as peribronchiolar cuffing (arrow, **16c**); differentials for this effect include edema, eosinophilic infiltrates, and bronchopneumonia.

iii. The eosinophilia in this case suggests a hypersensitivity response. Fecal examination for parasites and heartworm testing should be done, although the intensity of eosinophilia is unusual. If negative, bronchoscopy and BAL with cytologic examination and culture should be considered. However, eosinophilic bronchopneumopathy (pulmonary infiltrates with eosinophils) often remains of undetermined etiology, as was the case with this dog. The mass effect in this dog may represent an eosinophilic granuloma or abscess. Further evaluation was not permitted.

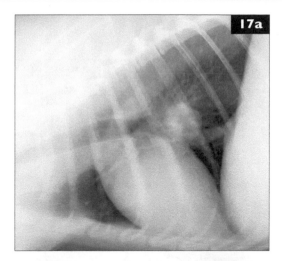

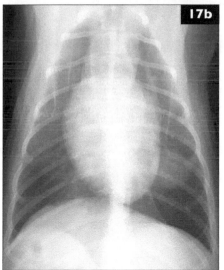

17 A 10-year-old spayed female Toy Poodle is presented for a 1-month history of a dry hacking cough throughout the day and night. She is otherwise healthy. Physical examination is normal. Thoracic radiographs (**17a, b**) are made.
i. What is the major finding?
ii. What are the differential diagnoses?
iii. What would the relevance of CT imaging be for a patient such as this?

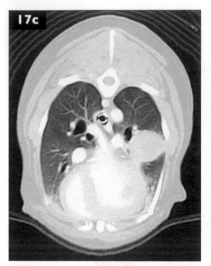

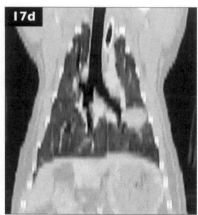

17 i. There is a spherical soft tissue/fluid opacity mass within the hilar region of the left caudal lobe. It is approximately two intercostal spaces wide, with discrete margins except for its cranioventral axial border. Other thoracic structures are unremarkable.

ii. The most common cause of a single lung mass in the dog is primary lung tumor. Other differentials include granuloma, abscess, and cyst.

iii. Although the tumor's histopathologic grade is important for making a prognosis, so too is identification of regional lymph node enlargement and involvement of other lung lobes. CT imaging has greater sensitivity for detecting both tracheobronchial lymphadenomegaly and pulmonary metastasis than radiography. It can also help with any surgical planning (**17c, d**). Bronchoalveolar carcinoma was diagnosed in this case.

18 A 3-year-old male Doberman Pinscher is presented for anorexia, weakness, and coughing of 10-day duration. The dog is lethargic and tachypneic. Mucous membranes are pale pink, with slightly slow capillary refill time. The HR is irregular and rapid. Pulses are weak and variable. The jugular veins are normal. There is a soft systolic murmur at the left apex. Thoracic radiographs indicate cardiomegaly with a moderate amount of pulmonary edema. An ECG is recorded (18, simultaneous leads I, II, and III at 25 mm/s, 1 cm = 1 mV).

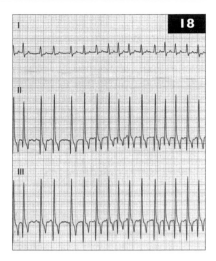

i. Describe the ECG findings.
ii. What is your assessment of this dog's problems?
iii. What are your initial therapeutic goals?

19 A 12-year-old male Greyhound has had recurrent respiratory distress episodes over the past month. The dog appears quiet, but fully responsive. Muffled heart and lung sounds are heard on thoracic auscultation. Chest percussion reveals a bilateral horizontal line of dullness. Jugular veins are distended. Brief thoracic ultrasound indicates pleural effusion and mild pericardial effusion. Thoracocentesis yields 400 ml of clear yellow fluid: SG, 1.020; total protein, 24 g/l (2.4 g/dl); albumin 15 g/l (1.5 g/dl); globulin 9 g/l (0.9 g/dl); alb/glob ratio, 1.67; cytologic examination, moderate cellularity (WBC count 60/µl) with excellent cell preservation, mixed cell population with numerous small lymphocytes, occasional neutrophils and a large population of foamy activated macrophages, scattered erythrocytes are seen, many macrophages show erythrophagia; occasional reactive mesothelial cells, but no overtly neoplastic cells are noted; there is a lightly basophilic proteinaceous background; enrichment culture and *Actinomyces/Nocardia* culture results are both negative.

Serum biochemistry shows mildly increased cholesterol (8.2 mmol/l [316.6 mg/dl]; normal 3.8–7.0 mmol/l [146.7–270.3 mg/dl]), urea (11 mmol/l [30.8 mg/dl]; normal 2–9 mmol/l [5.6–25.2 mg/dl]), and creatinine (176 µmol/l [2 mg/dl]; normal 27–124 µmol/l [0.3–1.4 mg/dl]), and moderately low albumin (15 g/l [1.5 g/dl]; normal 22–35 g/l [2.2–3.5 g/dl]); in-house 'dipstick' urinalysis (free-catch) shows marked proteinuria.

i. What type of fluid was drained from this patient?
ii. What are the differential diagnoses for this type of effusion?
iii. What additional tests would be indicated?

18 i. The HR is 200 bpm. The rhythm is atrial fibrillation (AF). Mean electrical axis is normal (~90°). Chaotic atrial electrical activation characterizes AF. There are no P waves because organized atrial depolarization is absent. Irregular ECG baseline undulations (fibrillation or 'f') waves occur instead. The ventricular rate is always irregular and often rapid, depending on AV conduction velocity and recovery time. QRS complexes usually appear normal with AF (unless abnormal intraventricular conduction coexists); minor variation in QRS amplitude is common.

ii. Clinical signs suggest pulmonary congestion and low cardiac output. Dilated cardiomyopathy is likely, although longstanding congenital disease affecting the left heart is possible. Atrial dilation predisposes to AF. AF can precipitate congestive failure with underlying cardiac disease. Advancing heart disease increases sympathetic activation, which accelerates AV conduction and ventricular rate. The disorganized atrial activation of AF prevents effective atrial contraction, which is especially important for optimal ventricular filling at high HRs. Therefore, onset of AF with uncontrolled ventricular rate (and loss of the 'atrial kick') impairs ventricular filling, reduces cardiac output, and promotes congestion.

iii. Rapidly reduce HR to improve cardiac filling and output (IV diltiazem) and improve oxygenation (IV furosemide, supplemental O_2). Further assessment and therapy should follow.

19 i. Fluid analysis suggests a longstanding transudate, which has attracted inflammatory cells into the pleural space ('modified transudate').

ii. Differential diagnoses include congestive heart failure, neoplasia, and thoracic organ injury such as diaphragmatic hernia or lung lobe torsion. Hypoalbuminemia (reduced oncotic pressure) exacerbates transudative effusions. Elevated central venous pressure and distended jugular veins can occur with large-volume pleural effusion as well as from right-sided heart failure or inflow obstruction.

iii. Urine protein/creatinine ratio should be measured on a cystocentesis sample; it was 2.7 in this case, indicating a protein losing nephropathy. Urine culture was negative. Renal biopsy would provide histologic diagnosis. Post-thoracocentesis radiographs and echocardiography are also advised to screen for cardiac or other intrathoracic disease.

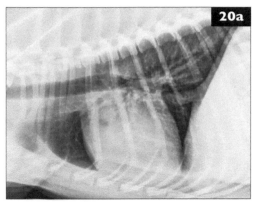
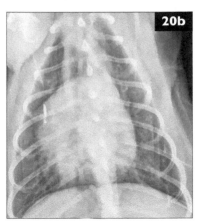

20 A 9-year-old 6 kg (13.5 lb) male neutered mixed breed dog is presented for a routine geriatric examination. No problems are reported at home. Physical examination is normal except for a soft systolic murmur heard best at the left apex. Early degenerative valve disease is suspected. Lateral (20a) and DV (20b) chest radiographs are obtained.

i. What is a 'vertebral heart score' (VHS)?
ii. How is VHS calculated?
iii. What is a normal VHS?
iv. Can the VHS be used in cats?

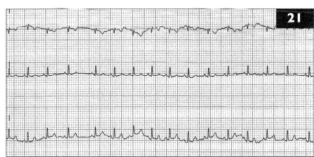

21 An 11-year-old female DSH cat is presented for cough and intermittent open-mouth breathing. The coughing began several months ago. During the coughing and breathing 'spells', she would extend her head parallel to the ground. Otherwise, the cat seems normal. An ECG is recorded (21; leads I, II, and III at 25 mm/s, 1 cm = 1 mV).

i. What is your ECG interpretation?
ii. Why do the QRS complexes occur irregularly?
iii. What is the clinical significance, if any?

20 i. VHS measures cardiac size compared to vertebral length. Because correlation between body length and heart size is good despite chest conformation, this relationship can help identify and quantify cardiomegaly.

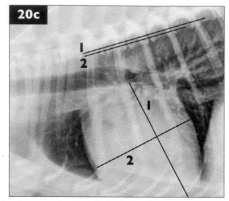

ii. On the lateral radiograph, measure cardiac long axis (1) from ventral border of the carina (left mainstem bronchus origin) to cardiac apex (20c). Measure short axis (2) perpendicular to L within the central one-third of the heart (at greatest cardiac width). Compare both 1 and 2 lengths with the thoracic spine beginning at the cranial edge of T4. Estimate each length to the nearest 0.1 vertebra (v); their sum is the VHS. In this dog, VHS is 10.2 v.

iii. A VHS between 8.5 and 10.5 v is normal for most dogs, but some breed variation exists. For example, in dogs with a short thorax (e.g. Miniature Schnauzers) an upper limit of 11 v is considered normal; up to about 9.5 v is normal in dogs with a long thorax (e.g. Dachshunds).

iv. Yes. Feline normal VHS on lateral view is 6.7 to 8.1 v (mean, 7.5 v). The DV/VD view can also be used in cats: an S dimension up to 4 v is normal (measured from T4 on lateral view).

21 i. The rhythm is sinus arrhythmia, with a HR of ~200 bpm. The mean electrical axis and complex measurements are normal.

ii. Sinus arrhythmia is the result of waxing and waning parasympathetic tone. Sinus arrhythmia is a common finding in normal dogs, but is not usually seen in the clinical setting in cats. Even though sinus arrhythmia may be noted in calm, resting cats, its presence in an excited cat (e.g. in the clinic) is often a result of elevated parasympathetic tone.

iii. Diseases that are associated with high parasympathetic tone generally involve the respiratory, gastrointestinal, or central nervous systems. The sinus arrhythmia in this cat is likely secondary to the respiratory disease (presumably feline asthma, although heartworm disease and pulmonary parasites would also be likely differentials in some regions). The sinus arrhythmia itself is of no clinical concern. This rhythm should be differentiated from other irregular heart rhythms such as frequent premature beats or atrial fibrillation. (**Note:** Cough is rarely a sign of congestive heart failure in cats.)

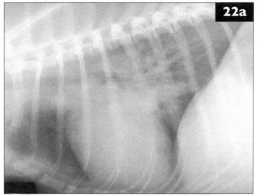

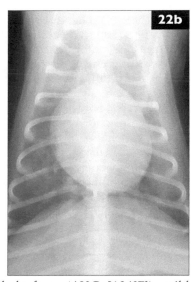

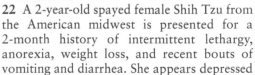

22 A 2-year-old spayed female Shih Tzu from the American midwest is presented for a 2-month history of intermittent lethargy, anorexia, weight loss, and recent bouts of vomiting and diarrhea. She appears depressed and thin. Physical examination findings include fever (40°C [104°F]), mild tachypnea (52 breaths/min), pale mucous membranes, multiple enlarged peripheral lymph nodes, and hepatosplenomegaly. Right lateral (**22a**) and DV (**22b**) views of the thorax are obtained.

i. Is there thoracic lymphadenopathy?
ii. Is there an abnormal lung pattern?
iii. What is your radiographic diagnosis?

23 A 4-year-old spayed female German Shepherd Dog has a recent history of weakness, with a possible syncopal episode. The owners say she started slowing down a couple weeks ago. She is taking no medications. The dog is alert and in good body condition. Body temperature is normal, as are respiratory rate and effort. The jugular veins are not distended, but occasional strong jugular pulsations are seen at a rate slower than the HR. Thoracic auscultation is unremarkable except for a slow, regular heart rhythm of 50 bpm. Femoral pulses are quite strong.

i. What differentials should be considered for the bradycardia?
ii. Would strong femoral pulsations be expected in this case?
iii. Does the intermittent jugular venous pulse provide a diagnostic clue? If so, how?
iv. What test should be done first?

22 i. There is no increased soft tissue volume in the areas of the sternal, cranial mediastinal, and tracheobronchial lymph nodes. Given the peripheral lymph node enlargement, radiographic and ultrasonographic evaluations of the thorax and abdomen are relevant to screen for other lymphadenomegaly.

ii. There is a diffuse unstructured interstitial pattern. This increases the overall opacity of the lung and makes the vascular edges less distinct as the contrast between vessel border and aerated lung is decreased.

iii. The unstructured interstitial pattern is non-specific; etiologic differentials could include lymphoma or other neoplasia, mycotic pneumonia, diffuse hemorrhage, and fibrosis. Lymphoma is a strong consideration in view of the lymphadenopathy and hepatosplenomegaly. However, these signs, along with the fever, interstitial lung pattern, gastrointestinal signs, and weight loss, suggest disseminated mycotic infection. A fine needle aspirate of the popliteal lymph node revealed a reactive cell population with *Histoplasma capsulatum* organisms phagocytized by macrophages.

23 i. Regular bradycardia at this HR is most likely an idioventricular escape rhythm, which usually accompanies complete (third degree) AV block, although sinus arrest or persistent atrial standstill are less common possibilities. Other causes of bradycardia usually produce an irregular rhythm, either because of intermittent AV block or fluctuations in sinus activation rate (e.g. sick sinus syndrome, markedly increased vagal tone, or slow sinoventricular rhythm from hyperkalemia). Normal dogs can have slow HRs at rest, but do not show clinical signs of low cardiac output with activity.

ii. Yes. Perception of arterial pulse strength depends largely on the difference between arterial systolic and maximal diastolic pressure (the 'pulse pressure'). A longer time between heart beats allows diastolic pressure to fall lower and cardiac filling to increase. This produces a greater stroke volume and wider (increased) pulse pressure.

iii. Bounding jugular pulse waves associated with only intermittent heart beats occur when atrial and ventricular contraction happens simultaneously (AV dissociation). These so-called cannon 'a' waves occur when the atria contract against closed AV valves, causing retrograde flow (toward the vena cavae and jugular veins). Complete AV block with a ventricular escape rhythm is the most common cause.

iv. An ECG.

24 A 4-month-old female DSH kitten has exercise intolerance and respiratory difficulty. A loud systolic murmur was found when the kitten was initially seen by a veterinarian 2 months ago, but the murmur is softer now. You suspect a congenital heart defect. Among other tests, an ECG is recorded (24a, leads as marked, 25 mm/s, 1 cm = 1 mV).
i. What is the HR and cardiac rhythm?
ii. Is the mean electrical axis (MEA) normal?
iii. What is a MEA?
iv. How is MEA determined?

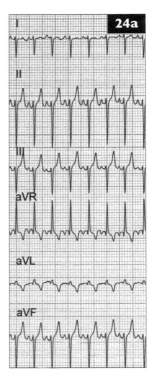

25 A 7-year-old castrated male DSH cat is presented for weight loss, lethargy, and breathing difficulty. Physical examination findings include tachycardia, mild depression, labored respiration, and increased respiratory sounds that are more pronounced during expiration. Pleural effusion is noted on thoracic radiographs. Approximately 200 ml of milky white fluid is removed via thoracocentesis. A sample of the fluid is shown (25, cytospin preparation, Wright's stain, 50× oil).

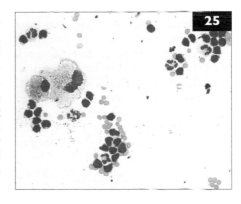

i. Based on the gross description and cytologic appearance, what type of pleural effusion is suspected in this case?
ii. What laboratory tests would help confirm the diagnosis?

24 i. 210 bpm, normal sinus rhythm.
ii. No. The MEA is deviated rightward and cranial.
iii. MEA describes the average direction of ventricular depolarization.
Major intraventricular conduction
disturbances or ventricular enlargement can cause an abnormal MEA.
iv. By convention, only frontal plane

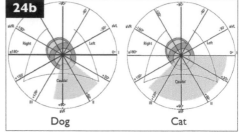

leads are used to estimate MEA. The lead axis orientation is defined by degrees
(from 0 to ±180°) around a circle (24b). Note that the positive pole of leads aVR
and aVL lies on the 'negative' side of the circle. Highlighted sectors indicate normal
MEA ranges. MEA can be estimated by either of these methods:

- Identify the lead with the tallest R (positive) wave. The MEA points toward
  the positive electrode of this lead.
- Identify the lead with the most isoelectric QRS (positive and negative
  deflections). Find the perpendicularly oriented lead on the diagram. If the QRS
  in this perpendicular lead is mostly positive, the MEA points toward this lead's
  positive pole; if it is mostly negative, the MEA points toward the negative
  pole. If all leads appear isoelectric, the MEA is indeterminate.

25 i. This fluid appears to be chyle. Chylous effusions contain chylomicrons and are
classically milky white on gross examination; they may acquire a pink tinge if
hemorrhage has also occurred. Cytologically, chyle typically contains mostly small
lymphocytes, with varying numbers of non-degenerate neutrophils and large mononuclear cells, which often contain clear cytoplasmic vacuoles from phagocytized
lipid. The fluid in this case also shows nucleated cells that are predominantly small
lymphocytes, with lesser numbers of non-degenerate neutrophils and macrophages
(containing numerous small, clear cytoplasmic vacuoles).

Chylous effusions can accumulate secondary to a variety of conditions, including
cardiac failure, trauma, thoracic neoplasia or infection, and chronic cough.
ii. Confirmation that an effusion is chylous is based on comparison of the
triglyceride and cholesterol content of the effusion with the corresponding
concentrations in serum. Chylous effusions have triglyceride concentrations
exceeding those in serum by a factor of >3:1. The cholesterol:triglyceride ratio in
chylous fluid is <1.

Pseudochylous effusion also occurs and is defined as a milky white, turbid fluid
that lacks chylomicrons. The milky white appearance of pseudochylous effusion is
related to the degradation of cellular membranes, with a high concentration of
cholesterol but low concentration of triglyceride.

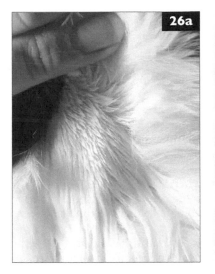

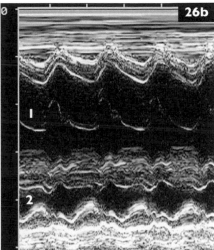

26 A 7-year-old female DSH cat is presented for further evaluation of pleural effusion. She is mildly tachypneic with increased respiratory effort. Her abdomen is distended with fluid. Lung sounds are muffled ventrally. HR is 220 bpm. A grade 3/6 systolic murmur is heard best at the right apex. After 130 ml of modified transudate are withdrawn by thoracocentesis her respiratory rate and effort improve; abdominocentesis yields 250 ml of similar fluid. An area over the jugular vein is shaved before venipuncture (26a). Echocardiography is done (26b, M-mode, ventricular level; 26c, color

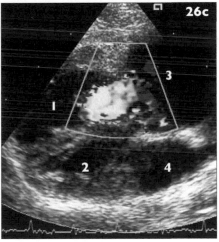

flow, right parasternal long axis in systole; 1 – RV, 2 – LV, 3 – RA, 4 – LA).
i. What is the significance of the physical finding shown in 26a?
ii. How would you interpret the echo images?
iii. What are your treatment recommendations at this time?
iv. How would you manage long-term therapy in this cat?

27 What is the recommended treatment for heartworm disease (HWD) in the dog?

26 i. Usually, increased right heart filling pressure causes jugular venous distension, but venous obstruction from cranial vena cava thrombosis or a cranial mediastinal mass can also cause distension. When both pleural and abdominal effusions of modified transudate exist, jugular distension is a strong indicator of underlying right heart failure, cardiac tamponade, or uncommonly, pericardial constrictive disease.

ii. There is marked RV and RA dilation consistent with chronic volume overload; the LV looks small. **26c** also shows severe tricuspid regurgitation. Considerations include longstanding congenital tricuspid dysplasia or feline arrhythmogenic RV cardiomyopathy, although arrhythmias or focal RV wall abnormalities were not noted in this cat. Additional views would help further evaluate tricuspid apparatus structure (thickened leaflets were observed here).

iii. Congestive heart failure therapy is indicated, including furosemide, an angiotensin-converting enzyme inhibitor, and pimobendan; spironolactone may also be helpful.

iv. Parameters to monitor include renal function, serum electrolytes, BP, respiratory rate and effort, and cardiac rhythm. Drainage of recurrent pleural effusion and intensified diuretic therapy may become necessary. Either atrial or ventricular tachyarrhythmias are likely to develop and may require additional therapy. A diet liked by the cat should be fed (ideally one reduced in salt).

27 Melarsomine dihydrochloride. 'Standard' therapy (2.5 mg/kg via deep epaxial lumbar intramuscular injection; repeat in 24 hours on opposite side) can be used in dogs with low risk for post-treatment pulmonary thromboembolism (i.e. class 1 disease; PTE). However, an alternative protocol is currently advised for all HW-positive dogs, not just those with more severe disease. The alternative protocol (one dose initially, then 4–6 weeks later, 'standard' adulticide therapy) reduces the risk of fatal PTE from sudden heavy worm kill. Strict rest for 4–6 weeks after therapy is important. If possible, prior treatment with a monthly HWD preventive drug and doxycycline (10 mg/kg q12h for 4 weeks; for *Wolbachia* organisms) is also suggested. Dogs with caval syndrome are not given adulticide until after worms are surgically removed.

If Melarsomine is currently unavailable, the American Heartworm Society recommends:
- Limit the infected dog's activity to reduce lung pathology.
- Carefully initiate preventative therapy.
- Administer doxycycline (protocol as above; repeat every 3 months until adultcide is available) to reduce pathology and infective potential of the worms.

See www.heartwormsociety.org for more information

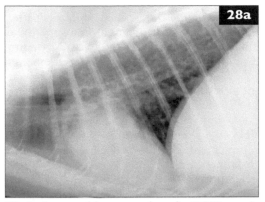

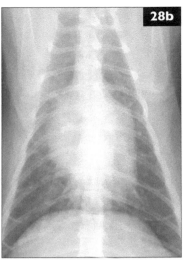

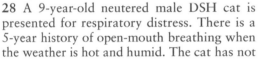

28 A 9-year-old neutered male DSH cat is presented for respiratory distress. There is a 5-year history of open-mouth breathing when the weather is hot and humid. The cat has not been receiving any medications. This most recent episode of respiratory distress appears to have responded to furosemide administration. A grade 2/6 systolic heart murmur is heard best at the left sternal border and more softly on the right. Thoracic radiographs (28a, b) are made.
i. What are the clinical differentials to be evaluated by the radiographic study?
ii. What radiographic changes are present?
iii. Are the radiographic changes more supportive of cardiac or pulmonary disease?
iv. What diagnostic procedure(s) should be done next?

29 A 10-year-old male neutered German Shorthair Pointer (29) is presented because of poor exercise tolerance when hunting and recent abdominal swelling. The dog is alert. Abnormal examination findings include ascites, ventrally muffled lung sounds, a soft left-sided systolic murmur, and dental disease. It is unclear whether jugular vein distension is present. Chest radiographs show equivocal cardiomegaly and moderate pleural effusion.

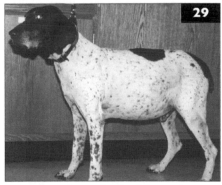

i. Would central venous pressure (CVP) measurement be useful in this case?
ii. What is CVP, and how is it measured?
iii. What can confound accurate CVP measurement?

28 i. Clinical differential diagnoses involving the thoracic cavity in this patient should include cardiac disease (e.g. hypertrophic or other cardiomyopathy, or previously undiagnosed congenital malformation) with congestive heart failure, pleural effusion (of any cause), and pulmonary diseases such as pneumonia and feline asthma.

ii. Moderate generalized cardiomegaly with a large LA is evident without associated enlarged pulmonary vessels. A diffuse bronchial pattern is also present. Pleural effusion is not evident.

iii. The radiographic cardiomegaly (VHS ~9.3 v) indicates cardiac disease. However, the pulmonary changes are more typical of chronic bronchial disease than pulmonary edema of congestive heart failure.

iv. The cardiomegaly and murmur indicate the need for additional cardiac assessment by echocardiography; in this case, hypertrophic cardiomyopathy with mild LV outflow tract obstruction was found. However, because of the diffuse radiographic bronchial pattern, further assessment for airway disease by hematology, heartworm testing, fecal examination, and BAL were recommended.

29 i. Yes. An elevated CVP suggests that right heart failure or pericardial disease (tamponade or constriction) underlies the effusions.

ii. CVP measures systemic venous (and right heart filling) pressure. Intravascular volume, venous compliance, and cardiac function influence CVP. Normal CVP is 0–8 (to 10) cmH$_2$O; respiration causes minor fluctuations. To measure CVP, aseptically place a jugular catheter that extends into or close to the RA. Connect it with extension tubing and a three-way stopcock to a fluid administration set. Attach a vertically-oriented water manometer to the stopcock; position the stopcock (representing 0 cmH$_2$O) at the (horizontal) level of the patient's RA. Turn the stopcock off to the animal, so the manometer fills with fluid. Then turn the stopcock off to the fluid reservoir, allowing fluid in the manometer to equilibrate with CVP. Take repeated measurements, with manometer and patient in the same position, during exhalation.

iii. Large-volume pleural effusion raises intrapleural pressure and, thus, CVP. Such effusions should be drained before measuring CVP. Inaccurate readings can also occur when the catheter tip is not within the RA or proximal vena cava, the stopcock is not at RA level, and body position varies.

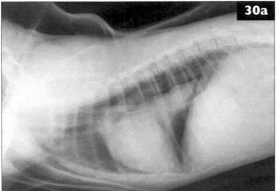

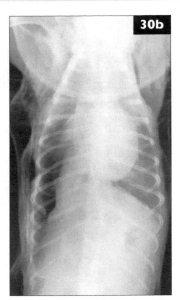

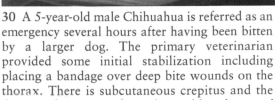

30 A 5-year-old male Chihuahua is referred as an emergency several hours after having been bitten by a larger dog. The primary veterinarian provided some initial stabilization including placing a bandage over deep bite wounds on the thorax. There is subcutaneous crepitus and the dog is tachypneic, tachycardic, and has decreased breath sounds on the right side. The body temperature is 37°C (99°F). Right lateral (30a) and DV (30b) thoracic radiographs are taken.

i. Does this dog have a pneumothorax?
ii. What are the types of pneumothorax?
iii. What are the mechanisms of pneumomediastinum?

31 A young dog is presented for surgical repair of a patent ductus arteriosus. A left thoracotomy exposes the region of the heart base and proximal great vessels. The surgical field is shown before the pericardium is incised (31). Cranial is to the left in the image.

i. What is the dark elongated structure overlying the heart?
ii. Where does it terminate?
iii. What clinical signs does it cause?

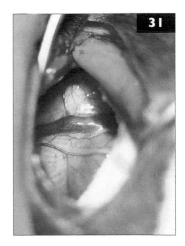

30 i. Yes. Soft tissue opacity in the right hemithorax, in the shape of collapsed lung lobes, is displaced from the thoracic wall. There are no vascular shadows in the right hemithorax. Radiographic detection of pneumothorax can be difficult with concurrent pneumomediastinum and subcutaneous emphysema, as here, because of the summation effect of subcutaneous air pockets. Look for increased lung soft tissue opacity, with distinct separation from the thoracic wall, rather than only regions of lucency.

ii. Pneumothorax is classified as 'open' or 'closed' and 'non-tension' versus 'tension'. With open pneumothorax, air enters the pleural space through a hole in the thoracic wall. The thoracic wall is intact with closed pneumothorax; free air leaks from the lung. Tension pneumothorax results from progressively increasing intrapleural pressure, similar to a one-way valve allowing air into the pleural space with each breath, without escape. Increasing intrapleural pressure compresses the lung and vasculature, leading to critical cardiopulmonary compromise. Non-tension pneumothorax does not cause a progressive increase in intrapleural free air and pressure.

iii. Pneumomediastinum develops from: pharyngeal, laryngeal, tracheal, or esophageal disruption; wounds involving cervical fascial planes; and peri-bronchiolar dissection of air within the lung to the pulmonary hilus. Pneumo-mediastinum is usually secondary to trauma or, occasionally, to infection with gas-forming organisms. Because the mediastinum communicates with cervical fascial planes, air can dissect in either direction. Pneumomediastinum can lead to pneumothorax if the mediastinal pleura ruptures; however, pneumothorax does not cause pneumomediastinum.

31 i. A persistent left cranial vena cava. This vessel is a remnant of the embryonic left cranial cardinal vein, which drains blood from the cranial part of the embryo in parallel with the right cranial cardinal vein. During normal development, the left cranial cardinal vein degenerates and disappears as an anastomosing vein (the left brachiocephalic vein) develops to carry venous blood from cranial left structures to the right cranial cardinal vein (which becomes the right brachiocephalic vein and cranial vena cava).

ii. The persistent left cranial vena cava courses lateral to the left AV groove and joins the great cardiac vein caudally to empty into the coronary sinus of the caudal RA.

iii. It causes no clinical signs, but may complicate surgical exposure of other structures at the left heart base.

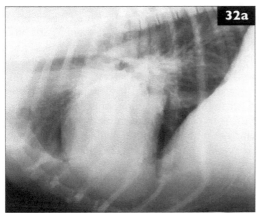

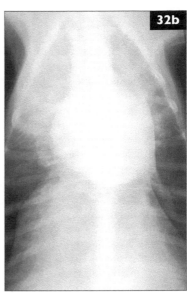

32 A 9-year-old spayed female Dobermann is presented for poor exercise tolerance, inappetence, and recent respiratory distress. She appears alert and well fleshed. HR is 160 bpm, sinus rhythm. A grade 2/6 systolic murmur and S_3 gallop sound are heard at the left apex. Breath sounds are harsh, but no crackles are heard. The rest of the examination is unremarkable. Lateral (32a) and DV (32b) chest radiographs are obtained.
i. Describe the radiographic findings.
ii. What is the most likely diagnosis?
iii. How would you proceed with this case?

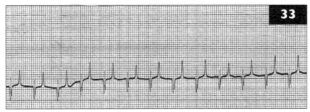

33 A 6-year-old male DSH cat is examined for recent onset of poor appetite, hiding, and increased vocalization. The owner says the cat seems to spend more time than usual at the litterbox. The cat appears lethargic; mucous membranes are pink and pulses strong. The abdomen is tense and painful on palpation; a large bladder is noted. HR is 120 bpm. A lead II ECG is recorded (33, 25 mm/s, 2 cm = 1 mV).
i. What is your ECG interpretation?
ii. What is your assessment of this case?
iii. How would you treat this cat?

32 i. The vertical orientation of the cardiac silhouette is typical for Dobermanns. However, cardiomegaly (VHS ~12.1 v), with moderate LA and LV enlargement, is evident. Peribronchial and mild hilar interstitial pulmonary infiltrates are present.
ii. Dilated cardiomyopathy, with early congestive heart failure (pulmonary edema).
iii. Additional baseline data, to confirm the diagnosis and identify concurrent abnormalities, would include an echocardiogram, ECG, BP measurement, serum biochemistries, CBC, and urinalysis. Therapy with furosemide, pimobendan, and an angiotensin-converting enzyme inhibitor is indicated. Furosemide dosage is titrated as needed to control edema. Other therapy that may be helpful could include spirono-lactone, a low-dose beta blocker (e.g. carvedilol; after pulmonary edema is resolved), and fish-oil (omega-3 fatty acid) supplement. Although few Dobermanns show marked clinical improvement to oral L-carnitine supplementation, a 3- to 6-month therapeutic trial is reasonable. Monitoring patient cardiopulmonary and metabolic status is important. Azotemia, hypotension, electrolyte disturbance, and refractory pulmonary edema are comon. Cardiac arrhythmias, especially ventricular tachy-arrhythmias and atrial fibrillation, often develop and require antiarrhythmic therapy.

Discussions with the owner about exercise and dietary salt restriction, monitoring resting respiratory rate, potential complications, and the relatively poor long-term prognosis with strong possibility of sudden death are important.

33 i. HR is 120 bpm. P waves are absent, QRS complexes are wide (0.06–0.07 seconds), and T waves appear tented. Sinoventricular rhythm is most likely. Other rhythm differentials could include either sinus arrest, sinoatrial block, or atrial standstill with a ventricular (or junctional, with aberrant intraventricular conduc-tion) escape rhythm.
ii. Presumptive diagnosis is urethral obstruction with severe hyperkalemia-induced ECG abnormalities; (K^+ was 10.2 mmol/l [10.2 mEq/l] in this cat). Hyperkalemia slows conduction velocity and alters refractory period. Experimental studies describe ECG changes associated with progressive hyperkalemia: T waves become narrow and sometimes symmetrically peaked (tented; serum K^+ ≥6 mmol/l); P waves flatten (K^+ ~7 mmol/l) then disappear (K^+ ≥8 mmol/l), producing a so-called sinoventricular rhythm; QRS complexes widen (K^+ >6 mmol/l); abnormal rhythms can occur (K^+ >10 mmol/l), with eventual asystole. However, with clinical hyperkalemia, these changes occur inconsistently, perhaps because of additional electrolyte derangements and acidosis.
iii. Regular insulin (0.25–0.5 U/kg IV) with glucose (2 g/U insulin, diluted to a 10% solution) is recommended for severe hyperkalemia from feline urethral obstruction. Once the obstruction is relieved, subsequent fluid therapy should include 2.5–5% dextrose. Sodium bicarbonate (1–2 mEq/kg, slow IV) could provoke hypocalcemia in cats with urethral obstruction and hyperphosphatemia.

34 An owner returned home to find her indoor cat breathing rapidly and markedly lame in both hindlimbs. The cat is an 8-year-old neutered male DLH mix. The cat can advance the right hindlimb, but cannot place the foot in a plantar position. The left limb is dragged behind. This image (34a) was taken during examination of the hindlimbs (right paw is to the left).

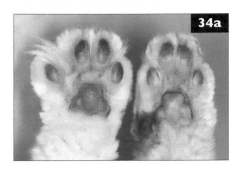

i. What condition is present?
ii. How could this lesion be confirmed?
iii. What underlying diseases are commonly associated with this?

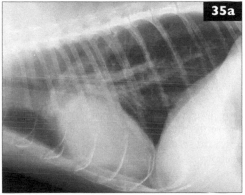

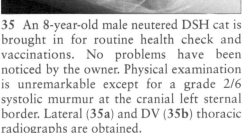

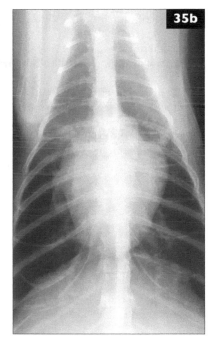

35 An 8-year-old male neutered DSH cat is brought in for routine health check and vaccinations. No problems have been noticed by the owner. Physical examination is unremarkable except for a grade 2/6 systolic murmur at the cranial left sternal border. Lateral (35a) and DV (35b) thoracic radiographs are obtained.

i. Describe the radiographic findings.
ii. What are your differential diagnoses?
iii. What are your recommendations to the owner?

34 i. Feline arterial thromboembolism (ATE) or saddle thrombus of the terminal aorta. The right hind foot pad appears pink and the toes are splayed, suggesting some residual motor activity. The left hind foot pad is pale, from poor perfusion. Such asymmetry in degree of vascular compromise is not uncommon.

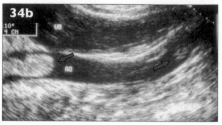

Both hind feet may feel cool compared with the forelimbs, although the left hindlimb in this cat is likely to feel cooler than the right. Femoral pulses are usually absent or markedly weak or asymmetric. Affected limbs also often have cyanotic nail beds and ischemic muscle contracture. Acute ATE usually causes severe pain.

ii. Ultrasonography may reveal a thrombus in the caudal abdominal aorta, as in this case (**34b**; large and small thrombi [small arrows] within distal aortic lumen, AO; UB, urinary bladder).

iii. Feline myocardial disease, especially hypertrophic, restrictive, and 'unclassified' cardiomyopathies. ATE also has occurred with other cardiac diseases and with systemic inflammatory conditions (e.g. neoplasia, viral infection, sepsis).

35 i. There is mild cardiomegaly (VHS ~10 v), with LV and atrial (especially left auricular) prominence. This imparts a slight 'valentine' shape to the cardiac silhouette (**35b**). The pulmonary parenchyma and vessels are unremarkable.

ii. Hypertrophic cardiomyopathy is strongly suspected. Other differentials for left heart enlargement and murmur suggestive of LV outflow obstruction include chronic hypertension, hyperthyroidism, previously undiagnosed congenital (sub)aortic stenosis, or another acquired ventricular outflow obstruction.

iii. An echocardiogram, BP measurement, and serum T_4 are indicated. CBC, serum biochemistries, and urinalysis are also recommended. In this case, BP and T_4 tests were normal; echocardiography showed LA enlargement and asymmetric LV hypertrophy with dynamic outflow obstruction (hypertrophic obstructive cardiomyopathy). Possible sequelae include arterial thromboembolism, congestive heart failure, and arrhythmias (exacerbated by stress, tachycardia, and LV outflow obstruction). Low-dose aspirin or clopidogrel is usually prescribed to reduce thromboembolic risk. Benazepril is recommended for clinical disease, but is of unclear benefit earlier. Atenolol may be helpful by reducing outflow obstruction and slowing HR. The owner is advised to monitor the cat's resting respiratory rate and effort, activity level, appetite, and attitude. Re-evaluation in 6–9 months is suggested unless problems arise sooner.

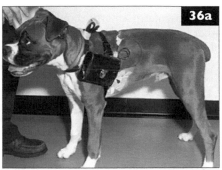
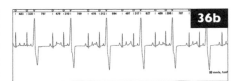
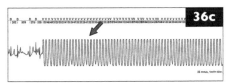

36 A 3-year old intact male Boxer began having syncopal episodes 3 weeks ago. After a brief run, he suddenly stopped, looked tired as well as pale and disorientated, and then collapsed unconscious after a few seconds. The dog spontaneously regained full consciousness after 8–10 seconds. Since then, the owner has observed four similar episodes, always during exercise. The dog is completely normal between the events and in good body condition. Physical examination is unremarkable. Hematology, serum biochemistry, and thyroid test results are normal. Echocardiography (including Doppler), ECG, thoracic radiographs, and abdominal ultrasonography are unremarkable.

A 24-hour (Holter) ECG recording is obtained to screen for episodic arrhythmias (36a) as the owner records the dog's activity in a diary. Samples from when the dog is alert (36b) and during another syncopal event (36c, red arrow) while exercising are shown.

i. What ECG abnormality is shown in 36b?
ii. What ECG abnormality is shown in 36c?
iii. What is the most likely diagnosis in this patient?
iv. How would you manage this case as well as advise the owner about prognosis?

37 A 14-year-old male Weimaraner is presented for recent abdominal swelling and a collapse episode early this morning. Ascites and a slow HR are identified on physical examination. An ECG is recorded (37, leads as marked, 25 mm/s, 0.5 cm = 1 mV).
i. What is your ECG interpretation?
ii. What test can be done to assess autonomic neural influence?
iii. How is this test done?
iv. If there is no response, what do you recommend?

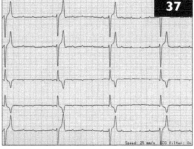

36 i. Sinus rhythm (120 bpm) with uniform ventricular premature complexes in a trigeminal pattern (ventricular trigeminy); that is, two normal complexes followed by a ventricular ectopic complex (indicated by 'V' in the top margin).
ii. Sinus rhythm is interrupted by rapid ventricular tachycardia at 450 bpm. Syncope occurred (red arrow) shortly after the onset of tachycardia.
iii. Arrhythmogenic RV cardiomyopathy (ARVC), or 'Boxer cardiomyopathy'. Ventricular tachyarrhythmias, usually with an upright configuration in lead II, are typical and often occur with excitement or exercise. Echo findings can be normal or show changes typical for dilated cardiomyopathy.
iv. ARVC is difficult to manage and no cure exists. Antiarrhythmic drugs (e.g. mexiletine with atenolol, sotalol, or amiodarone) are used to reduce ventricular tachyarrhythmia frequency and severity, and resulting clinical signs. This may improve quality of life; however, antiarrhythmic therapy may not reduce the risk of sudden death or increase life expectancy.

Some cases develop myocardial dysfunction and heart failure over time, so cardiac size and function should be monitored. An implantable cardioverter-defibrillator (ICD), used in people with life-threatening ventricular arrhythmias, could be considered in Boxer ARVC. However, the expense, programming challenges, and risk of inappropriate and painful electroshocks make ICD therapy problematic.

The prognosis is guarded, although some affected dogs survive for years. Sudden death is common. Affected animals should not be bred, as ARVC is thought to be inherited.

37 i. HR is 30 bpm. Sinus P waves are seen, but complete (third degree) AV block and a ventricular escape rhythm are evident. The slightly prolonged (0.05 second) P waves suggest LA enlargement. QRS complex measurements and mean electrical axis generally are not determined for idioventricular rhythms.
ii. The atropine response test. Atropine, a competitive muscarinic receptor antagonist, has little to no effect on bradyarrhythmias caused by intrinsic sinus or AV node disease.
iii. Record an ECG within 5–10 minutes after injection of atropine (0.04 mg/kg IV). If the HR does not increase by at least 150% or AV conduction improve, repeat the ECG 15–20 minutes after the injection; an initial vagomimetic effect can last over 5 minutes. Normal sinus node response is a rate increase to >135 bpm (usually to 150–160 bpm). However, a positive response (increased sinus rate and AV conduction) may not predict response to oral anticholinergic therapy.
iv. When there is no response to atropine challenge, medical therapy is unlikely to improve symptomatic bradycardia and artificial pacing is indicated.

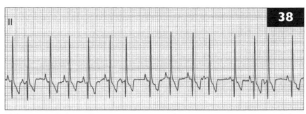

38 A 9-year-old spayed female Miniature Schnauzer is presented for evaluation of a heart murmur, cardiomegaly, and cough, which persists despite therapy with furosemide, enalapril, and theophylline. A mild increase in respiratory rate and effort is observed. A grade 3/6 murmur is heard at both left and right cardiac apical areas. Soft pulmonary crackles are heard. Femoral pulses are strong, but with occasional deficits. Systolic BP is 138 mmHg. Thoracic radiographs indicate marked LA enlargement and mild pulmonary infiltrates consistent with edema. A hemogram and serum chemistries are unremarkable. An ECG is recorded (38, lead II at 25 mm/s, 1 cm = 1 mV).

i. What is your ECG interpretation?
ii. How would you manage the case at this time?
iii. What are your recommendations for follow-up?

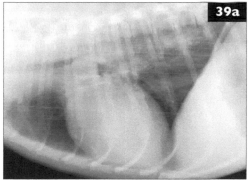
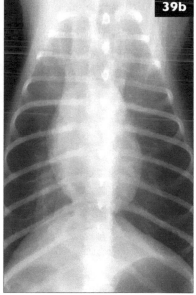

39 A 2-year-old male Miniature Poodle is presented for a history of coughing and gagging, which began over a year ago. Multiple medications have been used with no resolution. Physical examination is unre-markable except for a 2/6 systolic murmur over the mitral region. Lateral (39a) and DV (39b) thoracic radiographs are shown.

i. Is there radiographic evidence of heart disease?
ii. Are there any non-cardiac changes to account for the coughing and gagging?

38 i. The HR is 130 bpm, with sinus rhythm. There are several atrial premature complexes (APCs) preceded by negative P' waves (2nd, 5th, 9th complexes from the right). The QRS complex configuration suggests a normal mean electrical axis. Sinus P waves are wide (0.05–0.06 second), consistent with LA enlargement. QRS complexes are slightly wide (0.07 second) with prominent Q and upper limit R waves, suggesting LV enlargement. Chronic degenerative mitral valve disease (MVD) is the likely underlying diagnosis.

ii. The respiratory signs, LA enlargement, and pulmonary infiltrates are consistent with unresolved pulmonary edema. Furosemide therapy should be intensified, pimobendan added, and the enalapril dose optimized. Echocardiography is recommended to further characterize cardiac structure and myocardial function. APCs are common with MVD, but theophylline may be increasing their frequency. Discontinuation of theophylline is advised unless it clearly is required to manage the dog's cough. Exercise restriction, moderately-low salt diet, and monitoring of respiratory rate and effort are indicated.

iii. Serum electrolytes, renal function, heart rhythm, and pulmonary status should be monitored. Furosemide dosing is adjusted as needed to control edema. Spironolactone may also be helpful. If atrial tachyarrhythmias worsen, digoxin with or without diltiazem or a beta blocker is recommended.

39 i. There is no definitive cardiac enlargement, based on various methods of cardiac mensuration. Likewise the cardiac shape is normal. The radiographic interpretation is that the heart is within normal limits.

ii. The airways, lung, and esophagus should be carefully scrutinized for either primary or secondary changes. There is a small amount of air in the cranial thoracic esophagus, seen in the lateral view, from the thoracic inlet through the 4th intercostal space. Typical esophageal dilation is not evident in the DV view. The gastric and intestinal shadows are moderately gas filled, but not abnormally distended. The lung fields are normally radiolucent with the exception of a focal interstitial opacity in the right caudal lobe around the primary bronchial path.

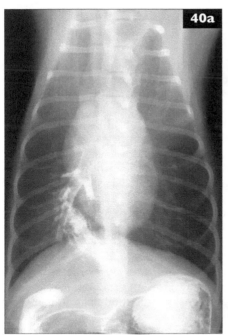
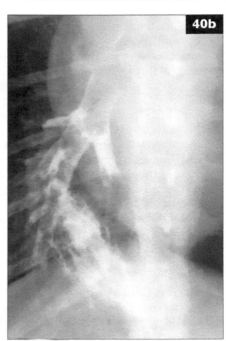

40 Further questioning regarding the dog in 39 reveals that the cough is much worse after drinking. A liquid barium swallow is done; DV views are shown (40a, b).
i. What is the radiographic diagnosis following the contrast study?
ii. Was it inappropriate to do the barium swallow?

41 A 7-year-old male DSH cat is presented for physical examination and vaccinations. The owner is concerned because a littermate has recently been diagnosed with hypertrophic cardio-myopathy. The cat is purring loudly during attempts at thoracic auscultation.
i. How can purring be discouraged during auscultation?
ii. Which thoracic region(s) must be

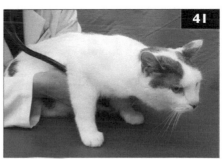

auscultated carefully for possible presence of a murmur in cats?
iii. After purring is stopped, a soft extra sound is heard at the left apex. What is this most likely to be?

40 i. The simultaneous opacification of the distal thoracic esophagus and right caudal and accessory lobe bronchi indicate an esophagobronchial fistula. Such fistulae occur only rarely in dogs and cats. Most are thought to result from esophageal foreign body penetration or chronic irritation. This diagnosis should be suspected when coughing is closely associated with drinking and eating; other considerations with this history include oropharyngeal dysphagia and esophageal disease with aspiration.

ii. No. Esophageal contrast radiography most consistently demonstrates the esophagobronchial connection. Optimal choice of contrast agent depends on whether communication with the lung only or with other thoracic regions, such as the mediastinum, is suspected. Barium aspiration into the trachea and bronchi is generally cleared effectively by coughing and normal mucociliary transport, with no significant residual effect. Barium in bronchioles and alveoli is cleared more slowly by macrophages and granuloma formation. Extensive alveolar deposition can compromise respiration. Barium causes a granulomatous reaction in the mediastinum.

The pulmonary response to aspirated iodinated contrast depends on ionicity; ionic products induce severe acute edema and inflammatory response, while non-ionic agents cause only a mild inflammatory response. An oral non-ionic product is recommended when potential for lung parenchymal contamination is high. If that study is negative, a barium contrast study is then recommended to confirm the negative study. Esophageal leaks visible only with barium contrast have occurred in people. Esophagobronchial fistula is best treated by affected lung lobe removal and esophageal closure.

41 i. Holding a finger over one or both nostrils; waving an alcohol-soaked cotton ball near the cat's nose; gently pressing on the larynx (cricoid cartilage); turning on a water faucet near the animal; or securely holding the cat away from the examination table and suddenly lowering (pretending to drop) him.

ii. The feline heart lies more horizontally in the chest compared with dogs, so it is important to auscultate the left and right sternal border regions, as well as left and right apical (near the precordial impulse) and basilar regions.

iii. An S_4 gallop sound. This diastolic sound (as well as the S_3) is not normally audible in cats (or dogs). The S_3 and S_4 are lower in frequency and usually softer than normal heart sounds (S_1 and S_2); they are easier to hear using the bell of the stethoscope (or light pressure with a single-sided chestpiece). An S_3 or S_4 sound is sometimes called a gallop rhythm, although it is unrelated to the heart's electrical rhythm. Gallop sounds indicate ventricular diastolic dysfunction. The S_4 is heard with increased ventricular thickness and stiffness (e.g. hypertrophic cardio-myopathy). Heart failure and increased LA pressure intensify gallop sounds.

42 An 11-year-old male Rhodesian Ridgeback has a large intrathoracic mass with severe pleural effusion. CT reveals that the mass involves the left cranial lung lobe and extends into the right lung. The left cranial lung lobe, which is torsed, is removed via left lateral thoracotomy. Because the mass also involves the right hemithorax, the dog is repositioned for right lateral

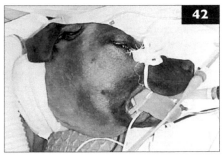

thoracotomy. Partial lobectomy of the right middle and caudal lung lobes is necessary to remove the mass. Mechanical ventilation is used postoperatively to assist recovery (42).

i. What are the primary indications for ventilation therapy, especially in a case such as this?

ii. Which general indication has the better prognosis for survival to hospital discharge?

iii. Describe the mechanical ventilation mode that combines both spontaneous and ventilator-initiated breaths, and its advantage.

43 What parameters indicate when it is reasonably safe to begin weaning a patient with pulmonary dysfunction from mechanical ventilation?

44 An 8-year-old male Great Dane is presented for lethargy of 2-week duration and abdominal distension. The dog is alert and normothermic. Mucous membranes are pink, capillary refill time is 3 seconds, femoral pulses are unremarkable, and mild jugular distension is seen. HR and rhythm and respirations are normal. Ascites is evident. Heart sounds are quite soft and lung sounds

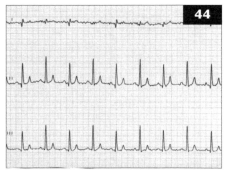

are normal on auscultation. An ECG is recorded (44, leads as marked, 50 mm/s, 1 cm = 1 mV).

i. What is your ECG diagnosis?

ii. Does the ECG provide an indication of the dog's underlying problem?

iii. If so, what is the explanation for this finding?

42 i. Primary indications for ventilation therapy are (1) hypoventilation and (2) hypoxemia unresponsive to O_2 administration. This dog is likely to have both hypoventilation (surgical pain) and hypoxemia (lung injury). Mechanical ventilation can also be helpful by decreasing the work of breathing.

ii. Dogs treated with mechanical ventilation for hypoventilation have a better prognosis than those requiring ventilator therapy for other causes of hypoxemia.

iii. With deep sedation and neuromuscular control, the ventilator initiates all breaths. However, a more physiologic ventilator mode is intermittent mandatory ventilation, where the patient can trigger breaths and the ventilator initiates additional breaths to ensure delivery of the prescribed minute volume. Synchronized intermittent mandatory ventilation (SIMV) is a variation where the ventilator is programmed to override (not initiate) a mechanical ventilation cycle when the patient attempts a spontaneous breath. This synchronization avoids competition between the patient and ventilator, and allows the patient to assume more of the work of breathing when able. Therefore, SIMV is commonly used to begin weaning the patient from the ventilator.

43 Positive end-expiratory pressure <4 cm H_2O, normal minute volume and peak airway pressure, inspired O_2 concentration <40%, arterial PO_2 >80 mmHg, and arterial PCO_2 <50 mmHg are parameters evaluated in determining when to begin weaning from the ventilator.

44 i. HR is 140 bpm, with normal sinus rhythm. Some baseline muscle tremor artifact is evident. The electrical axis is normal. P wave duration is 0.05 second, but this is acceptable in giant breeds. Other complex measurements are normal. Electrical alternans is present.

ii. Yes. Electrical alternans occurs most often with large-volume pericardial effusion.

iii. Electrical alternans is a recurring, beat-to-beat alteration in the size or configuration of the QRS complex (and sometimes T wave). It results from the heart's swinging motion, back and forth on alternating beats, within the pericardial fluid. This motion changes the cardiac orientation within the torso, which affects the ECG appearance. Electrical alternans may be more evident at HRs between 90 and 140 bpm or in certain body positions (e.g. standing). Other ECG changes sometimes seen with pericardial disease and effusion include diminished amplitude QRS complexes (often less than 1 mV in dogs) and ST segment elevation suggesting an epicardial injury current (not seen in this case). Sinus tachycardia is common with cardiac tamponade. Various tachyarrhythmias also occur in some cases.

This dog had a large amount of pericardial effusion causing cardiac tamponade, hemangiosarcoma involving the RA wall, and pulmonary metastases.

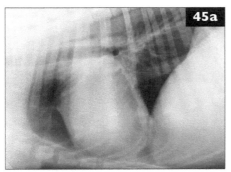

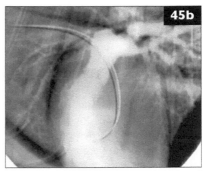

45 A second opinion is sought by the owner of a 1-year-old male German Shepherd Dog. A murmur was recently heard by a veterinarian when the dog was presented for routine vaccination. A lateral radiograph (45a) and angiocardiogram (45b) are shown.
i. Based on the information given, what abnormality is present?
ii. How can the severity of this be assessed?
iii. What are the management options for this case?

46 A 30 kg (66 lb), young adult male German Shepherd Dog of unknown age is presented for an enlarging abdomen and decreased activity of 3 weeks duration. The owners note that the dog groans when he moves and with petting. His appetite is good. On physical examination, a ballottable fluid wave is present in the abdomen. Body temperature is 38.9°C (102°F). HR is 120 bpm with a slightly irregular rhythm. Femoral pulses and precordial impulses are weak. Jugular distension is evident. Heart sounds are very soft; no murmur is heard and lung sounds are normal. Lateral (46a) and DV (46b) thoracic radiographs are obtained. Echocardiography is not available.

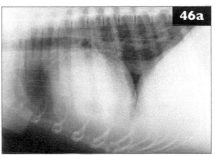

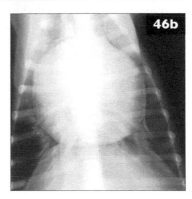

i. Describe the radiographic findings.
ii. What are your differential diagnoses?
iii. How would you manage this case?

45 i. RV enlargement is seen (**45a**). Contrast injection into the RV reveals a thickened, fused pulmonic valve (inverted 'Y' shape, **45b**) typical for valvular pulmonic stenosis. Mild RV hypertrophy and main PA dilation are secondary to the stenosis.

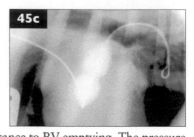

ii. By the systolic pressure difference (gradient) between RV and PA. RV systolic pressure increases above normal because of increased resistance to RV emptying. The pressure gradient (instantaneous) is estimated from peak PA outflow velocity (via spectral Doppler echocardiography) and the Bernoulli equation (pressure gradient = 4 × peak velocity^2). Pressure gradient (peak to peak) can be measured directly during cardiac catheterization; this is lower than that estimated by Doppler in the awake animal.

iii. Balloon valvuloplasty, recommended for severe valvular pulmonic stenosis, can create a larger orifice by tearing valvular adhesions (**45c**; indentation of inflated balloon from stenotic valve prior to tearing). Marked reduction in pressure gradient is often achieved, although valvuloplasty is not helpful in some cases and even contraindicated in others. Beta-blocker therapy may be prescribed to reduce HR and myocardial O_2 requirement, as well as increase diastolic filling and myocardial perfusion, if balloon valvuloplasty is unsuccessful or not pursued.

46 i. There is marked, generalized cardiomegaly with tracheal elevation (**46a**). The heart has a round, globoid appearance on DV view. Pulmonary vessels and parenchyma appear normal. Mild caudal vena caval dilation and ascites are evident.

ii. Large pericardial effusion with cardiac tamponade is likely considering the globoid cardiac silhouette without identifiable heart contours. Other causes of a large, rounded heart with signs of right-sided failure include dilated cardiomyopathy and congenital tricuspid dysplasia with severe tricuspid insufficiency. However, the muffled heart sounds, lack of murmur, and loss of caudodorsal cardiac contours make these less likely here. Pericardioperitoneal diaphragmatic hernia is another differential, although the heart shadow appears distinct from the diaphragm on DV and right heart failure would be unexpected.

iii. Clinical and radiographic signs are most consistent with cardiac tamponade. Medications for congestive heart failure (e.g. furosemide, enalapril) are likely to further impair cardiac filling and forward output. Pericardiocentesis is indicated and should be done right away. Even if only partial removal of the effusion is accomplished, reduced intrapericardial pressure should improve cardiac filling and output. Electrocardiography is indicated to identify the arrhythmia and to monitor rhythm during pericardiocentesis. If possible, referral for echocardiography and further evaluation is recommended.

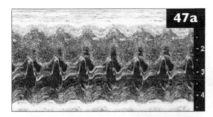

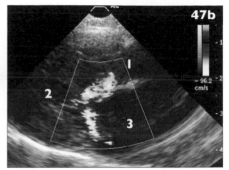

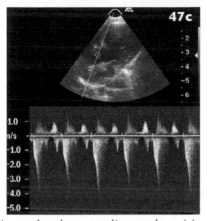

47 A 3-year-old male neutered DSH cat is referred because of a heart murmur. He is alert, in good body condition, and has no clinical signs. Physical examination is normal, except for a systolic grade 3/6 heart murmur, heard best over the left apex and radiating to the right side.

Hematologic and serum biochemical test results are unremarkable. Systolic BP is normal (135 mmHg). Thoracic radiographs show cardiomegaly, without venous engorgement or evidence for pulmonary edema. Echocardiography is performed. M-mode image at the mitral level (47a), color flow Doppler in systole from right parasternal LV outflow view (47b, 1 – aorta, 2 – left ventricle, 3 – left atrium), and continuous wave Doppler interrogation of the LV outflow tract from left apical position (47c) are shown. Measurements from M-mode images are (reference values in brackets):

	Diastole (mm)		Systole (mm)	
IVS	6	(3–5.5)	9	(4–9)
LV chamber	15	(10–20)	7	(4–11)
LV wall	7	(3–5.5)	10	(4–10)
LA	23	(6–12)		
Aorta	11	(7–12)		
LV FS	53%	(40–66%)		

i. Based on the echocardiographic examination, what is the working diagnosis?
ii. What echocardiographic abnormalities are shown?
iii. What clinical management can be advised for this case?

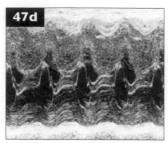

47 i. M-mode measurements indicate mild/moderate LV and IVS hypertrophy, with marked LA enlargement. Hypertrophic cardiomyopathy is likely, as systemic hypertension and hyperthyroidism are absent. The murmur and findings shown in the figures (described below) support a working diagnosis of hypertrophic obstructive cardiomyopathy (HOCM).

ii. Mitral valve systolic anterior motion is seen (47a, d). The anterior (septal) mitral leaflet is pulled toward the IVS (arrow), which contributes to dynamic LV outflow obstruction in mid systole. Secondary mitral regurgitation (from mitral leaflet displacement) and increased LV outflow turbulence (47b) explain the murmur.

Severity of dynamic obstruction can be estimated by Doppler peak LV outflow velocity (47c), here ~4 m/s (pressure gradient of ~64 mmHg). When optimal Doppler alignment is not possible (as in this case), the true resting gradient is underestimated. The LV outflow velocity spectrum's shape shows abrupt acceleration in mid systole; this concave, asymmetrically-shaped waveform is typical for dynamic obstruction.

iii. Treatment for asymptomatic HOCM is controversial. Anecdotal improvement in physical activity has occurred after beta blocker or diltiazem therapy. Beta blockers can reduce LV outflow obstruction acutely, but controlled long-term studies are lacking. The efficacy of angiotensin-converting enzyme inhibitors is also unclear. Furosemide is not indicated without congestive failure.

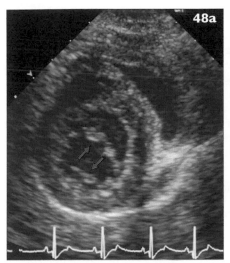

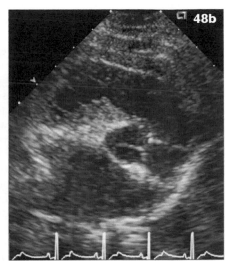

48 A 9-year-old male Miniature Schnauzer is reluctant to jump on and off the furniture. The owner observes no other abnormalities. The dog's HR is 100 bpm. A soft systolic murmur is heard at the left apex. Mild lumbar pain is detected, but no neurologic deficits. The rest of the examination is normal. Chest radiographs and ECG are unremarkable. An echocardiogram is done; LV dimensions from M-mode imaging are 3.44 cm (end diastole) and 2.04 cm (systole). Two-dimensional right parasternal short axis views at mitral valve (48a) and aortic (48b) levels, and a long axis 4-chamber view in systole (48c) are shown

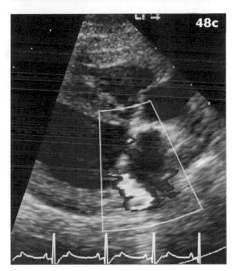

i. What are the echo findings?
ii. What is your diagnosis?
iii. How would you manage this case?

49 How should AV reciprocating tachycardia, associated with ventricular pre-excitation, be treated?

48 i. There is moderate mitral valve thickening (arrows, 48a). Ventricular proportions look normal. LA enlargement is minimal at this time. Color flow examination demonstrates mild mitral regurgitation (48c). M-mode LV dimensions and FS (40.7%) are normal. FS is calculated from the LV dimensions as (LV diastolic − LV systolic)/LV diastolic × 100.

ii. Early degenerative mitral valve disease (endocardiosis).

iii. There are no clinical signs of heart failure and minimal to no evidence for hemodynamic compromise (normal heart size and function). This dog would be classified as stage B1 heart failure according to the modified American Heart Association/American College of Cardiology staging system. Specific cardiac medications are not clearly indicated at this time. Potential benefits of low-dose beta blocker or other therapy are under investigation. Routine health maintenance care, management of lumbar pain (in this case), avoidance of high salt intake, client education about early signs of cardiac decompensation, and cardiac evaluation in 6–12 months are recommended.

49 If a vagal maneuver is not effective, drugs that slow conduction or prolong the refractory period of the bypass tract, AV node, or both may terminate the tachycardia. Diltiazem (or verapamil), procainamide, lidocaine, or a beta blocker (slowly IV) can be tried; amiodarone or a class IC antiarrhythmic agent are alternatives. However, if atrial fibrillation was pre-existing, amiodarone, sotalol, or procainamide is recommended for the tachycardia. Although digoxin slows AV conduction, it can decrease the accessory pathway's refractory period, so it is avoided with ventricular pre-excitation. Intracardiac electrophysiologic mapping with ablation of the accessory pathway(s) has successfully abolished refractory AV reciprocating tachycardia in some dogs. (See also case 130.)

50 A 5.5-year-old intact male Shih Tzu is presented for episodes of respiratory stridor and labored breathing over the past 6 months. The episodes involve sudden-onset, noisy ('roaring') inspiratory sounds, with the dog appearing uncomfortable, rigid, and slightly cyanotic. They occur unpredictably and are often triggered by exercise or excitement. The respiratory distress is short lived;

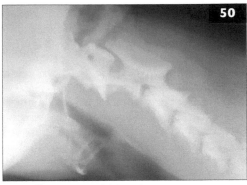

complete resolution of clinical signs generally occurs within minutes.

On presentation, the dog is slightly overweight, alert, and fully responsive. Physical examination is unremarkable. No facial deformities are observed, both nostrils appear patent, and visual inspection of the throat and neck palpation are unremarkable. Hematology, serum biochemistry, and arterial blood gas test results are all normal. Thoracic radiographs are unremarkable. A lateral radiograph of the laryngeal area is shown (50).

i. What differential diagnoses could cause the episodic inspiratory stridor and cyanosis in this dog?

ii. What abnormality can be observed on the radiograph of the neck region?

iii. Are there additional tests that can be recommended for a definitive diagnosis?

iv. What are the available therapeutic options?

51 A 5-year-old male DSH cat is presented for recent onset of anorexia, lethargy, weight gain, and trouble breathing. The cat's mucous membranes are pink with normal capillary refill time. The HR is 180 bpm with a regular rhythm; no murmur is heard. Lung sounds are somewhat muffled. Femoral pulses are normal.

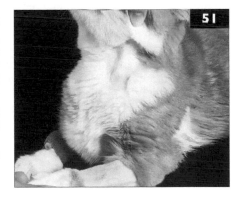

i. What physical abnormality is shown (51)?

ii. What can cause this?

iii. What test(s) should you do next?

50 i. Stridor is a loud musical sound caused by turbulent air flow in the upper airways, usually associated with obstruction. Sometimes, stridor is audible only when the animal breathes deeply (e.g. with exercise or excitement). It usually occurs during inspiration. Anatomic deformities that partially obstruct the upper airway, common in brachycephalic dogs, can cause stridor. These include stenotic nares, extended (elongated) soft palate, laryngeal deformities (including everted saccules), and hypoplastic trachea. Functional abnormalities (e.g. tracheal collapse, laryngeal paralysis), as well as upper airway obstruction from a foreign body, tumor, abscess, or severe mucosal edema, can also cause stridor.

ii. The radiograph shows an elongated soft palate, which impinges on the laryngeal opening (*aditus laryngis*).

iii. Soft palate entrapment at the larynx can be seen by visual inspection of the pharyngeal and laryngeal area during deep sedation or general anesthesia. The examination should also include retrograde rhinoscopy to exclude potential disorders in the nasopharyngeal area (e.g. choanal mass or foreign body) and careful inspection of the pharynx and tonsillary crypts.

iv. Surgical resection of the elongated soft palate is the treatment of choice. Some cases may require prior clinical stabilization (i.e. sedation, cage rest, O_2 supplementation, antibiotic and anti-inflammatory treatment) before surgery.

51 i. Marked jugular vein distension.

ii. Jugular veins become distended when pressure within rises. Persistent jugular distension, with the head in a normal erect position, is usually associated with right-sided congestive heart failure, cardiac tamponade or, rarely, constrictive pericardial disease. When there is no obstructive lesion between jugular vein(s) and RA, the appearance of the jugular veins provides an indication of right heart filling pressure.

Occasionally, jugular vein distension without pulsation occurs because of disease that obstructs blood flow through the cranial vena cava, proximal jugular veins, or RV inflow region. This can occur from thrombosis or other intravascular mass lesion, or from external compression of the vena cava.

Although not well seen in the photograph, this cat also had subcutaneous edema of the ventral jaw, thoracic inlet, and forelimbs. These findings comprise the 'cranial caval syndrome', which is usually caused by venous obstruction within the cranial thorax (e.g. cranial mediastinal mass or cranial vena caval thrombosis).

iii. Thoracic radiographs are indicated to evaluate the cranial mediastinum as well as other thoracic structures. Thoracic ultrasonography can also demonstrate presence of a mediastinal mass or venous thrombosis. Needle aspirate of a mass lesion or any pleural effusion may provide an etiology. (See also case **52**.)

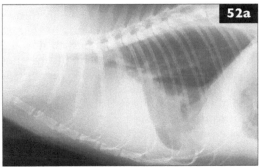

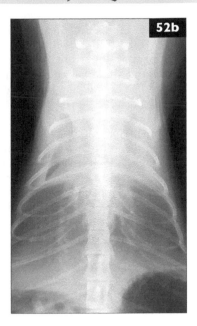

52 Lateral (52a) and DV (52b) thoracic radiographs are obtained on a 5-year-old DSH cat with anorexia, lethargy, respiratory difficulty, marked jugular vein distension, and cranial subcutaneous edema (see case 51).
i. What is your radiographic interpretation?
ii. List the main differential diagnoses.
iii. How would you proceed with this case?

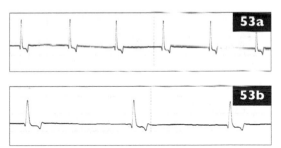

53 A 6-year-old male intact English Bull Terrier is presented after a 3-day history of lethargy and episodic collapse during daily walks. During these episodes the dog trembled but never lost consciousness or sphincter control. Previous history is unremarkable. The dog is slightly lethargic, but fully responsive and in good body condition. Physical examination suggests mild dehydration, with tacky mucous membranes but normal capillary refill time. Femoral pulses are strong and regular at a rate of 50/minute. Thoracic auscultation is unremarkable. ECG recordings at 25 mm/s (53a) and 50 mm/s (53b) are shown.
i. What is your ECG interpretation?
ii. What are the possible underlying causes?
iii. What other tests would be indicated for this patient?

52 i. The cardiac silhouette is obscured by a moderate amount of pleural effusion. The cranial thorax is filled with soft tissue/fluid opacity. The partially atelectic cranial lung lobes are displaced caudally and the trachea is pushed dorsally, indicating a cranial mediastinal mass lesion is present rather than pleural fluid alone. The caudal lung lobes and vessels appear normal. A large amount of gas in the stomach (aerophagia) is consistent with respiratory distress.

ii. The most common causes of a cranial mediastinal mass lesion are lymphoma and thymoma, although a granulomatous or other lesion is also possible. Large cranial mediastinal masses compress the cranial vena cava, which raises venous pressure in the cranial body and promotes the cranial subcutaneous edema as well as jugular vein distension seen in this case. Pleural effusion is often concurrent.

iii. Definitive diagnosis is needed to guide specific therapy. Needle aspirate of the mass and pleural fluid may yield a cytologic diagnosis. If not, a biopsy is indicated (ultrasound-guided or surgical). Lymphoma was diagnosed in this cat.

53 i. The figures show a slow HR (60 bpm), flat baseline, no obvious P waves, and slightly widened QRS complexes. These features suggest lack of atrial electrical activity (atrial standstill). It is unclear if the QRSs are escape complexes. Atrial fibrillation (AF) is another cause of absent P waves, but AF causes baseline undulation ('f' waves) and irregular AV conduction, which produces a chaotic ventricular rhythm.

ii. Moderate to severe hyperkalemia can cause atrial standstill by inhibiting atrial muscle depolarization. However, sinus node activity generally persists and is conducted via internodal pathways to the AV node and then into the ventricles (sinoventricular rhythm).

Persistent atrial standstill (silent atria) results from atrial myocardial disease. It is characterized by atrial mural fibrosis and thinning, conduction failure, and atrial enlargement; an escape rhythm is required to stimulate the heartbeat. This disease is most common in English Springer Spaniels. In other cases, atrial standstill can be secondary to cardiomyopathy or myocarditis.

iii. Serum electrolytes should be measured immediately and hyperkalemia, if present, treated at once. Hypoadrenocorticism and urinary obstruction are common causes of hyperkalemia; appropriate diagnostic tests are done as indicated. If serum potassium is normal, additional tests should include thoracic radiographs and echocardiography. Serum cardiac troponin I concentration may indicate active myocardial damage. (See also case **54**.)

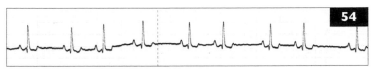

54 After initial examination, the following serum biochemical results are obtained on the dog with collapsing episodes described in 53:

Parameter	Result	Reference range
Urea	13.1 mmol/l (36.7 mg/dl)	2.5–9.6 mmol/l (7–26.9 mg/dl)
Creatinine	189 µmol/l (2.1 mg/dl)	44–159 µmol/l (0.5–1.8 mg/dl)
Total protein	76.0 g/l (7.6 g/dl)	52.0–82.0 g/l (5.2–8.2 g/dl)
Albumin	38.0 g/l (3.8 g/dl)	23.0–40.0 g/l (2.3–4.0 g/dl)
Globulin	38.0 g/l (3.8 g/dl)	25.0–45.0 g/l (2.5–4.5 g/dl)
Albumin/globulin ratio	1.0	0.50–1.50
Alanine transferase	32.0 U/l	10–100 U/l
Alkaline phosphatase	81.0 U/l	23–212 U/l
Glucose	7.0 mmol/l (126 mg/dl)	4.1–7.9 mmol/l (74–142 mg/dl)
Sodium (Na)	135 mmol/l (135 mEq/l)	144–160 mmol/l (144–160 mEq/l)
Potassium (K)	8.4 mmol/l (8.4 mEq/l)	3.5–5.8 mmol/l (3.5–5.8 mEq/l)
Na/K ratio	16.0	>27
Calcium	3.0 mmol/l (12 mg/dl)	1.90–3.0 mmol/l (7.6–12 mg/dl)
Phosphorus	1.7 mmol/l (5.3 mg/dl)	0.81–2.20 mmol/l (2.5–6.8 mg/dl)
Cholesterol	8.4 mmol/l (324 mg/dl)	2.8–8.3 µmol/l (108–320 mg/dl)
Basal cortisol	<28 nmol/l (<1 µg/dl)	28–250 nmol/l (1–9 µg/dl)
Post adreno-corticotropic hormone (ACTH) cortisol	<28 nmol/l (<1 µg/dl)	50–660 nmol/l (1.8–23.9 µg/dl)

An ECG (**54**, 25 mm/s) is recorded after initial therapy.
i. What caused the presenting clinical signs and ECG abnormalities in this dog?
ii. What initial treatment is indicated?
iii. What is your interpretation of the ECG shown here?

55 How is heartworm disease (HWD) severity graded?

54 i. Hyperkalemia caused the relatively slow HR and lack of P waves on initial ECG (see case 53). Besides hyperkalemia, the dog's hyponatremia and reduced Na/K ratio suggest hypoadrenocorticism (Addison's disease). This was confirmed by low pre- and post-ACTH cortisol concentrations. Reduced circulating volume associated with this disease can cause dehydration, prerenal azotemia, and weakness.

ii. Initial therapy is aimed at correcting hypovolemia, electrolyte imbalances, and metabolic acidosis. In some cases, aggressive IV 0.9% saline administration is adequate. However, for severe or non-responsive hyperkalaemia, concurrent administration of regular insulin (0.5–1.0 U/kg) plus dextrose (2 g/U insulin used) in the IV fluid is indicated. Alternatively, a slow IV bolus of Na bicarbonate (1–2 mEq/kg) or 10% calcium gluconate (2–10 ml) can be given. Serum potassium should be monitored closely. Once a diagnosis of hypoadrenocorticism is confirmed, mineralocorticoid and glucocorticoid therapy is initated.

iii. Sinus arrhythmia at a rate of 100 bpm is present. P waves are clearly seen now and the QRS complex duration is shorter. This ECG was recorded 24 hours after initiation of fluid therapy; serum K concentration was 6.1 mmol/l (6.1 mEq/l).

55 Class 1: Asymptomatic/mild HWD. Clinical signs: none or only occasional cough, fatigue with exercise, or mildly reduced condition. No radiographic or laboratory abnormalities.

Class 2: Moderate HWD. Clinical signs: as for class 1. Radiographic signs may include RV and mild PA enlargement, circumscribed perivascular and/or mixed alveolar/interstitial infiltrates. Laboratory abnormalities may include mild anemia (PCV 0.2–0.3 l/l [20–30%]), +/- mild (2+) proteinuria.

Class 3: Severe HWD. Clinical signs may include constant fatigue, persisent cough, dyspnea, cachexia, or other signs of right-sided heart failure (ascites, jugular distension and pulse). Radiographic signs include RV +/- RA enlargement, severe PA enlargement, circumscribed to diffuse mixed patterns of pulmonary infiltrates, +/- signs of pulmonary thromboembolism. Laboratory abnormalities include anemia (PCV <0.2 l/l [<20%]), other hematologic abnormalities, or proteinuria (>2+). Class 3 dogs should be stabilized before adulticide treatment (use alternate melarsomine protocol).

Class 4: Caval syndrome. Shock-like condition following RV inflow obstruction by a mass of worms. Signs as for class 3 with acute collapse or weakness, often with pallor, dyspnea, hemoptysis, hemoglobinuria, and bilirubinuria. Intravascular hemolysis, azotemia, abnormal liver function with increased enzyme activity, and dissemination intravascular coagulation are common.

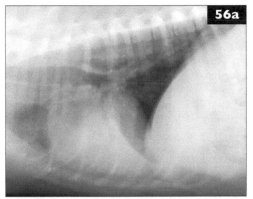

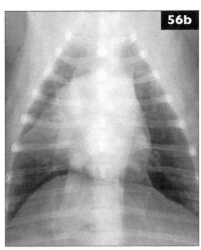

56 A 6-year-old neutered male West Highland White Terrier was rescued from a fire 5 days ago. At that time the dog showed some difficulty breathing, but lung sounds and thoracic radiographs were normal. He had been treated with supplemental O_2 for 4 days and seemed to be improving clinically. However, thoracic auscultation now reveals increased breath sounds and occasional crackles. Left lateral and DV radiographs are obtained (56a, b).

i. What radiographic changes are present, and what is the radiographic diagnosis?
ii. What is the pulmonary pathophysiology of smoke inhalation?

57 A 4-year-old castrated male Yorkshire Terrier is presented for episodes of respiratory distress. After physical examination and other clinical tests, a surgical treatment is recommended. This intraoperative photograph (57) demonstrates the lesion responsible for the respiratory distress. Cranial is to the left in this photograph.

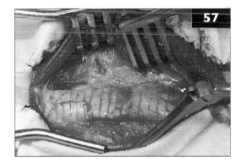

i. What is the cause of the dog's historical respiratory distress?
ii. What preoperative diagnostic tests would be useful to document this diagnosis?
iii. Assuming that the lesion is present only in the location demonstrated in the photograph, during what phase of respiration would the respiratory distress be most prominent?
iv. If respiratory distress is severe when the dog is initially presented, what treatments should be done to stabilize the animal, and with what priority?

56 i. The right middle lung lobe demonstrates well-defined cranial and caudal lobar borders, effacement with the mid-right cardiac border, and air bronchogram formation (56c, arrows). A small volume of air is in the mid-thoracic esophagus. The radiographic diagnoses are right middle lobe alveolar pattern and mild aerophagia. Differentials to be considered include secondary bacterial pneumonia, aspiration pneumonia, and partial atelectasis secondary to bronchial obstruction.

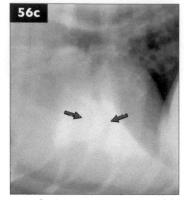

ii. Thermal injury, gases, and irritant particulate products generated by the fire damage the airways and lung parenchyma. Hypoxia, release of inflammatory mediators, and, potentially, airway occlusion occur in variable combinations related to the duration of exposure and the type of combustible materials. The radiographic changes are due to pulmonary edema and pneumonia.

Thoracic radiographs are often normal at presentation. During the first 24–36 hours, pulmonary interstitial to alveolar radiographic patterns can develop. These relate to the increased mucosal secretions, mucosal sloughing, and secondary bacterial infection that are later sequelae.

57 i. Tracheal collapse. Weakened cartilaginous rings and/or redundancy of the dorsal tracheal membrane usually underlie the narrowing of the tracheal lumen that occurs. Cervical, intrathoracic, or both regions of the trachea can be involved.
ii. The standard tests for diagnosing this condition are (1) cervicothoracic radiographs taken during both inhalation and exhalation, (2) cervicothoracic fluoroscopy, and (3) tracheoscopy.
iii. The image shows the cervical trachea from a ventral midline approach. Tracheal collapse limited to the cervical trachea causes inspiratory dyspnea.
iv. If respiratory distress is severe on presentation, the dog should be sedated, placed in a quiet O_2-rich environment, and monitored closely. If sedation fails to reverse the respiratory distress, deeper sedation or anesthesia should be employed for endotracheal intubation. Oxygen is delivered through the endotracheal tube and ventilation is provided as necessary. Once all vital parameters are stable under deep sedation or anesthesia, the dog is allowed to recover slowly. If the dog cannot be extubated without respiratory distress recurring, emergency surgical correction or intraluminal stent placement may be necessary. A temporary tracheostomy tube may be placed if definitive correction is not available; however, this technique may complicate definitive correction.

58 A 4-year-old Yorkshire Terrier with episodic respiratory distress is diagnosed with tracheal collapse (see case 57). This intraoperative photograph demonstrates the lesion and the surgical treatment employed. Cranial is to the left in this photograph.

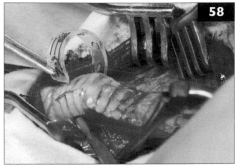

i. What diagnostic modality is used to grade this condition, and what are the four grades?
ii. Of what biomaterial is the implant being employed in the photograph made?
iii. What muscle bellies are being retracted by the Weitlaner retracter?
iv. What iatrogenic complication can occur with this technique, and what can be done to treat the complication?

59 An 8-year-old neutered female Ragdoll cat weighing 3.5 kg (7.7 lb) is presented for labored breathing of sudden onset approximately 12 hours earlier. The cat lives mainly indoors and is fed a commercial maintenance diet. The cat appears distressed, with open-mouth breathing, an extended neck, abducted elbows, and increased abdominal effort. Thoracic percussion revealed a bilateral horizontal line of dullness. The HR is elevated (250 bpm). Systolic BP is 70 mmHg (normal 120–170 mmHg). Initial thoracic imaging indicates pleural effusion is present. Thoracocentesis yields 200 ml of fluid (59). The cat's respiratory rate and pattern improve dramatically after thoracocentesis. Fluid analysis: tryglcerides, 16.96 mmol/l (1501 mg/dl); cholesterol, 3.6 mmol/l (139 mg/dl); total protein, 39.8 g/l (3.98 g/dl); albumin, 21.8 g/l (2.18 g/dl); globulin, 18.0 g/l (1.8 g/dl); alb/glob

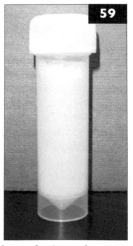

ratio, 1.21; macroscopic examination, white, opaque fluid; cytologic evaluation, moderate cellularity (5.0×10^9/l) with good cell preservation, neutrophils (14%), lymphocytes (56%), macrophages (30%); occasional mesothelial cells and plasma cells seen; no evidence of neoplasia; no bacteria identified; results of both aerobic and anaerobic culture, negative.
i. What type of fluid was aspirated from the chest of this patient?
ii. List some abnormalities that can cause this.
iii. What additional diagnostic tests are indicated?

58 i. Tracheoscopy is used to grade the degree of collapse as 25% collapse (grade 1), 50% collapse (grade 2), 75% collapse (grade 3), or near total collapse (grade 4).
ii. The prosthetic tracheal ring in the photograph was made from a polypropylene syringe barrel; however, commercially manufactured polypropylene tracheal ring prostheses are available in a variety of sizes. Prosthetic tracheal rings have also been fashioned from polyvinyl chloride drip chambers of intravenous administration sets.
iii. Prosthetic tracheal rings are applied to the cervical trachea via a ventral midline surgical approach from the larynx to the manubrium. The sternohyoideus muscles are separated on the midline, and these are the muscle bellies that are being retracted by the self-retaining retractors in the photograph.
iv. The major iatrogenic complication of this surgical technique is damage to the recurrent laryngeal nerves located in the peritracheal fascia. The resultant laryngeal paralysis may be treated by cricoarytenoid laryngoplasty. Intraluminal tracheal stenting avoids iatrogenic recurrent laryngeal nerve injury, but the cervical portion of the trachea may be better served by extraluminal ring prostheses, while intraluminal stenting is better for intrathoracic tracheal collapse.

59 i. The appearance of the pleural fluid, as well as its cytologic and biochemical features, indicate a chylous effusion. Most effusions in cats and dogs are bilateral, as in this case, because the right and left pleural cavities communicate through mediastinal fenestrations.
ii. Increased pressure within (or permeability of) the thoracic duct system allows chyle to leak into the pleural space. Mediastinal neoplasia (especially lymphoma in cats) can cause lymphatic obstruction and inflammation and lead to chylous effusion. Any process that increases systemic venous pressure (e.g. right-sided heart failure from cardiomyopathy, dirofilariasis, or pericardial disease, as well as cranial vena caval thrombosis) can result in chylothorax. Trauma is another potential cause of chylothorax, especially in outdoor cats. Congenital lymphatic malformation can also predispose to chylous effusion. When no underlying cause can be identified, idiopathic chylothorax is diagnosed.
iii. Diagnostic tests should include thoracic radiographs (after thoracocentesis) to evaluate cardiac size and shape, the lungs, cranial mediastinum, and other visible structures. Echocardiography is useful to screen for underlying cardiac disease, and may show evidence for cardiomyopathy, mediastinal or intrathoracic mass lesion, or other abnormality. Routine hematologic, biochemical, and heartworm tests are also recommended. Lymphangiography can demonstrate lymphangiectasia and areas of obstruction.

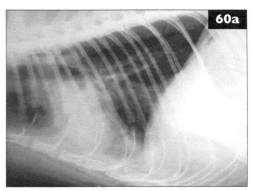

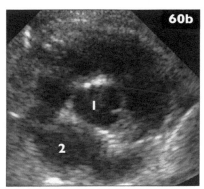

60 The cat in 59 developed chylothorax. It lived mainly indoors and there was no history of trauma. A lateral chest radiograph taken after thoracocentesis is shown (60a). An echocardiogram was also done; a right parasternal short axis view at the level of the heart base is shown (60b). All other echo views were unremarkable; concurrent ECG monitoring showed sinus rhythm at approximately 250 bpm. Hematology and serum biochemistry test results were unremarkable. Tests for feline immunodeficiency virus, feline leukemia virus, and heartworm disease were negative. 1 – aorta, 2 – left atrium.
i. What is the most likely cause of chylothorax in this case?
ii. What are the treatment options and prognosis?

61 A 4-month-old female purebred cat exhibits lethargy, fever, weight loss, respiratory difficulty, and constipation. The kitten is thin, febrile (39.4°C [103°F]), and tachypneic. Thoracic radiographs reveal pleural effusion. Thoracocentesis yields a turbid, yellow fluid with a cell count of 8760/µl, protein content of 45 g/l (4.5 g/dl), and pH of 6.0. A photomicrograph of a direct smear of the fluid is shown (61, Wright's stain, 500× oil).

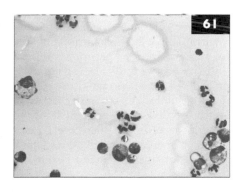

i. How would you classify this fluid based on fluid characteristics as well as cytologic findings?
ii. Based on fluid evaluation, as well as the signalment and clinical findings, what is the most likely diagnosis?
iii. What antemortem diagnostic tests are available to confirm this, and what are their limitations?

60 i. Mild residual pleural effusion, without venous congestion or pulmonary edema, is present (**60a**). Normal atrial size (**60b**) and other normal echo findings suggest a non-cardiac origin for the effusion. Lack of evidence for a mediastinal mass, thrombus, or other cause of increased cranial vena caval pressure or lymphatic disruption, with no known trauma, suggests an idiopathic chylothorax, although neoplasia cannot be fully excluded.

ii. Medical management is attempted before considering surgery. Chylothorax of identifiable and treatable cause may resolve. However, no treatment for idiopathic chylothorax is consistently effective, although spontaneous resolution after several weeks or months is reported rarely.

Thoracocentesis is repeated as necessary; a chest tube is placed in patients with rapid fluid accumulation or traumatic chylothorax. Electrolytes are monitored with frequent thoracocentesis. Medical therapy can include a low-fat diet (to reduce lymph flow) and administration of rutin (a natural bioflavonoid that inhibits inflammation and fibrosis and promotes macrophage activation). Octreotide, a synthetic analogue of somatostatin, may reduce gastrointestinal secretions and decrease thoracic duct lymphatic flow.

Surgical intervention (i.e. thoracic duct ligation, pericardectomy, and omentalization of the thoracic cavity) is recommended in patients that do not respond to medical management.

61 i. This fluid is classified as an exudate, based on both the high nucleated cell count (>5000/µl) and the high total protein (>30 g/l [>3.0 g/dl]). Cytologic examination also reveals a highly proteinaceous effusion (basophilic, stippled background with protein crescents) with increased cellularity. Cells are composed of a mixture of neutrophils and macrophages with a few small lymphocytes. The cytologic diagnosis was therefore proteinaceous effusion with moderate neutrophilic, macrophagic inflammation.

ii. Feline infectious peritonitis (FIP) is the most likely cause, although this is a difficult disease to diagnose definitively antemortem.

iii. FIP is a feline corona virus (FCoV). Many other coronaviruses (including non-pathogenic FCoV) are antigenically similar to the pathogenic FCoV. As a result, antibody titers and even PCR tests are not specific for FIP. Results of these diagnostic tests are therefore considered together with clinical and historical findings in order to reach a presumptive diagnosis.

The best antemortem test for FIP is biopsy, where the diagnosis can be confirmed by histopathology. The characteristic lesion in FIP (both effusive and dry form) is pyo-granulomatous vasculitis. In this case the diagnosis of FIP was confirmed at necropsy.

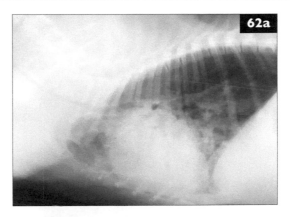

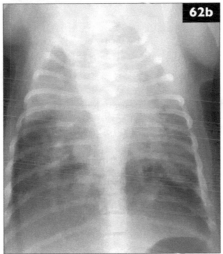

62 A 4-month-old female English Bulldog develops respiratory difficulty that progresses to dyspnea over the course of 4 days. She is febrile. A hemogram reveals a degenerative left shift with toxic neutrophils. Right lateral (62a) and DV (62b) radiographs are taken.

i. Describe the radiographic abnormalities.

ii. What are your radiographic diagnoses?

iii. What, if any, is the correlation between the two major findings?

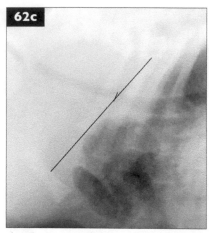

62 i. A ventral bilateral soft tissue pulmonary opacity is present. Well-defined air bronchograms of the left cranial lobe are summated (superimposed) with the cardiac shadow in the lateral view. A strong lobar border sign is evident between the right cranial and middle lobes in the DV view at the 6th intercostal space. The soft tissue opacity is heterogeneous between the heart and diaphragm. The dorsal portions of the caudal lobes are hyperinflated. The trachea is narrower than normal, with a tracheal diameter:thoracic inlet ratio of 0.06. The landmarks for the tracheal diameter:thoracic inlet ratio are shown (62c). Bulldogs with a ratio less than 0.13 are likely to have a hypoplastic trachea.
ii. Hypoplastic trachea and bronchopneumonia.
iii. Tracheal hypoplasia is a congenital anomaly reported most commonly in Bulldogs. Although bronchopneumonia was the most common coexisting acquired disease found in a study of 103 dogs with radiographically defined hypoplasia, it was present in only seven of the dogs. It was thought that tracheal hypoplasia did not predispose the dogs to bronchopneumonia. The authors concluded that tracheal hypoplasia can be well tolerated when not coexisting with other respiratory or cardiovascular disease.

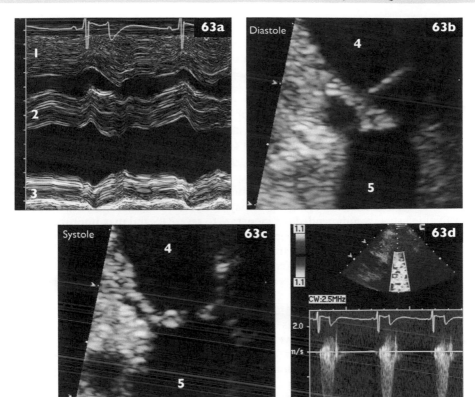

63 A 6-year-old male neutered Wire Haired Fox
Terrier is presented for evaluation of a cardiac
murmur present since puppyhood, but possibly louder now. The dog has shown no
clinical signs and is bright and alert. Physical examination is normal except for a
grade 4/6 systolic murmur heard best at the left cardiac base. Echocardiography is
performed; images shown are M-mode at the ventricular level (63a), right
parasternal short axis close-up in diastole (63b) and systole (63c), and continuous
wave Doppler in the same position (63d). 1 – RV wall, 2 – IVS, 3 – LV wall, 4 – RV
outflow tract, 5 – PA.

i. What is evident from 63a?
ii. Describe the findings in 63b–d.
iii. What are your recommendations to the owner?

64 What is angiostrongylosis, and how is it transmitted?

63 i. Severe RV wall hypertrophy (1.2 cm, diastole, compared to LV wall of 0.8 cm) is most striking. IVS thickening is present, but exaggerated by adjacent tricuspid valve echos. This RV hypertrophy indicates chronic, marked RV systolic pressure overload (e.g. severe pulmonic stenosis or pulmonary hypertension).
ii. The abnormally thickened pulmonic valve (**63b**) exhibits systolic 'doming' with incomplete opening (**63c**) because of fused, malformed leaflets. Diagnosis is congenital valvular pulmonic stenosis (PS). Maximal pulmonary systolic velocity is 5 m/s (**63d**); estimated RV to PA systolic pressure gradient (PG) is 100 mmHg (modified Bernoulli relationship, PG= $4 \times v^2$).
iii. PS with Doppler-derived gradient over 80–100 mmHg is considered severe. PS sequelae can include RV and atrial enlargement, tricuspid regurgitation, myocardial ischemia, arrhythmias, and right-sided congestive failure or sudden death, especially with severe stenosis. However, signs may not develop for several years. Balloon valvuloplasty is recommended for moderate to severe PS and may improve clinical signs and survival. This palliative procedure is most successful with simple pulmonic leaflet fusion, although significant systolic pressure gradient reduction is possible with some dysplastic valves. Exercise is also restricted for moderate to severe PS. Beta blocker therapy may help reduce myocardial ischemia and arrhythmias.

64 Nematodes of the genus *Angiostrongylus* can parasitize several species. *A. vasorum* most often affects dogs as well as foxes, wild canidae, and other species. This parasite is found in western Europe and the UK, eastern Canada (Newfoundland), and portions of South America and Africa; its distribution appears to be spreading. *A. vasorum* requires an intermediate host (slug or snail) in which L_1 larvae mature to an infective L_3 stage. The final host becomes infected by ingesting the intermediate or a paratenic (frog) host. L_3 penetrate the host's intestine, migrate to mesenteric lymph nodes where they mature to the L_5 stage, then travel via lymphatic flow to the right heart and PAs. Adult worms are ~20–30 mm long. The prepatent period is about 1–3 months. The adult females' eggs hatch in the pulmonary capillaries; L_1 larvae pass through alveolar and bronchial walls, are coughed up, swallowed, and excreted in the feces. Infected dogs may pass larvae for several years. Respiratory signs (cough, tachypnea, dyspnea) usually predominate, but other common manifestations can relate to a coagulopathy of variable severity, pulmonary hypertension, neurologic abnormalities, as well as non-specific gastrointestinal signs, lethargy, or weight loss.

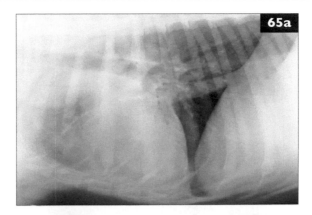

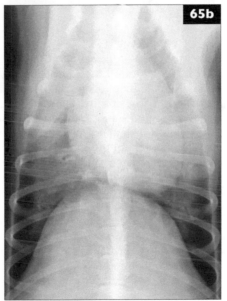

65 A 2-year-old male mixed breed dog weighing 41 kg (90 lb) was presented for depression and hemoptysis of 1-day duration. Cephalic intravenous sedation was used to assess the oral cavity and larynx; no abnormalities were found. The following day, the limb used for injection is found to be swollen and bruised. Right lateral (65a) and DV (65b) thoracic radiographs are taken.

i. What are the radiographic findings, and what is your diagnosis?

ii. What additional diagnostic tests will you use to confirm your diagnosis?

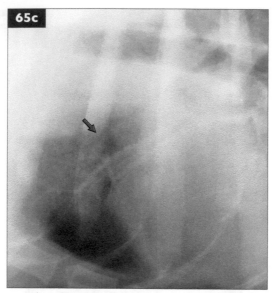

65 i. The right cranial and middle lung lobes and the cranial segment of the left cranial lobe are of increased soft tissue opacity. There is a distinct lobar border sign between the right cranial and middle lobes, an air bronchogram (65c, arrow) involving the right cranial lobar bronchus, and effacement of the right cranial border of the heart. The ventral border of the cranial mediastinum shows a ventrally directed convex contour, but there is no shift of the trachea in either view. The radiographic diagnosis is cranial and middle lung alveolar–interstitial pattern with etiologic differentials of pulmonary hemorrhage, bronchopneumonia, and aspiration pneumonia.

ii. With a history of acute hemoptysis and postvenipuncture ecchymosis there is concern for an acquired coagulopathy, such as from anticoagulant rodenticide toxicity. Tests for hemostasis are indicated. Prothrombin time was found to be >120 seconds (normal 5–12 seconds) in this dog; partial thromboplastin time was 45 seconds (normal 9–19 seconds). Further questioning of the owner revealed exposure to brodificoum.

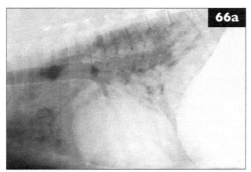

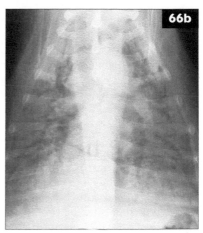

66 A 14-year-old spayed female Labrador Retriever is presented about 9 hours after water submersion and subsequent resuscitation. Major clinical signs are generalized depression and tachypnea. Wheezes and crackles are heard on thoracic auscultation. Initial pulse oximetry reading is 85%. Lateral (66a) and DV (66b) thoracic radiographs are taken approximately 36 hours after hospital admission; earlier radiography was deemed unsafe based on patient instability.

i. What are the radiographic findings, and are these typical in drowning cases?

ii. What are the principal pathophysiologic differences between freshwater and saltwater drowning?

iii. What is the principal therapeutic goal for drowning patients, and how is this achieved?

iv. What is the role of antibiotic therapy in treating drowned patients?

v. What is the prognosis for dogs that submerge in freshwater?

67 A 7-year-old male Persian cat with labored breathing and poor appetite has a respiratory rate of 50 breaths/min, HR of 180 bpm with an irregular rhythm, and a grade 2/6 systolic murmur at the cranial left sternal border. You record an ECG (67, leads as marked, 25 mm/s, 1 cm = 1 mV).

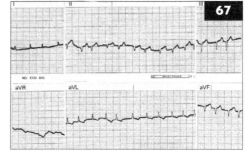

i. What is your ECG diagnosis?

ii. Do these findings suggest any particular cardiac abnormalities?

iii. What would you do next for this case?

66 i. There is a widespread alveolar pattern with prominent air bronchograms. This is typical in the early pathophysiologic stages post drowning, although radiographic signs may lag behind clinical signs. A mixed interstitial-bronchial pattern may coexist or may remain as the alveolar pattern resolves.

ii. Low-tonicity freshwater is rapidly absorbed from the airways, leading to hypervolemia, hyponatremia, and sometimes hemolysis (with hyperkalemia, hemoglobinemia, and hemoglobinuria). However, fluid redistribution can occur quickly, leading to pulmonary edema and hypovolemia with normal electrolyte concentrations. High-tonicity saltwater draws fluid from the intravascular space to increase pulmonary fluid accumulation. Freshwater interferes with surface tension properties of pulmonary surfactant by altering its ionic composition. Saltwater washes out some surfactant without changing the properties of remaining surfactant.

iii. Hypoxemia must be reversed with O_2 therapy and, if necessary, positive end-expiratory pressure or continuous positive airway pressure.

iv. Antibiotics do not affect survival in drowned animals and can lead to resistant organisms if bacterial pneumonia develops; therefore, antibiotic use should be restricted to documented infections.

v. The prognosis for dogs drowning in freshwater is good as long as respiratory failure does not ensue. Prolonged submersion and delayed resuscitation contribute to poorer prognosis.

67 i. The HR is 160 bpm. The rhythm is atrial fibrillation (AF); note the lack of P waves and rhythm irregularity. There is a left axis deviation (approximately –60°). The QRS complexes are slightly wide at 0.04–0.05 second.

ii. Almost all cats that develop AF have serious underlying cardiac disease with marked atrial enlargement. A certain 'critical mass' of atrial tissue is needed to sustain AF, which generally requires atrial dilation in animals of small body size. The left axis deviation of the QRS complexes (left anterior fasicular block pattern) suggests LV hypertrophy. Based on the ECG findings, the most likely differential diagnosis is hypertrophic or perhaps restrictive cardiomyopathy; other considerations include hyperthyroidism (although this cat is fairly young), chronic severe hypertension, or longstanding congenital disease (e.g. subaortic stenosis or mitral dysplasia).

iii. Chest radiographs and echocardiography are recommended, along with BP measurement and a routine laboratory database. This cat had hypertrophic cardiomyopathy with pulmonary edema. For cats with hypertrophic cardiomyopathy and AF, diltiazem or a beta blocker is used without digoxin. Furosemide, benazepril, and low-dose aspirin were also prescribed.

68 A 4-year-old male Labrador Retriever from the central USA is presented for persistent fever, despite antibiotic treatment, and chronic cough. The cough seems to respond to prednisone, but returns once the prednisone is discontinued. The dog is bright, alert, and responsive. Body temperature is 40°C (104.1°F). HR is 152 bpm and respiratory rate is 60 breaths/min. Lung sounds are described as harsh. Mandibular, right prescapular, and popliteal lymph nodes are somewhat enlarged. Thoracic radiographs show a diffuse interstitial nodular pattern and a 4 × 4 cm indistinct pulmonary mass in the left caudodorsal lung lobe. The cardiac silhouette, pulmonary vasculature, and remaining structures are within normal limits. An arterial sample is obtained for blood gas analysis (see below).

Test	Result	Normal	Units
pH	7.483	7.31–7.42	
PCO_2	20.0	29–42	mmHg
PO_2	56.8	85–95	mmHg
HCO_3	14.7	17–24	mmol/l
Base excess	-6.1		mmol/l
Total CO_2	15.3		mmol/l
% Saturation	92.3		%

i. What is your interpretation of the blood gas results?
ii. What is the alveolar-arterial (A–a) gradient?
iii. What does this mean?
iv. Identify the most likely causes for this dog's problems.

69 A 10-year-old spayed female Boston Terrier is presented for signs of right-sided heart failure; pericardial effusion with cardiac tamponade is suspected. An echocardiogram is done (**69**, 1 – RV, 2 – LV, 3 – LA). A cardiac mass lesion is not identified. Pericardiocentesis is done; definitive diagnosis of malignancy is not possible based on cytologic characteristics. Thoracotomy for subtotal pericardectomy is planned.

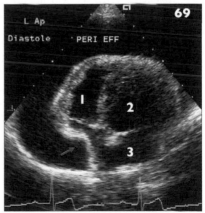

i. Is cardiac tamponade present?
ii. What are the likely causes of the pericardial effusion?
iii. What intercostal space is preferred for open thorax pericardectomy, and why?
iv. What would be the advantages of thoracoscopy for treating this case?
v. What would be the disadvantages of thoracoscopy for treating this case?

68 i. Marked hypoxemia with primary respiratory alkalosis and compensatory metabolic acidosis.

ii. The A–a gradient is the difference between the partial pressures of O_2 in the alveolus (PAO_2) and arterial blood (PaO_2). PAO_2 is estimated as fraction of inspired O_2 (FiO_2) $\times$ ($P_{barometric}$ - P_{H_2O}) – $PaCO_2/R$. R is the respiratory exchange quotient (O_2 uptake per CO_2 produced), which is assumed to be 0.8. For animals breathing room air at sea level: $PAO_2 = 150$ mmHg – $PaCO_2/0.8$. In this dog, estimated PAO_2 is 125 and A–a gradient is 68.2 mmHg.

iii. The A–a gradient helps separate the effect of hypoventilation on measured PaO_2. In normal lungs, PAO_2 should essentially equal O_2 tension in the pulmonary capillaries and, therefore, in arterial blood (PaO_2). An A–a gradient ≤10 mmHg is considered normal. Ventilation/perfusion (V/Q) abnormalities, shunt, and impaired gas diffusion increase the A–a gradient; hypoventilation does not increase the gradient because PAO_2 is also decreased. A–a gradients >15 mmHg usually indicate some degree of V/Q mismatch. The marked A–a gradient and hypoxemia in this dog indicate severe pulmonary dysfunction.

iv. Systemic fungal disease, lymphoma, or other metastatic neoplasia would be most likely. Blastomycosis was diagnosed in this dog.

69 i. Yes. Cardiac tamponade occurs when intrapericardial fluid pressure exceeds normal right heart filling pressure. This is indicated by collapse of the RA wall (arrow) in this diastolic image.

ii. Pericardial effusion in dogs is usually caused either by neoplasia or idiopathic pericarditis. Hemangiosarcoma, usually involving the right auricular appendage or other right heart structure, is the most common cardiac tumor. Aortic body tumor is second most common and more likely in brachycephalic dogs. Mesothelioma occurs occasionally. Pericardial effusion also occurs secondary to right-sided heart failure, LA tear, coagulopathy, uremia, and infection from a migrating foreign body, among other causes.

iii. Thoracotomy at the right 5th intercostal space is preferred for subtotal pericardectomy. This approach allows better visualization for identification and possible excision or biopsy of a RA mass, compared with a left-sided approach.

iv. Thoracoscopic surgery provides a minimally invasive approach for peri-cardectomy. Major advantages, in the hands of an experienced operator, include excellent visualization with less postoperative morbidity than with thoracotomy.

v. The major disadvantages to a thoracoscopic procedure include increased patient risk with biopsy or excision of a RA mass, if encountered. Also, a smaller area of pericardium is excised compared to a subtotal pericardectomy performed via thoracotomy.

70 A 10-year-old spayed female Boston Terrier develops signs of right-sided heart failure. Cardiac tamponade is identified by echocardiography and pericardiocentesis is performed. No cardiac mass lesion is visible by echocardiography. Further imaging by CT also fails to identify a cardiac mass, but demonstrates a 1.5 cm pulmonary mass located peripherally in the left cranial lung lobe, as well as sternal lymphadenomegaly. A thoracotomy is planned to biopsy the lung mass (70)

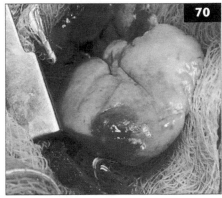

and lymph nodes and to perform subtotal pericardectomy.
i. What are your differential diagnoses for the mass shown?
ii. What finding would suggest a poor prognosis associated with this mass?
iii. Which intercostal space would be preferred for thoracotomy to access this mass?

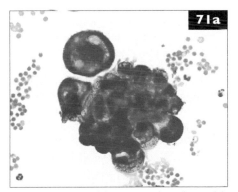
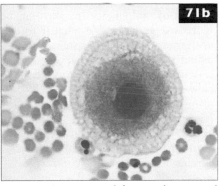

71 A 10-year-old castrated male Golden Retriever is presented for weakness and abdominal distension. Physical examination findings include ascites, muffled heart sounds, and distended jugular veins. Thoracic radiographs show an enlarged, slightly rounded cardiac silhouette. Pericardial effusion is documented by echocardiography. Pericardial fluid samples stained with Wright's stain are shown (71a, direct smear, 50× oil; 71b, cytospin preparation, 100× oil).
i. Based on the appearance of this fluid, list the most relevant cytologic differentials.
ii. What additional tests would be useful?

70 i. The most likely diagnosis for this mass is primary pulmonary adeno-carcinoma; other primary lung tumors include squamous cell carcinoma, anaplastic carcinoma, and adenoma. Topographically, primary lung carcincomas are described as bronchogenic, bronchoalveolar, or alveolar. The histologic diagnosis in this case was bronchogenic carcinoma.

Other considerations could include a metastatic pulmonary neoplasm or fungal granuloma; however, multiple lung masses would be more characteristic of these conditions than a single mass. Rarely, a pulmonary cyst or abscess could create a similar appearance.

ii. The most consistent predictor of remission and survival time for primary lung tumors is the presence or absence of metastasis to tracheobronchial lymph nodes. In this case, a tracheobronchial lymph node was positive for bronchogenic carcinoma, although enlargement was more obvious in the sternal lymph nodes, which also contained metastatic bronchogenic carcinoma.

iii. The left 5th intercostal space was chosen for the surgical approach here, because this space allows convenient access to the base of the left lung lobes in case a complete pulmonary lobectomy is required.

71 i. Note the cohesive cluster of basophilic, pleomorphic, round to polygonal cells in **71a**, and the large mesothelial cell with macronucleolus in **71b**. Segmented and pyknotic neutrophils are also present (**71b**). Cells in this fluid display numerous criteria of malignancy (marked anisocytosis and anisokaryosis, multinucleation, increased and variable nuclear to cytoplasmic ratio, and macronucleoli). Their appearance is most consistent with mesothelial cell origin, making mesothelioma a primary differential. However, another relevant differential is marked mesothelial cell hyperplasia, which occurs secondary to chronic fluid accumulation within body cavities. Reactive mesothelial cells also exhibit many criteria of malignancy, thereby mimicking neoplasia. Finally, although many cells in this sample appear to be mesothelial (large round cells with abundant basophilic cytoplasm and a pericellular corona), cytologic appearance alone cannot differentiate malignant mesothelial from malignant epithelial neoplasia. Therefore, metastatic carcinoma/adeno-carcinoma must also be considered.

ii. A thorough physical examination and careful imaging of the thorax and abdomen are warranted to identify any discrete masses. A CBC, chemistry panel, and urinalysis may help determine other organ involvement. Finally, histopathology is likely the most useful diagnostic tool to distinguish between cytologic differential diagnoses. In this case, malignant mesothelioma was diagnosed via histopathology at necropsy.

72   An 8-year-old neutered male Springer Spaniel is referred for a cough of 3-month duration. Initially, the cough was dry, harsh, and occasionally accompanied by retching. Two weeks later the cough had become productive and the dog appeared lethargic. One week before referral, the dog rapidly became depressed, dyspneic, and febrile (39.8°C [103.6°F]). Amoxicillin–clavulanate was prescribed and all clinical signs except the cough improved greatly.

At presentation the dog is bright, alert, fully responsive, and moderately overweight. Rectal temperature is normal. A cough can be elicited easily by tracheal palpation. On auscultation, rhonchi are heard occasionally during coughing. No other abnormalities are detected. Hematology and routine serum biochemistry tests are normal. Fecal examination is negative for gastrointestinal parasites and lungworms. Thoracic radiographs are obtained under general anesthesia with the lungs manually inflated (DV view shown, 72a).

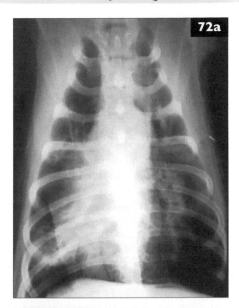

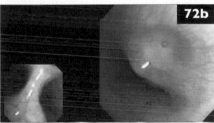

Bronchoscopy (72b) and BAL are performed. No bronchial foreign body is observed. BAL fluid contains many well-preserved cells, including numerous well-differentiated ciliated columnar epithelial cells, a large population of pyknotic neutrophils, numerous foamy activated alveolar macrophages, and scattered goblet cells and small lymphocytes. Free cilia, mucus, and mucin granules are noted in the background. No infectious agents are seen. There is no significant aerobic or anaerobic bacterial growth.

i. What is the clinical interpretation of the radiographic abnormalities?

ii. Which abnormalities are evident on the bronchoscopy image and BAL cytology?

iii. What is your diagnosis?

iv. How would you manage this case?

73   What is the modified American Heart Association/American College of Cardiologists (AHA/ACC) heart failure staging system?

72 i. A diffuse bronchial pattern with some bronchiectasis is seen. The right middle lung lobe appears consolidated. The caudal right lobe contains a mixed interstitial/alveolar pattern. Bronchopneumonia is suspected based on history and physical findings. The bronchial pattern is consistent with chronic bronchial disease, which can predispose to secondary infection.

ii. Bronchial mucosal edema and hyperemia, with excessive mucus production are seen. Several mucus plugs were found in primary and secondary bronchi, especially on the right (72b). BAL cytology indicates a neutrophilic bronchitis; prior antibiotic therapy likely accounts for the negative culture results.

iii. Chronic bronchitis (CB). An episode of secondary infection probably occurred, although not confirmed. Other CB complications can include occult parasitism and mycoplasmal infection. CB is often recognized only when advanced. Its causes are poorly understood; bronchial damage from chronic environmental irritant exposure, as well as genetic factors, may predispose to CB.

iv. Goals are to control coughing, relieve airway obstruction, and slow disease progression. Inhaled irritant (e.g. cigarette smoke, mold) exposure should be minimized. Saline nebulization, coupage, and mild exercise help mobilize bronchial mucus. Inhaled steroids (e.g. fluticasone) reduce local airway inflammation and excessive mucus production, with minimal systemic side-effects. Secondary bacterial infection is a potential complication with CB.

73 This method of heart failure (HF) staging is based on an AHA/ACC system. The guidelines focus on the importance of early diagnosis and progressive nature of cardiac disease. Because edema and effusions are not always clinically evident, this classification does not emphasize the term 'congestive', although patient fluid status is important. The four stages are:

A Patient 'at risk' for developing heart disease, but cardiac structural abnormality is not yet apparent.

B Structural cardiac abnormality (e.g. murmur) is evident, but no clinical signs of HF have occurred.
  B1: Normal heart size (no or minimal signs of hemodynamic compromise).
  B2: Cardiac remodeling and enlargement are now evident.

C Structural cardiac abnormality, with past or present clinical HF signs.

D Persistent or end-stage heart failure, signs refractory to standard therapy.

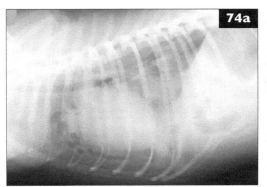

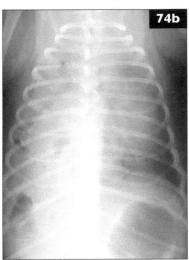

74 A 2-year-old neutered male mixed breed dog weighing 8.6 kg (19 lb) was hit by a car 2 days ago. Initial post-trauma evaluation was unremarkable, but since then the dog has vomited several times and appears uncomfortable. Physical examination reveals a tense, painful abdomen, but no other abnormalities. Combination thorax and cranial abdomen radiographs are made (74a, b).

i. What are the radiographic findings?
ii. What is the radiographic diagnosis?

75 A 13-year-old female Golden Retriever was seen by another veterinarian for lethargy, labored breathing, vomiting, and anorexia. Pleural effusion was identified. Furosemide (50 mg q12h) and enalapril (15 mg q24h) were prescribed. Today the dog is bright, alert, and panting. Body temperature is 38.5°C (101.4°F) and HR is 120 bpm. Lung sounds are normal on auscultation; heart sounds are soft, but no murmur is heard. Blood for CBC and serum chemistries is obtained. Thoracic radiographs indicate moderate cardiomegaly with minimal pleural effusion. An ECG is recorded (75, leads as marked, 25 mm/s, 0.5 cm = 1 mV).

i. What is your ECG interpretation?
ii. Are any underlying abnormalities suggested by the ECG?
iii. What test(s) do you recommend next?

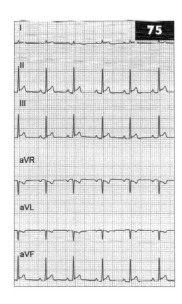

74 i. There is increased soft tissue/fluid opacity to the thoracic cavity. Additionally, circular and tubular-shaped gas-filled structures are evident, particularly in the cranioventral and right lateral regions, extending to the 3rd intercostal space. The ventral and right half of the diaphragm, much of the cardiac border, and the caudal vena cava are effaced. Within the cranial abdomen is a gas shadow, located cranioventrally, with poor delineation of the ventral hepatic border.
ii. The radiographic diagnosis is traumatic right-sided diaphragmatic hernia with intrathoracic displacement of small bowel and, probably, portions of the liver. The radiographic appearance here is diagnostic for diaphragmatic hernia. No further diagnostic imaging is needed in this patient. In less obvious cases, barium oral contrast to define the position of the gastrointestinal tract, abdominal ultrasound, and positive-contrast celiography are additional diagnostic imaging procedures that can be used to establish the diagnosis of diaphragmatic hernia.

75 i. The HR is 100 bpm, with sinus rhythm. The electrical axis and complex measurements are normal. The ST segment is slightly elevated (~0.2 mV) in the caudal leads.
ii. The ST segment begins at the end of the QRS complex ('J' point) and blends into the T wave (without clear demarcation) in dogs and cats. ST segment deviation from the isoelectric baseline can result from abnormal ventricular repolarization (from myocardial ischemia or other injury) or be secondary to abnormal depolarization (from ventricular hypertrophy, aberrant conduction, or certain drug effects). ST segment elevation >0.15 mV in dogs (>0.1 mV in cats) or depression >0.2 mV in dogs (>0.1 mV in cats) is considered abnormal. ST segment elevation in the caudal leads (II, aVF, III) can occur with pericarditis, LV epicardial injury, right ventricular ischemia/endocardial injury, transmural infarction, myocardial hypoxia, and digoxin toxicity, or secondary to ventricular hypertrophy or conduction disturbance.
iii. Echocardiography is indicated. Cardiac biomarker assay could be helpful, if echocardiographic findings are equivocal. Increased circulating cardiac troponin I indicates myocardial cell membrane injury or necrosis. Plasma brain natriuretic peptide, or its precursor NT-proBNP, is a non-specific functional marker of cardiac disease, especially chronic ventricular dysfunction.

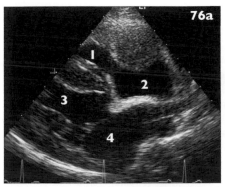
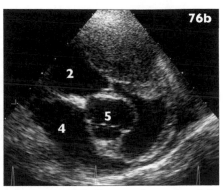

76 An echocardiogram is done on the dog in case 75. Images from the right parasternal long axis (76a) and short axis (76b) views are shown. 1 – RV, 2 – RA, 3 – LV, 4 – LA, 5 – Ao.
i. What is shown in the images?
ii. What is the most likely etiology?
iii. What are your recommendations?

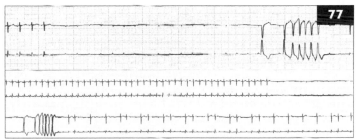

77 A 10-year-old spayed female DSH cat develops episodes of 'falling over'. The cat would seem to be acting normally, then suddenly stop moving, appear dazed, fall onto its side, and shortly thereafter jump upright quickly and appear normal again. The owner is especially concerned because the cat has fallen off furniture, stair rails, and from the top of the refrigerator. Physical examination is unremarkable. A 24-hour ambulatory ECG (Holter) is recorded (77). Two channels are recorded simultaneously. The top part (with visible grid) is an enlarged segment from the longer time period shown at the bottom.
i. What ECG rhythms are seen on this Holter ECG?
ii. Could the clinical signs be attributed to ECG events in this cat?
iii. What other tests would be helpful?
iv. What are the management options?

76 i. A large, soft tissue mass has invaded the lateral right AV junction. The mass may partially obstruct right ventricular inflow, contributing to the pleural effusion. A small pericardial effusion is present.

ii. Hemangiosarcoma (HSA) is the most common heart tumor in dogs. Cardiac HSA usually involves right heart structures, most often the right auricular appendage. Depending on location or size, cardiac tumors can cause impaired cardiac filling from pericardial effusion and tamponade, inflow or outflow obstruction, arrhythmias, myocardial dysfunction, or a combination. Middle-aged to older dogs are affected most often; 10–15 year olds have the highest occurrence rate. Spayed females appear to have greater risk than intact females. Golden Retrievers have a higher risk for HSA than the general dog population.

iii. The prognosis is poor. Risks of metastasis and tumor bleeding with cardiac tamponade are high. This mass's size and location preclude surgical excision; biopsy might be possible. Most cardiac tumors are resistant to chemotherapy, but some show temporary response. Subtotal pericardiectomy could prevent cardiac tamponade, and secondary thoracic metastasis does not appear to affect survival time. Balloon pericardiotomy is not recommended because HSA can bleed excessively if abraded during the procedure. Supportive care is given, with pericardiocentesis for signs of tamponade.

77 i. The first four complexes in the upper strip are normal sinus complexes. Nineteen non-conducted P waves follow without ventricular activity. This is high-grade second degree AV block (multiple non-conducted P waves in succession). A ventricular escape complex finally occurs, followed by a short paroxysm of ventricular tachycardia. Intermittent second degree AV block follows (bottom strip).

ii. High-grade second degree AV block, with prolonged ventricular asystole, can cause syncope as cardiac output falls. Ventricular escape activity can be delayed when AV block is sporadic, as in this case.

iii. Echocardiography is indicated to screen for organic heart disease. Hypertrophic (or other) cardiomyopathy can be associated with heart block, as can myocardial ischemia, infarction, fibrosis, and infiltrative disease.

iv. Pacemaker implantation is generally indicated for symptomatic AV block. However, the transvenous approach has been associated with pleural effusion development in cats. Anticholinergic drugs are often unhelpful. Diltiazem and atenolol can worsen AV block. Interestingly, many cats with complete AV block are asymptomatic because of a consistent ventricular escape rate high enough to sustain normal (indoor) activity. This cat's owner refused further tests and treatment. Eventually the cat stopped collapsing and was reportedly doing well several years later when an ECG showed complete AV block with steady ventricular escape rhythm.

78 A 4-year-old spayed female mixed breed dog developed fever, anorexia, greenish mucoid stools, and raspy lung sounds approximately 36 hours following a dental procedure. The dog is febrile, tachycardic, and tachypneic on physical examination. Thoracic radiographs reveal pleural effusion and a possible focal opacity in the left caudodorsal lung field. Thoracocentesis is attempted, but only about 2 ml of a red, cloudy fluid is obtained. Samples are submitted for cytologic evaluation (78, cytospin preparation using Wright's stain, 100× oil) and culture/sensitivity.

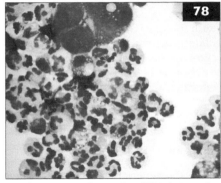

i. Give a cytologic diagnosis based on the findings in the figure.
ii. In view of the patient's history, what considerations should be given to selection of an antimicrobial agent(s)?

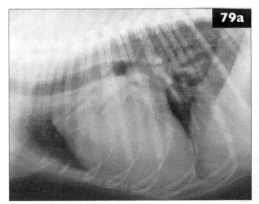
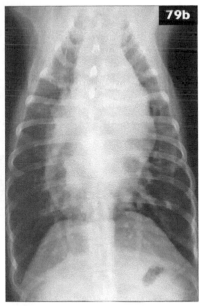

79 A newly adopted 5-month-old female Australian Shepherd Dog is seen for routine health examination. She has a loud cardiac murmur. Chest radiographs are obtained (79a, lateral; 79b, DV).
i. Describe the radiographic findings.
ii. What is your diagnosis?
iii. What are your recommendations?

78 i. Increased numbers of neutrophils (predominantly degenerate in appearance) with phagocytized bacteria of mixed morphology (short rods, chaining to filamentous rods) are present, as well as some reactive large mononuclear cells. The cytologic diagnosis is neutrophilic inflammation with bacterial sepsis.

ii. The history of a recent dental procedure raises the concern for anaerobic bacterial infection. Therefore, a broad-spectrum antibiotic and/or one with specific anaerobic activity should be chosen while awaiting culture/sensitivity results. Antimicrobial therapy can then be changed if necessary. In this particular case, both *Escherichia coli* and *Bacteroides* spp. were isolated from the pleural fluid sample, and a diagnosis of embolic pneumonia with secondary pyothorax was made.

79 i. Cardiomegaly (VHS ~13.7 v) with left heart prominence is seen. There is a large 'ductus bump' in the cranial descending aorta (large arrow, **79c**), as well as a left auricular (LAu) bulge (small arrow) and a small main PA (arrowhead) bulge. The slight apex shift towards the right hemithorax is incidental. Enlarged pulmonary lobar arteries and veins indicate pulmonary overcirculation.

ii. Left-to-right shunting patent ductus arteriosus (PDA) without congestive heart failure (CHF) at present. The triad of PA, aortic, and LAu bulges (sometimes nicknamed 'PAL') on DV view is a classic finding, but infrequently seen all together. Dogs with PDA are often asymptomatic when first diagnosed, although reduced exercise ability, tachypnea, or cough is sometimes reported. PDA prevalence is much greater in females than males.

iii. Auscultation should confirm the characteristic continuous murmur; hyperkinetic arterial pulses are also typical. Nevertheless, echocardiography is recommended to screen for concurrent defects or valve insufficiency, confirm PDA diagnosis, estimate pressure gradient across the ductus, and evaluate myocardial function. PDA closure is recommended, either by a transcatheter occlusion procedure or open-chest surgery. Without ductal closure, gradual myocardial function deterioration, arrhythmias, and CHF are expected. After ductal closure, life span is usually normal.

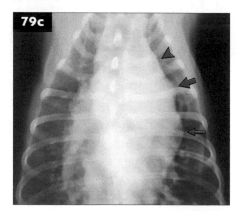

79c

80 A 5-month-old Australian Shepherd Dog is examined for a loud cardiac murmur. An ECG is recorded as part of the diagnostic evaluation (80, leads as marked, 25 mm/s, 1 cm = 1 mV).

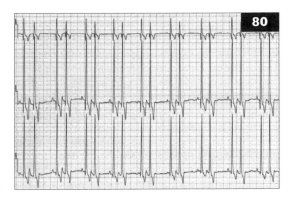

i. What is your ECG interpretation?
ii. Are any enlargement criteria evident?
iii. What conditions are most likely to cause these findings?

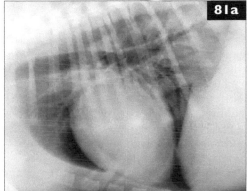
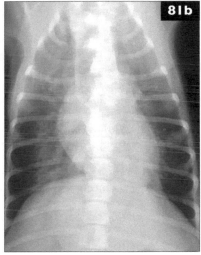

81 A 4-month-old female mixed breed dog weighing 11.4 kg (25 lb) was found hanging from a deck by its leash after being unobserved for 15–30 minutes. The dog was unconscious, but was resuscitated by the owner. On presentation, the dog is alert and responsive. Lung sounds are increased on the right side. Right lateral (81a) and DV (81b) radiographs are made.

i. What is the concern relative to the thoracic cavity in this patient?
ii. Are there radiographic abnormalities present, and if so, what are they?

80 i. HR is 140 bpm, with sinus rhythm and atrial premature complexes in a bigeminal pattern (a premature complex follows each sinus complex). The premature P' waves are superimposed on preceding T waves. Sinus P waves (0.05 second) and QRS complexes (0.08 second) are widened; markedly increased R wave amplitude (4.8 mV) is seen in lead II. Other measurements and electrical axis are normal.

ii. Yes. Wide P waves suggest LA enlargement. Increased R wave amplitude with normal electrical axis is the classic LV dilation pattern; QRS widening can occur with ventricular enlargement or intraventricular conduction disturbance.

iii. Congenital patent ductus arteriosus or mitral dysplasia with severe valve insufficiency would be most likely in young dogs. Acquired (degenerative) mitral valve insufficiency is another common cause of markedly increased R wave amplitude and widened P waves. Atrial tachyarrhythmias, including frequent premature beats, atrial tachycardia, and atrial fibrillation, are more likely when atrial enlargement develops. The arrhythmia was not specifically treated in this case as it did not persist or worsen. More frequent atrial premature beats or paroxysmal atrial tachycardia can be treated with diltiazem, a beta blocker (e.g. atenolol), or digoxin, or a combination of digoxin and diltiazem or beta blocker.

81 i. Strangulation causes fixed upper airway obstruction. This can result in the development of non-cardiogenic (negative pressure) pulmonary edema. During strangulation, intense negative intrathoracic pressure develops. This leads to increases in venous return, pulmonary blood volume, and pulmonary capillary hydrostatic pressure, along with concurrent decreases in pulmonary interstitial hydrostatic pressure. These changes culminate in increased fluid leakage across pulmonary capillary membranes. A hypoxia-induced hyperadrenergic state may further contribute to the increased pulmonary vascular volume and capillary permeability.

In addition to the air flow obstruction, compression of the cervical arteries and veins further compromises central nervous system viability. If the strangulation is associated with a fall or suspension from a substantial height, hyoid fracture, laryngeal or tracheal injury, and cranial cervical spine injury may be possible and complicate the clinical signs.

ii. A bilaterally symmetric caudal dorsal alveolar pulmonary pattern is present. The changes are most intense in the central and dorsal peripheral zones of these lobes. The lateral and ventral peripheral regions are relatively spared. These findings are typical of non-cardiogenic pulmonary edema.

82 A 2-year-old Springer Spaniel living on a farm developed an intermittent, moist cough about 1 month ago. Anorexia, lethargy, and a 10 kg (22 lb) weight loss have since occurred. Treatment with cephalexin and enrofloxacin were helpful, but not curative; those antibiotics were discontinued yesterday. The dog appears moderately depressed. Body temperature, HR, and respirations are within normal limits, but mucous membranes are pale and capillary refill time is slightly prolonged (~3 seconds). Harsh lung sounds and pulmonary crackles are heard bilaterally. Tracheal palpation elicits a moist cough. Prescapular lymph nodes and the left popliteal lymph node are moderately enlarged. A hemogram shows mild anemia (hematocrit 0.33 l/l [33.5%]) and leukocytosis (WBC 39.26 × 10⁹/l [10³/µl]), with a mature neutrophilia (34.55×10^9/l [10^3/µl]) and monocytosis (1.96×10^9/l [10^3/µl]). Serum biochemistries and urinalysis are unremarkable. Thoracic radiographs reveal mixed bronchiolar–alveolar infiltrates, especially in ventral regions, with a concurrent nodular interstitial pattern. There is a

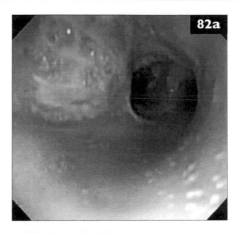

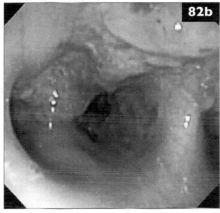

pronounced increase in perihilar opacity and the dorsal tracheal margin appears thick and undulating. The cardiac silhouette is normal (VHS 10.6 v). Needle aspirates of the enlarged peripheral lymph nodes are non-diagnostic. Bronchoscopy (82a, b) is performed. BAL cytology shows mostly degenerate and pyknotic neutrophils with rare macrophages; no infectious agents are identified.

i. What findings are shown in the bronchoscopic images?
ii. What differential diagnoses should be considered?
iii. How would you proceed with this case?

83 What is sildenafil, and what are its cardiopulmonary indications?

82 i. The airway mucosa appears diffusely thickened with areas of ulceration. A mass-like thickening is present in the trachea. Thick mucoid secretions were also seen.

ii. The weight loss, lymphadenopathy, and hemogram abnormalities suggest chronic systemic inflammatory response. Given the radiographic findings, differentials include fungal or parasitic pneumonia (in endemic regions) or neoplasia such as lymphoma. The ventral alveolar pattern suggests possible concurrent aspiration pneumonia. The tracheal thickening could represent a granuloma, abscess, polyp, or neoplasia such as lymphoma. BAL cytology indicates purulent exudate of unknown etiology; previous antibiotic therapy may have suppressed evidence of bacterial cause.

iii. BAL fluid should be cultured and the tracheal thickening biopsied. Fungal antigen testing or fecal tests for pulmonary parasites may be helpful. Lung biopsy may be necessary for definitive diagnosis. Supportive care would include broad-spectrum antibiotic therapy while awaiting culture results, nebulization to improve airway hydration, and coupage to help mobilize secretions. In this dog, cultures for aerobic and anaerobic bacteria, mycoplasma, and fungal growth were negative. *Blastomyces* spp. antigen and Baermann fecal tests were negative. Biopsy showed necrotic cellular debris, many neutrophils, and no infectious agents. Stratified squamous epithelium, atypical for the trachea, suggested a metaplastic/dysplastic response. Although not clearly malignant, neoplasia was suspected. Lung biopsy was not permitted.

83 It is a selective phosphodiesterase-5 inhibitor that enhances nitric oxide-dependent pulmonary vasodilation by increasing cyclic guanosine monophosphate concentrations. Sildenafil has been used to treat severe pulmonary hypertension (e.g. from chronic respiratory disease or congenital shunts); it may also be helpful in managing dogs with pulmonary hypertension from chronic left-sided heart failure. Doses of 0.5–2.0 (or even up to 3.0) mg/kg q12h or q8h appear to be well-tolerated in dogs and have resulted in decreased Doppler-estimated PA pressures as well as improved clinical signs and exercise tolerance. Adverse effects can include cutaneous flushing and nasal congestion. Other adverse effects reported in people include headache, priapism, and myalgia.

84 A 7-year-old female mixed breed dog weighing 33 kg (72 lb) is presented as an emergency several hours after being hit by an automobile. The major presenting signs are increased respiratory effort and tachycardia. Lung sounds are absent over the left caudal lung field and there is abdominal pain on palpation. Thoracic and abdominal radiographs are consistent with the abnormality seen in these intraoperative photographs (84a, initial appearance; 84b, after tissue manipulation). The dog was stabilized for approximately 36 hours prior to ventral midline celiotomy.

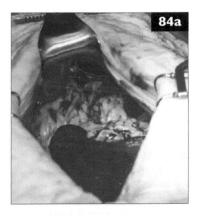

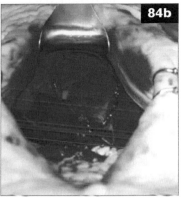

i. What is the diagnosis?

ii. What is the rationale for waiting 36 hours before performing surgery? Should such a delay be routine for dogs with this diagnosis?

iii. What is the name of the retractor illustrated in these photographs, and how does it help or hinder the surgery?

iv. Should the edges of the damaged structure be trimmed before repairing it with sutures? Why or why not?

v. Why is this condition susceptible to re-expansion pulmonary edema, and what is done to minimize the chance of this complication?

85 A new client presents a 16-month-old spayed female Rottweiler for vaccination. The owner thinks the dog's exercise tolerance is reduced lately. As a puppy, a soft murmur had been noted, but it was thought of little concern. The dog is alert, with a coarse haircoat and slight build. Body temperature is normal, HR is 120 bpm, and respirations are 30/min. Mucous membranes are pink. Femoral pulses are slightly weak. Precordial palpation and jugular veins are normal. On auscultation, a murmur is heard in both systole and diastole; the point of maximal intensity is at the left base. The systolic murmur is louder, but it seems to taper quickly and the second heart sound (S_2) can be heard. Lung sounds are normal.

i. What is/are the likely cause(s) of the murmur?

ii. What test(s) would you recommend next?

iii. Could the murmur noted when the dog was young be related to the present condition?

84 i. Traumatic diaphragmatic hernia (**84a**: omental fat and part of the liver lie across the diaphragmatic tear; **84b**: after abdominal contents are repositioned).
ii. Surgical correction is indicated as soon as the animal is stable. It required 36 hours to stabilize this case for surgery, but this long a delay should not be routine. Although older literature reports higher mortality rates when surgery occurs within 12 hours of trauma compared with later, more recent literature suggests that patient stability is the key factor.
iii. A Balfour retractor. While this instrument is helpful for abdominal exploration, it can interfere with diaphragmatic repair.
iv. The rent edges should not be trimmed, except to excise obviously necrotic tissue. Trimming causes unnecessary bleeding and re-initiates the inflammatory process. Necrotic areas are excised to minimize inflammatory reaction and avoid placing sutures in tissue that will not heal.
v. Rapid lung re-expansion by manual or mechanical positive-pressure ventilation physically stresses the pulmonary microvasculature, which is relatively inflexible due to lung collapse. Pulmonary capillaries become leaky from this iatrogenic trauma and reperfusion injury may also ensue, leading to pulmonary edema. Re-expansion pulmonary edema can be avoided by gently applying positive-pressure ventilation and allowing the lungs to re-expand slowly and naturally.

85 i. A murmur heard in both systole and diastole is most often a 'continuous' murmur, characteristic for patent ductus arteriosus. However, the rapidly tapering systolic component and audible S_2 in this case is not typical for a continuous murmur. Rather, it is the so-called 'to-and-fro' murmur, comprised of mid-systolic (ejection) and diastolic decrescendo murmurs. With the to-and-fro murmur, the ejection murmur component tapers in late systole, allowing the S_2 to be heard as a distinct sound. The most common cause of a to-and-fro murmur is the combination of subaortic stenosis (SAS) and aortic insufficiency. Continuous (machinery) murmurs increase in intensity throughout systole and continue through S_2 into diastole. They result from a continuous pressure gradient throughout the cardiac cycle. Occasionally, holosystolic and diastolic decrescendo murmurs occur together (e.g. with ventricular septal defect and aortic insufficiency).
ii. Chest radiographs and Doppler echocardiography are indicated to assess cardiac and pulmonary structures. Because infective endocarditis is a likely cause of aortic insufficiency, CBC, serum chemistries, and other laboratory tests (e.g. cultures, titers) are indicated to search for etiology and other sequelae of endocarditis.
iii. Yes. Considering the dog's age and breed, congenital SAS with secondary aortic endocarditis is likely.

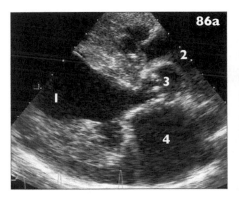

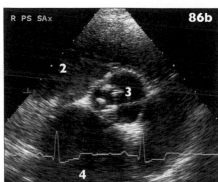

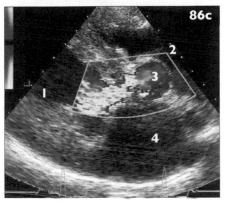

86 Chest radiographs and an echo-cardiogram are obtained on the dog in case 85. Radiographs show moderate cardiomegaly, with LA and LV prominence. Echocardiographic findings from the right parasternal position are shown (86a, long axis in systole; 86b, short axis in diastole; 86c, long axis in diastole). 1 – LV, 2 – RA, 3 – Ao, 4 – LA.

i. Describe the abnormalities seen in the figures.
ii. What is your diagnosis?
iii. What do you recommend to the owner of this dog?

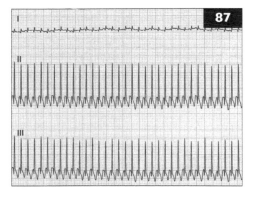

87 A 3-month-old Labrador Retriever with a cardiac murmur, is weak and slightly tachypneic on presentation. Mucous membranes are pale, HR is rapid, and pulses are weak. An ECG is recorded (87, leads as marked, 25 mm/s, 1 cm = 1 mV).
i. What is your ECG interpretation?
ii. What would you do next for this case?
iii. What congenital heart defect is most likely in this case?

86 i. LV hypertrophy suggests chronic systolic pressure overload. The subaortic region is narrowed. Hyperechogenicity of the septum and subendocardial LV wall is consistent with myocardial fibrosis. There are several bright nodules on the aortic valve leaflets. The LA is moderately dilated.

ii. Congenital subaortic stenosis (SAS), likely severe. The aortic leaflet nodules suggest aortic valve endocarditis, probably chronic as there was no fever or history of systemic illness. SAS predisposes to aortic valve endocarditis because of jet lesion injury to the valve. Severe SAS often leads to compromised myocardial perfusion, ischemia, and fibrosis. Concurrent aortic or mitral valve regurgitation also imposes a volume overload on the LV. Complications include arrhythmias, syncope, congestive failure, and sudden death.

iii. Exercise restriction and beta blockade (e.g. atenolol) are recommended with the aim of reducing myocardial O_2 demand and arrhythmias. Prophylactic antibiotic therapy is advised prior to procedures likely to cause bacteremia (e.g. dentistry). A broad-spectrum bactericidal antibiotic was recommended for 6–8 weeks in this case because endocarditis was suspected. Therapy for heart failure may be needed. Related dogs should be screened for SAS.

87 i. HR is 370 bpm, with sustained supraventricular tachycardia (SVT, note narrow, upright QRS complexes). Underlying mechanisms can include re-entry involving an accessory pathway and/or AV node, or an ectopic automatic focus in atrial or junctional tissue.

ii. Rapid SVT compromises hemodynamic stability. Stress and activity should be minimized. A vagal maneuver may slow or interrupt the tachycardia and aid in identifying its mechanism. Vagal maneuvers involve carotid sinus massage (gentle continuous pressure over carotid sinus region caudodorsal to larynx) or bilateral ocular pressure (over closed eyelids) for 15–20 seconds. The latter technique is contraindicated in animals with ocular disease. Although a vagal maneuver may initially be ineffective, if the rhythm disturbance persists after antiarrhythmic drug administration, repeating it may help. IV fluid administration helps support BP and reduce sympathetic tone; caution is needed if congestive heart failure is suspected. IV diltiazem is the drug of first choice for SVT. If ineffective, alternatives include lidocaine (occasionally effective), propranolol or esmolol slowly IV (with caution because of negative inotropic effect), IV procainamide, amiodarone or sotalol (PO), or IV digoxin (not usually recommended).

iii. Tricuspid dysplasia (TD). Heritability has been shown in Labrador Retrievers. Ventricular pre-excitation may be more prevalent with TD.

88 A 4-month-old female Chow Chow is presented for examination. She had been acting normal and eating well, but lately seems to be getting out of breath more easily when playing. The puppy is alert, excited, and panting. A systolic heart murmur, loudest at the cranial right sternal border, and increased breath sounds are heard on auscultation; otherwise the physical examination is unremarkable. Among other procedures, a selective angiocardiogram is done (88a).

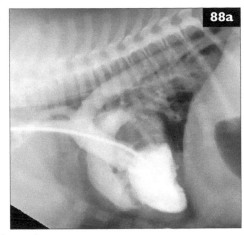

i. Where is the catheter positioned?
ii. What abnormality is shown in this image?
iii. Are the dog's physical examination findings consistent with this?
iv. What are the long-term consequences of this abnormality?

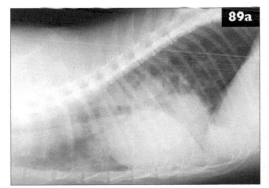

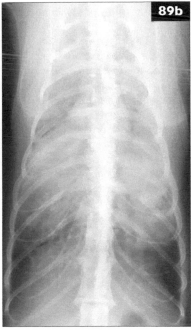

89 A 5-year-old neutered male DSH cat is presented with a 2-week history of rapid breathing that is becoming worse. A diagnosis of feline asthma is suspected. Right lateral (89a) and DV (89b) radiographs are shown.
i. Are the radiographic changes consistent with feline asthma?
ii. What are other differentials for these changes?

88 i. The catheter was inserted into a carotid artery and passed through the ascending aorta into the LV (88b). 1 – LV, 2 – Ao, 3 – RV outflow tract, 4 – PA.

ii. Radiopaque dye injected into the LV flowed to the aorta, but also into the RV outflow tract and PA, indicating a left-to-right shunting ventricular septal defect (VSD).

iii. Yes. The usual VSD location is in the membranous part of the septum, just below the aortic valve and septal tricuspid leaflet. Turbulent flow through the VSD is thus oriented from left base toward the right and ventrally.

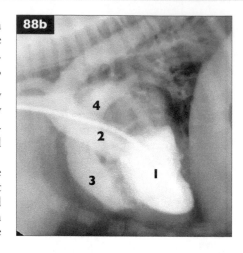

iv. Smaller (restrictive) defects are often well tolerated and without clinical signs; some even close spontaneously. Moderate- to large-size defects lead to left heart volume overload and, sometimes, pulmonary edema. Very large VSDs also cause RV enlargement, with both ventricles as a common chamber. Pulmonary hypertension with shunt reversal is more likely with very large defects. Aortic regurgitation also occurs with some VSDs, likely because of inadequate aortic root support. Aortic regurgitation imposes an additional LV volume load.

89 i. The distribution and intensity of the pulmonary opacity in the hilar and cranial regions are not typical of feline asthma. Common radiographic findings of asthma are thickened bronchial walls, lung hyperinflation from air trapping, and collapse of the right middle lung lobe. This patient has severe parenchymal disease as evidenced by the air bronchogram summated (superimposed) with the heart in the lateral view.

ii. Pneumonia and pulmonary edema are more differentials. This patient did not respond to diuretic therapy or antibiotics. The cat did not survive and was found to have pyogranulomatous pneumonia with lipid-filled macrophages in the alveoli. Lipid globules surrounded by inflammatory cells were randomly distributed in the pulmonary parenchyma. Aspiration of lipid was the suspected cause.

90 A 4-year-old male neutered DSH cat is presented for sudden development of tachypnea with increased abdominal effort. HR is 160 bpm, with a regular rhythm. Bilateral jugular pulsation is noted on examination. Both femoral pulses are strong and regular. Wheezes and crackles, loudest over the cranial lung region, are heard on thoracic auscultation. Cardiac auscultation and other examination findings are normal. Systolic BP is 125 mmHg. Serum biochemical tests show mildly elevated blood urea (10.3 mmol/l [28.9 mg/dl]; normal 3.5–8.0 mmol/l [9.8–22.4 mg/dl]). Chest radiographs show generalized cardiomegaly (VHS 9.5 v) with mild pleural effusion, pulmonary venous congestion, caudal vena cava distension, and a patchy alveolar pattern. An echocardiogram is obtained (2-D right parasternal long axis view, 90a; M-mode at ventricular level, 90b). 1 – RV, 2 – RA, 3 – LV, 4 – LA.

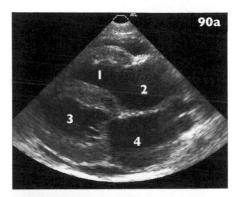

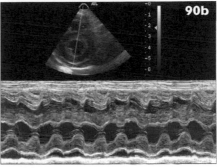

i. What is your interpretation of the radiographic findings?
ii. What abnormalities are shown on the echo images?
iii. What therapy would you use at this time?

91 What is sotalol, and when is it indicated?

90 i. The radiograph findings are consistent with biventricular congestive heart failure.

ii. The 2-D image shows biatrial enlargement (LA = 2.1 cm) and suggests biventricular hypertrophy. LV and IVS hypertrophy is confirmed on M-mode (**LF1b**). LV chamber size and systolic function are normal. Mild pericardial and pleural effusions were also seen.

Echo measurements:

	Diastole (cm)	Systole (cm)
IVS	0.9	0.9
LV chamber	1.4	0.7
LV wall	0.8	1.0
FS	50%	(40–66%)

Hypertrophic cardiomyopathy (HCM) is diagnosed when other causes of LV hypertrophy (e.g. fixed LV outflow obstruction, hypertension, hyperthyroidism, acromegaly) are absent. HCM, the most common feline myocardial disease, is characterized by idiopathic LV hypertrophy (symmetric or asymmetric) without LV dilation. Both ventricles are involved in some cases. Hypertrophy increases ventricular stiffness and, consequently, filling pressure, which can lead to pulmonary venous congestion and effusions.

iii. Congestive signs are treated with furosemide PRN. For long-term therapy, oral furosemide is given at the lowest effective dose. Although angiotensin-converting enzyme inhibitor, diltiazem, or beta blocker therapy is often prescribed, convincing evidence for long-term benefit is presently lacking. Spironolactone may reduce the hypokalemia from long-term furosemide therapy. Antiplatelet therapy is also recommended.

91 Sotalol HCl is a non-selective beta blocker with class III antiarrhythmic effects at higher doses (via repolarizing K+ channel blockade). It is used mainly for ventricular tachyarrhythmias. Its beta-blocking effects (from the l-isomer) are important to sotalol's antiarrhythmic effectiveness. Sotalol has minimal hemodynamic effects, although it can cause hypotension or worsened myocardial function. Sotalol can be proarrhythmic (as can all antiarrhythmic agents), although clinically used doses in dogs may mainly produce beta-blocking effects. Other adverse effects can include depression, nausea, vomiting, diarrhea, and bradycardia. Occasional anecdotal reports exist of aggression that resolved after discontinuing sotalol.

92 A 2-year-old male Lhasa Apso is presented for progressively worsening exercise intolerance and weakness. The dog's tongue appears bluish after mild to moderate activity. No murmur is heard, but right-sided heart enlargement is evident radiographically. A sample of the dog's blood spun in a hematocrit (Hct) tube is shown (92).

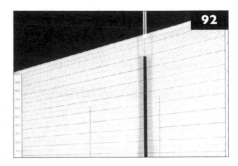

i. What can cause such a high Hct reading?
ii. What are the consequences of erythrocytosis (polycythemia)?
iii. How could erythrocytosis be managed in this case?
iv. What adverse effects are common with this therapy?

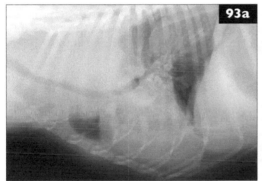

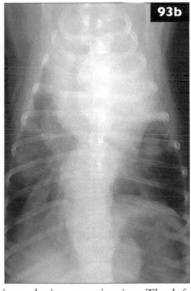

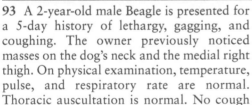

93 A 2-year-old male Beagle is presented for a 5-day history of lethargy, gagging, and coughing. The owner previously noticed masses on the dog's neck and the medial right thigh. On physical examination, temperature, pulse, and respiratory rate are normal. Thoracic auscultation is normal. No cough can be elicited, although the dog gags several times during examination. The left submandibular lymph node is prominent. Several subcutaneous masses are found on various parts of the body. Both third eyelids are protruding. Right lateral (93a) and DV (93b) radiographs are taken.
i. What are the causes of ventral deviation of the thoracic trachea?
ii. How can the radiographic changes be correlated with the history and physical examination findings?

92 i. Primary erythrocytosis (polycythema rubra vera) occurs independent of erythropoietin (Epo). Increased Epo production causes secondary erythrocytosis. Tissue hypoxia (e.g. from right-to-left shunt, pulmonary disease, high altitude) normally stimulates renal Epo release. Some (Epo-producing) tumors cause inappropriate erythrocytosis. The cyanosis suggests underlying tissue hypoxia.

ii. Mucous membranes may be bright red at rest, but readily become cyanotic with hypoxemia. Erythrocytosis increases blood viscosity, which reduces turbulence, so cardiac murmurs are softer or even inaudible. Increased viscosity and resistance to flow can impair tissue perfusion despite a higher O_2-carrying capacity. Manifestations of hyperviscosity include behavioral changes, seizures, and exercise intolerance.

iii. Options are periodic phlebotomy (e.g. 5–10 ml blood/kg) or hydroxyurea (40–50 mg/kg PO q48h or 3 times a week), with phlebotomy if necessary. Target Hct is where hyperviscosity signs are minimized, usually ~60%. Systemic vasodilating drugs should be avoided and exercise restricted. For tetralogy of Fallot (the diagnosis in this dog), palliative surgery to increase pulmonary blood flow is possible.

iv. Signs of hypoxia are exacerbated if Hct decreases too far. If phlebotomy causes hypotension, isotonic fluid replacement helps. Hydroxyurea's adverse effects include anorexia, vomiting, bone marrow suppression, alopecia, and pruritus; dose reduction may help. CBCs should be monitored q1–2weeks initially, then q4–8weeks.

93 i. The most common cause of ventral deviation of the thoracic trachea is a dilated esophagus. This can develop for various reasons. The anatomic structures dorsal to the trachea are the esophagus, fascial tissue of the mediastinum, tracheobronchial lymph nodes, longus coli muscle, cervicothoracic ganglion, and thoracic vertebrae. The esophagus is the structure most frequently affected by disease that will cause sufficient enlargement to displace the trachea. However, enlargement of other tissues in the area dorsal to the trachea (e.g. caused by an abscess, granuloma, or tumor) may also displace the trachea.

ii. The compressive effect of the craniodorsal mediastinal mass is the likely cause of both the gagging and coughing. The thoracic tracheal diameter is visibly reduced compared to that of the cervical trachea. Third eyelid protrusion can be caused by a number of conditions including Horner's syndrome. It is possible that the mass is impinging on, or causing inflammation or entrapment of, the second-order neurons of the thoracic sympathetic trunk.

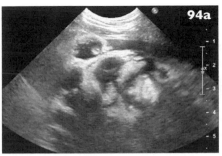
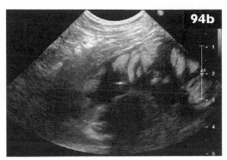

94 A cranial dorsal thoracic mass is identified radiographically in the dog in **93**. These 2-dimensional ultrasound images (**94a, b**) of the cranial dorsal mediastinal region are obtained.
i. What is your assessment?
ii. What are the advantages of ultrasound evaluation in this patient?

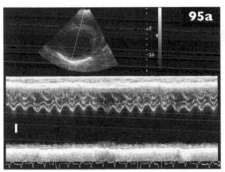
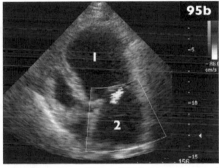

95 A 7-year-old male intact Doberman Pinscher weighing 43 kg (95 lb) is presented for sudden onset of dyspnea. Previous history is unremarkable. Physical examination reveals weak femoral pulses and a systolic heart murmur, grade 3/6, loudest over the left apex. Systolic BP is 70 mmHg. Serum biochemical tests show mildly elevated BUN (8.3 mmol/l [23.2 mg/dl]; normal 3.5–7.0 mmol/l [9.8–19.6 mg/dl]) and creatinine (135 µmol/l [1.5 mg/dl]; normal 0–130 µmol/l [0-1.47 mg/dl]). Urine SG is 1.050. Thoracic radiographs show cardiomegaly (VHS 13 v; normal <10.7 v), pulmonary venous congestion, and severe pulmonary edema. An ECG shows sinus rhythm with a HR of 160 bpm and frequent polymorphic ventricular premature complexes. Echocardiography is carried out (**95a, b**). 1 – LV, 2 – LA.
i. What echocardiographic abnormalities are seen in this dog?
ii. What is your overall assessment of this case?
iii. What additional biochemical tests could be useful in assessing this case?
iv. Outline your initial management plan for this dog.

94 i. The displacement of the lung from the thoracic wall creates an excellent window for ultrasound assessment and guided sampling of the soft tissue/fluid mass effect. The images show multiple round hypoechoic masses and a larger region of heterogeneous echogenicity. Ultrasound sampling of both areas yielded cytology consistent with lymphoma. This is an unusual radiographic presentation for enlargement of either cranial mediastinal lymph nodes or thymus because of the dorsal location of the mass effect.

ii. In most patients, survey ultrasonographic evaluation can be done without sedation or anesthesia. It allows characterization as to whether a mass is solid or cavitary and fluid filled, as well as its adjacency to critical structures. For example, the mass was very close to major thoracic vessels in this patient. Although the sonographic features of masses uncommonly yield a definitive etiologic diagnosis, the direct visualization of the mass allows guided sampling for cytology and culture and harvest of tissue cores for histopathologic evaluation. Screening of the patient for any clotting deficiency is recommended before any biopsy procedure. Depending on patient size and temperament, as well as the mass's size and proximity to critical vessels or organs, sedation or anesthesia may be needed for guided sampling.

95 i. The LV is dilated and wall motion markedly reduced (LV FS = 9%, **95a**), indicating poor contractility. Other findings include ventricular rounding (reduced sphericity index), LA dilation, and increased mitral E-point–septal separation (12 mm; (normal <7 mm). Mild mitral regurgitation (**95b**) is likely secondary to valve annulus dilation.

ii. The most likely diagnosis is dilated cardiomyopathy (DCM); other differentials include myocardial failure from chronic mitral regurgitation (although the valve is not thickened), previously undiagnosed congenital shunt, dietary deficiency (i.e. taurine, L-carnitine), tachycardia-induced cardiomyopathy, or myocardial ischemia/infarction. Congestive heart failure, systemic hypotension, prerenal azotemia, and ventricular tachyarrhythmia are also present.

iii. Although not necessary for diagnosis in this case, cardiac troponin I and NT-pro-BNP can indicate active myocardial insult and ventricular distension, respectively. Both parameters were elevated (cTnI: 0.78 ng/ml; reference range <0.15) (NT-pro BNP: 2928 pmol/l; reference range 0–210).

iv. Supplemental O_2 and IV furosemide (bolus or CRI) are indicated for severe pulmonary edema; dosing is guided by patient response. Dobutamine infusion will help support myocardial contractility and systolic BP. Oral pimobendan and angiotensin-converting enzyme inhibitor are given as soon as possible. BP and heart rhythm should be closely monitored. Antiarrhythmic and other supportive therapy may be needed.

96 A 2-year-old neutered male Persian cat acutely began open-mouth breathing about an hour ago. He was normal prior to this. However, about 9 months ago he had a similar episode. The cat is alert and in good condition. Mucous membranes are pink. Physical abnormalities appear limited to the open-mouth breathing and a mild serous nasal discharge. Heart and lung sounds are normal. Supplemental O_2 is administered and an IV catheter is placed. After a short time resting in an O_2 cage he appears comfortable and now has only mild tachypnea. Thoracic radiographs are obtained and indicate a mild, diffusely distributed bronchointerstitial pattern. Hemogram, serum chemistry, and urinalysis results are non-contributory. The cat is briefly anesthetized for otic and oropharyngeal examinations, which are normal, and bronchoscopy. Images from the trachea (**96a**) and right middle bronchus (**96b**) are shown.

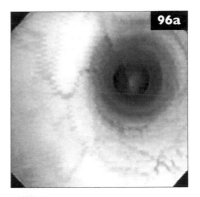
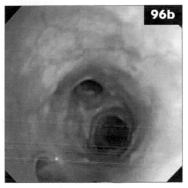

i. Describe the bronchoscopic findings.
ii. What are your differential diagnoses?
iii. Is BAL indicated in this case?
iv. What cytologic findings would you expect with feline idiopathic bronchitis?
v. How would you manage this case?

97 A 5-year-old, male cat is presented for acute hindlimb paralysis and crying (**97**). On examination, his hindlimbs were cool and femoral pulses were absent. Palpation of his hindlimbs elicited a pain response. Hindlimb nail beds were cyanotic and did not bleed on trimming. Chest radiographs showed

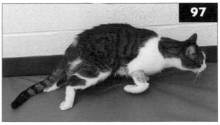

normal lung fields and LA enlargement; echocardiography documented LV hypertrophy consistent with hypertrophic cardiomyopathy.

i. What caused these clinical signs?
ii. How would you manage this case initially?
iii. What is the prognosis?

96 i. The trachea appears fairly normal. The bronchial mucosa (**96b**) is inflamed, with patchy pale and slightly raised areas, thought to represent edema. Other bronchi appeared similar.
ii. Causes of airway inflammation generally include allergic, parasitic, and infectious airway disease. Infiltrative disease is possible. but less likely.
iii. Yes. BAL, and bronchial brushing, samples should be examined cytologically and cultured. BAL can aid in diagnosing small airway, alveolar, and/or pulmonary interstitial diseases. However, BAL is not advised for patients in respiratory distress because it transiently exacerbates hypoxemia.
iv. Eosinophilic inflammation, suggesting a hypersensitivity response, is most common with feline idiopathic bronchitis or feline asthma; pulmonary parasites and heartworm disease (in endemic regions) should be ruled out. Over time a mixed inflammatory response can develop. However, some cats with idiopathic bronchitis have a (usually non-degenerative) neutrophilic inflammatory response.
v. If BAL cultures and parasite tests are negative, a glucocorticoid and bronchodilator (see cases **99** and **100**) are usually helpful. Potential inhaled irritants or allergens (e.g. litter, smoke, carpet cleaners, household aerosols) should be avoided. For acute respiratory distress, supplemental O_2 with a rapid-acting glucocortioid (e.g. prednisolone sodium succinate, to 10 mg IV or IM; or dexamethasone sodium phosphate, to 2 mg/kg IV) and terbutaline (0.01 mg/kg SC) or albuterol (via metered dose inhaler) are recommended.

97 i. Arterial thromboembolism (ATE) at the distal aorta. Tissue ischemia causes acute, painful hindlimb paresis with loss of palpable femoral pulses. Hypothermia, tachypnea, and azotemia are common. Feline cardiomyopathies are associated with increased ATE risk. Mechanisms include poor intracardiac blood flow, altered coagulability, or local endothelial injury.
ii. Initial goals include stabilizing the cat and preventing thrombus extension and additional ATE. Supportive care is given to optimize tissue perfusion and manage congestive heart failure (if present). An analgesic (e.g. hydromorphone or buprenorphine) is indicated. Heparin can reduce additional clot formation. Unfractionated heparin (initially IV, then SC) is used to prolong aPTT to 1.5–2.5 times pretreatment level. Alternatively, a low-molecular weight heparin has less risk for bleeding, but optimal dosage is unclear. Dalteparin sodium (100–150 U/kg SC q8–24h) and enoxaparin (1 mg/kg SC q12–24h) have been used. Fibrinolytic therapy is problematic and rarely used. When platelet count is adequate, low-dose aspirin or clopidogrel helps reduce platelet aggregation. Renal function and serum electrolyte concentrations should be monitored.
iii. Limb function can improve within weeks and some cats are clinically normal within a couple of months. However, recurrent ATE is common and long-term prognosis is generally poor.

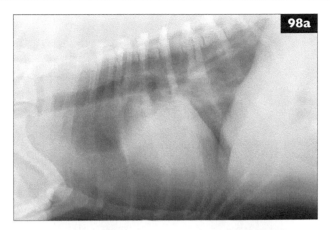

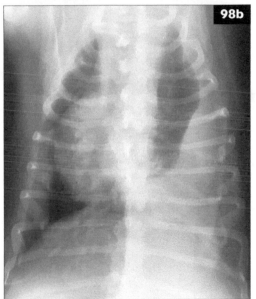

98 A 4-year-old male Dachshund is presented with the complaint of coughing, especially after drinking and eating. Coughing began 5 weeks ago. Five months previously, the dog underwent spinal surgery for a ruptured intervertebral disk. Physical examination is normal. Right lateral (98a) and DV (98b) thoracic radiographs are taken.

i. What clinical differentials are suggested by the history and complaint?
ii. What are the radiographic findings and your radiographic diagnosis?
iii. What will you do next to confirm your suspected diagnosis?

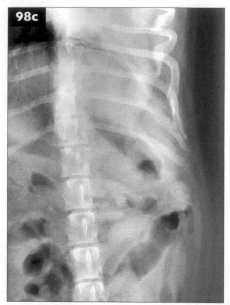

98 i. Differentials include dysphagia with laryngotracheal aspiration, pharyngitis/laryngitis, esophagitis, megaesophagus, and esophageal–bronchial fistula.

ii. Most of the left hemithorax is occupied by uniform soft tissue/fluid opacity that displaces the left lung from the thoracic wall and effaces the left cardiac border and left half of the diaphragm. The heart is shifted rightward (opposite of the effect expected when positioning shifts the sternum leftward) and is displaced dorsally, with fat opacity between the cardiac border and sternum. The trachea parallels the spine, the left diaphragmatic crus is poorly defined, and no air bronchograms, pleural fissure lines, or esophageal dilation are evident. Radiographic diagnosis: left-sided thoracic mass effect. Differentials include enlarging pulmonary mass, pleural mass, and left-sided diaphragmatic hernia.

iii. Abdominal radiographs to assess if the solid organs are appropriately located, thoracic ultrasound to further characterize the opacity, or CT. Enlargement of the left cranial abdomen in the VD view (**98c**) shows absence of the splenic head; no splenic tail was visible in the lateral view. Ultrasound showed a diaphragmatic defect with spleen adjacent to the heart. Surgical exploration confirmed splenic herniation through a tear in the left side of the diaphragm.

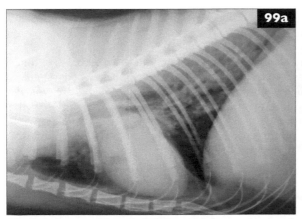

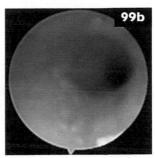

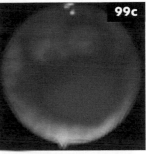

99 A 1.5-year-old male DSH cat had an episode of respiratory distress 2 days ago. Intense abdominal effort, open-mouth breathing, and wheezing occurred for about 10 minutes, then his breathing slowly returned to normal. The moderately over-weight cat is now alert and fully responsive. Physical examination reveals mildly increased abdominal effort during expiration. Rhonchi and wheezes are heard on thoracic auscultation. Gentle tracheal palpation easily triggers a cough. Hematology and serum biochemistry test results are normal.

The cat is anesthetized for thoracic radiography (99a) followed by bronchoscopy. The bronchial mucosa is edematous and bleeds easily at the touch of the scope (99b, c). Plugs of tenacious mucus obstruct some bronchi. BAL samples contain a large well-preserved mixed-cell population with many eosinophils. Occasional neutrophils and moderate numbers of foamy, activated alveolar macrophages are seen, along with scattered, well-differentiated ciliated columnar epithelial cells. No infectious agents, parasite eggs, or larvae are seen. Culture yields no significant bacterial growth.

i. What are the radiographic findings in this cat?
ii. What is your diagnosis?
iii. How would you manage this case?

100 Describe options for bronchodilator therapy.

99 i. A diffuse bronchial pattern and mild lung overinflation are seen. The cardiac silhouette is normal and there is no venous congestion or interstitial/alveolar pattern to suggest heart failure.

ii. The bronchial pattern and airway mucosal inflammation with excessive mucus and numerous eosinophils, as well as foamy activated macrophages, suggest airway hypersensitivity ('feline asthma'). Acute paroxysmal respiratory signs are typical in this condition. The cat's auscultatory findings suggest bronchospasm as well as accumulation of airway secretions.

iii. Reduction of airway inflammation, usually by long-term corticosteroid administration, is crucial. Administration by inhalation (e.g. fluticasone) avoids systemic side-effects and delivers the steroid directly to the airways. A dedicated spacer (e.g. 'Aerokat Feline Aerosol Chamber') designed for inhalation therapy is helpful. A bronchodilator is also important to reduce bronchospasm. Oral or injectable forms (e.g. terbutaline) can be used, but inhaled bronchodilators (e.g. albuterol, salbutamol) administered via the dedicated spacer seem more efficient and provide more rapid response in dyspneic cats.

Environmental triggers/irritants, including cigarette smoke, dust (including litter dust), and aerosols (e.g. deodorants, cleaning products), should be avoided when possible. Nebulization and coupage can help loosen and mobilize deep airway secretions. Obese cats may benefit from a reducing diet, as excessive fat can impair respiratory function.

100 Methyxanthine bronchodilators (theophylline and related drugs) and β_2-adrenoceptor agonists (e.g. terbutaline, albuterol) are usually used. Theophylline can also reduce respiratory muscle fatigue, increase mucus clearance, and reduce inflammation. Adverse effects include cardiac arrhythmias, sinus tachycardia, gastrointestinal upset, nervousness, and seizures. Long-acting theophylline preparations are usually effective administered twice daily. Plasma concentration measurement can guide dosing. Therapeutic (peak) concentrations are thought to be 5–20 mcg/ml. Collect samples at 4–5 hours (long-acting formulations) or 1.5–2.0 hours (immediate release theophylline) post dosing. A β_2-agonist can be used instead of, or occasionally in combination with, a methylxanthine agent. Adverse effects include arrhythmias, sinus tachycardia, nervousness, and occasionally hypotension. Albuterol administered by metered dose inhaler using a spacer and anesthetic mask can be effective, especially in cats. (See Drugs used for cardiac and respiratory diseases, pp. 255–261, for doses.)

101 A 7-year-old male mixed breed dog weighing 18.6 kg (41 lb) is presented for lethargy of 6-day duration, occasional coughing, and increased respiratory effort (especially during expiration). The dog has also been anorexic for the past 24 hours. Because there had been possible exposure to rat poison, the dog had been treated by vitamin K injection, but no improvement occurred. The dog is not receiving

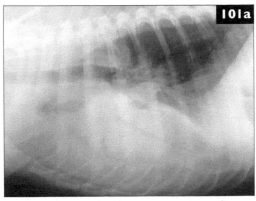

101a

heartworm preventive. Lung sounds are decreased. Thoracocentesis indicates chylous effusion. A right lateral thoracic radiograph is shown (101a).
i. What is the salient abnormality in the lateral radiograph?
ii. What is the imaging diagnosis?

102 A 1-year-old spayed female Bichon Frise is presented for a persistent, non-productive cough of 5-week duration and one known episode of collapse 2 days ago. The dog is bright, alert, and responsive. An irregular heart rhythm at 88 bpm is noted during initial examination; heart and lung sounds are normal. Mucous membranes color and capillary refill time are normal, as are arterial pulses and precordial palpation. The dog vomits shortly after blood samples are drawn for routine CBC and serum chemistry analysis, and then it collapses with apparent respiratory arrest. HR is ~12 bpm and membranes are cyanotic. An endotracheal tube is placed and O_2 administered with manual ventilation. Spontaneous respirations soon resume and HR increases. A short time later, after the dog is extubated, an arterial sample is obtained for blood gas analysis (see below).

Test	Result	Normal	Units
pH	7.25	7.31–7.42	
PCO_2	34.4	29–42	mmHg
PO_2	65.8	85–100	mmHg
HCO_3	14.6	17–24	mmol/l
Base excess	-12.7		mmol/l
Total CO_2	15.7		mmol/l
% Saturation	89.9		%

i. What is your interpretation of the blood gas results?
ii. What are the major causes of hypoxemia?
iii. What are your other diagnostic recommendations?

101 i. Well-defined air bronchograms are evident in the mid-ventral thorax. The cranial air bronchogram is directed ventrally towards the sternum. The caudal bronchogram is longer and angles towards the ventral diaphragm. A mild vesicular gas pattern is associated with the longer air bronchogram. Neither has visible connection with the trachea. There is also pleural effusion.

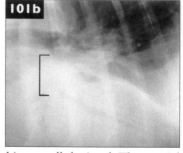

ii. Left cranial lung lobe torsion. Normally in a right lateral view, the left cranial lobe bronchus and origin of cranial and caudal subdivision bronchi are well depicted. The cranial segment bronchus should course cranially towards the manubrium; the caudal segment bronchus should course directly ventrally, not caudoventrally. The air bronchogram is well demonstrated in this dog, but visible connection with the common bronchus is lacking (bracketed area, **101b**). The common trunk bronchus tapers off from the trachea (summated [superimposed] with 5th ribs). Lung surrounding the peripheral portions of these air bronchograms has a mild vesicular gas pattern.

Radiographic features most suggestive of lung lobe torsion are vesicular emphysema in a lobe of soft tissue opacity and narrowed, blunted, and/or abnormally oriented lobar bronchus. Pleural effusion is a common but less specific finding. CT imaging is useful for presurgical diagnostic confirmation of lung lobe torsion.

102 i. Arterial hypoxemia is evident. The pH indicates acidosis. With respiratory acidosis, the $PaCO_2$ is elevated; bicarbonate increases in an attempt to compensate. However, HCO_3 is decreased here, indicating metabolic acidosis; the low normal $PaCO_2$ likely reflects partial respiratory compensation. PaO_2 <60 mmHg causes dangerously low hemoglobin (Hb) saturation. Cyanosis is visible when over 50 g/l (5 g/dl) of Hb becomes unsaturated (non-oxygenated). Cyanotic animals with normal hematocrit likely have PaO_2 <50 mmHg.

ii. Causes of hypoxemia usually involve either alveolar hypoventilation, pulmonary ventilation/perfusion (V/Q) mismatch with varying degrees of venous admixture (perfusion of non-ventilated areas; shunt), anatomic right-to-left shunt, or a combination of factors. Hypoventilation increases $PaCO_2$; with V/Q abnormalities, $PaCO_2$ can be low or normal. Impaired alveolar gas diffusion or low O_2 content of inspired air uncommonly causes hypoxemia. Reduced blood O_2-carrying capacity (e.g. anemia, hemoglobinopathy) also causes tissue hypoxia, even with normal PaO_2.

iii. Chest radiographs. If unremarkable, then airway fluoroscopy and/or bronchoscopy are recommended. Although the irregular heart rhythm is probably sinus arrhythmia, an ECG may identify AV block or other abnormality. Blood test results should help indicate if hypoxemia is chronic (erythrocytosis) or another cause for metabolic acidosis besides the arrest.

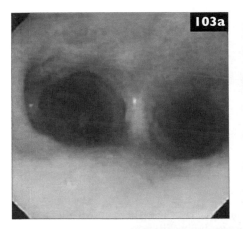

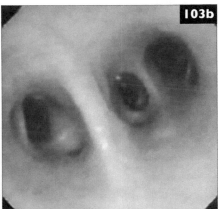

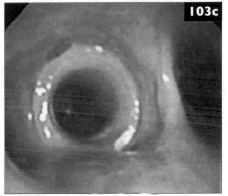

103 Chest radiographs of the dog in case **102** show normal cardiac size (VHS 10.0 v), pulmonary vessels, lung fields, and major airways. A thin pleural fissure line is noted near the right middle lobe. Pronounced sinus arrhythmia is seen on ECG, but HR exceeds 100 bpm during the recording; electrical axis and complex measurements are normal. Echocardiographic examination and routine serum chemistry and hemogram test results are unremarkable. The next day, bronchoscopy is done; images from the carina (**103a**), left main bronchus (**103b**), and region of the right middle lobar bronchus (**103c**) are shown.

i. What is your assessment of the bronchoscopic images?

ii. Could this explain the dog's hypoxemia, bradycardia, and collapse, as well as cough?

iii. How would you follow-up this patient?

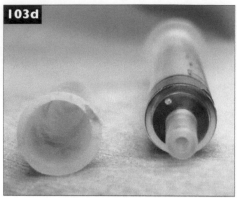

103 i. Mild mucosal edema and erythema is seen at the carina and within the right bronchus (103a, c). A whitish circular foreign body (FB) is in the right middle lobar bronchus (103c). This plastic, cone-shaped FB (the tip from a caulk tube, 103d) was freely moveable, slipping in and out of the bronchial orifice during attempts at removal with forceps. The airways to the left lung lobes appeared normal and there was no sign of tracheal collapse.

ii. Yes. Besides the physical presence of the FB being a cough stimulus, it was thought that the FB probably moved into the right main bronchus or trachea during coughing and/or vomiting, creating greater airway obstruction and causing hypoxemia and collapse. Severe bradycardia can result from marked increases in vagal tone related to underlying pulmonary or airway disease; the vomiting likely exacerbated this.

iii. Culture of airway washings obtained at the time of bronchoscopy is indicated. Appropriate antibiotic therapy is warranted, especially if coughing or other signs persist. Recheck examination and thoracic radiographs in 1–2 weeks are recommended because residual infection or inflammation is possible. No further coughing or episodic bradycardia occurred in this case after the foreign body was removed.

104 A 10-year-old male indoor-outdoor DSH cat is presented as an emergency after 2 days of lethargy and inappetence. There was no known trauma, but the cat does hunt mice and birds. The cat is tachypneic, with open-mouth breathing. Mucous membranes are extremely pale. There are multiple areas of subcutaneous hemorrhage on both thorax and abdomen. Increased breath sounds are heard on auscultation, but no cardiac

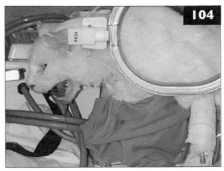

murmur. His hematocrit is 0.1 l/l (10%) and total protein is 50 g/l (5 g/dl). Supplemental O$_2$ is provided (104).

i. When presented with a cat in respiratory distress from unknown cause, what are your initial considerations?

ii. Based on the physical findings and hematocrit, what are your differential diagnoses?

iii. What additional tests or therapy do you recommend at this time?

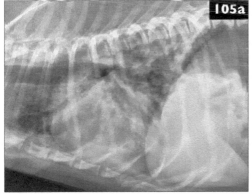

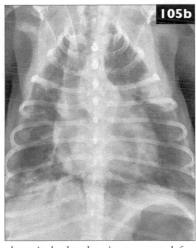

105 An 11-year-old male Maltese was treated for an episode of pancreatitis during the holiday season. Recovery was rapid and uneventful. Two days after discharge from the hospital, the dog is presented for acute respiratory distress. Thoracic radiographs are obtained (105a, b).

i. What radiographic abnormalities are seen?

ii. What are the likely causes of the acute respiratory signs?

iii. How should this case be managed?

104 i. Severe respiratory distress (orthopnea) is evident; the cat crouches in a sternal position with elbows abducted, neck extended, and mouth open (drooling) gasping for air. Considerations include airway obstruction (e.g. acute asthma), severe intrapulmonary disease (e.g. edema, pneumonia, hemorrhage, neoplasia), or pleural space disease (pleural fluid, pneumothorax, intrathoracic mass lesion, diaphragmatic hernia). Respiratory pattern and auscultatory findings help point to the underlying mechanism. (See also case 1 and Further reading.)

ii. Subcutaneous hemorrhage with severe anemia suggests trauma or coagulopathy, with time for fluid translocaton into the vasculature. Pulmonary hemorrhage and hemothorax along with anemia intensify respiratory distress. Rodenticide toxicity is a strong possibility (and was verified here). Cats can be poisoned secondarily by eating rodents that have ingested anticoagulant rodenticides. Other causes of coagulopathy include disseminated intravascular coagulation, severe thrombocytopenia, and hepatic failure.

iii. PT and aPTT should be measured. Prolongation of PT greater than that of aPTT strongly suggests anticoagulant rodenticide toxicity; vitamin K_1 therapy should be started (e.g. 5 mg/kg SC initially). Transfusion with fresh whole blood is also indicated here. Chest radiographs are useful; pleural fluid/blood may need to be aspirated to improve ventilation. Additional supportive care is given as indicated.

105 i. A moderate diffuse interstitial to alveolar lung pattern is seen, predominantly in the caudoperipheral regions (especially the right). A focal area of increased opacity is in the caudal portion of the left cranial lobe. The left heart appears mildly enlarged. The heavy interstitial pattern partially obscures pulmonary vessels, but no obvious pulmonary venous congestion is seen. The gas-distended stomach suggests dyspnea with aerophagia.

ii. Non-cardiogenic pulmonary edema from acute respiratory distress syndrome (ARDS) is likely. Although acute heart failure (e.g. from ruptured mitral chordae tendineae) is possible and can produce atypical edema distribution, more evidence of LA enlargement and pulmonary venous congestion is expected with chronic mitral valve disease. ARDS is a syndrome of acute capillary permeability disruption. It is associated with numerous illnesses including sepsis, aspiration of acidic gastric secretions, inhalation injury, multiple transfusions, shock, pancreatitis, microbial pneumonia, drug reaction or overdose, and major trauma or surgery.

iii. Supplemental O_2, other supportive measures, and treatment for underlying abnormalities are provided. Diuretics may help initially, but are of little benefit in the later phases of ARDS. Overzealous fluid therapy can worsen pulmonary edema and hypoxemia, so only the smallest volume needed to maintain cardiac output and arterial BP is given. Corticosteroids are of unconfirmed benefit.

106 Brief physical examination of the dog in case 105 presented for acute respiratory distress reveals good body condition, severe tachypnea and dyspnea, a soft systolic murmur at the left cardiac apex and harsh lung sounds on inspiration and expiration.

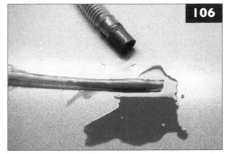

Supplemental O_2 via an oxygen chamber and a 4 mg/kg IM furosemide injection are initially administered. Chest radiographs show interstitial and alveolar lung infiltrates, especially in the caudal and peripheral regions, and mild left heart enlargement. Pulmonary vessels are not clearly delineated because of the heavy interstitial pattern, but there is no obvious pulmonary venous congestion (see 105a, b). There is no improvement after initial therapy; respiratory arrest occurs shortly thereafter. An endotracheal tube is placed and fluid (shown) is aspirated from the airway.

i. What is your working diagnosis/es in this case?
ii. What would you do next?
iii. How can the fluid help identify the underlying pathology?

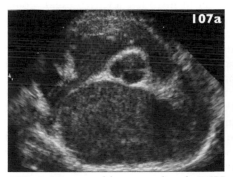
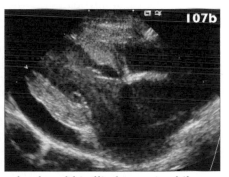

107 A 10-year-old neutered male DSH cat developed hindlimb paresis while at a boarding facility. The cat ambulates abnormally and has no pain response in either hindlimb. Femoral pulses are not palpable, but his extremities are warm and dorsal pedal pulses are identified. A gallop sound and grade 2/6 systolic murmur are heard on auscultation. Chest radiographs show marked cardiomegaly without pulmonary edema. Right parasternal short axis (107a) and long axis (107b) echocardiographic images are shown.

i. What abnormalities are seen on the echo images?
ii. What does this indicate?
iii. How would you manage this case?

106 i. Pulmonary edema is likely, but is it non-cardiogenic or cardiogenic in origin? The lack of obvious venous congestion, caudal/peripheral distribution of pulmonary infiltrates, and minimal cardiomegaly on radiographs speak against acute cardiogenic edema (although still possible). Non-cardiogenic edema can develop with ARDS, electric shock, or seizure activity. Diffuse pulmonary neoplasia or other infiltrative disease is also possible. Pancreatitis has been associated with ARDS. Given the otherwise unremarkable historical, ARDS was the working diagnosis.

ii. Emergency therapy was initiated with a positive-pressure ventilator using 100% O_2. Another 4 mg/kg bolus of furosemide was administered IV. A bronchodilator was also used. At this time, no specific treatment is available for ARDS other than assisted ventilation and other supportive care. In this case there was no response to emergency therapy.

iii. Analysis of edema fluid suctioned from the airways can help differentiate ARDS from cardiogenic edema. The ratio of edema fluid (E) protein content to plasma (P) protein content is 79–90% for ARDS; for cardiogenic pulmonary edema it is typically <50%. This dog's edema fluid E:P ratio was 86%. ARDS patients often deteriorate rapidly. This dog died from respiratory failure.

107 i. The LA is severely dilated (~2.6 cm). Spontaneous echo contrast (swirling 'smoke') is visible within the LA and LV. Pericardial effusion and mild LV hypertrophy are also present (LV wall ~ 0.6 cm, diastole).

ii. The LA size suggests severe LV diastolic dysfunction (e.g. from restrictive or hypertrophic cardiomyopathy), although mitral insufficiency, if present, could contribute to LA enlargement. Spontaneous contrast is thought to result from blood stasis with cellular aggregates and be a harbinger of thromboembolism (TE). Pericardial effusion can occur from advanced cardiomyopathy in cats.

iii. This cat has clear lungs and some hindlimb collateral circulation. Treatment is aimed at preventing further TE, optimizing cardiovascular function, and supportive care as needed. Low-molecular weight heparin (LMWH) was used in this cat (enoxaparin, 1 mg/kg SC q12h). LMWH only minimally affects coagulation times; its effect can be monitored indirectly by anti-Xa activity. When platelet numbers are adequate, concurrent low-dose aspirin (e.g. 5 mg/cat q72h) or clopidogrel (18.75 mg/cat PO q24h) can be added. An angiotensin-converting enzyme inhibitor and diltiazem are also recommended. This cat was managed medically for another 1.5 years, then died after his 4th arterial TE event.

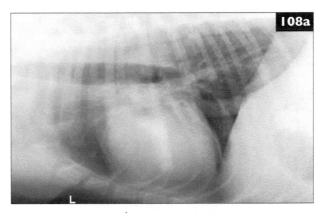

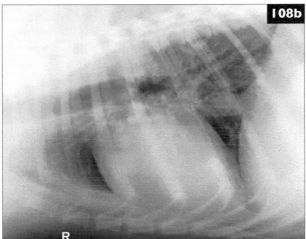

108 A 1-year-old neutered male Alaskan Malamute is presented with a 3-month history of coughing with intermittent hemoptysis. The dog has been living in the Mississippi river valley region of the USA. He has an inducible cough with mid-tracheal palpation, and coughs up bloody mucus during the examination. CBC and serum chemistries are normal. Left (108a) and right (108b) lateral thoracic radiographs are shown.
i. How would you characterize the radiographic lesions?
ii. What are the etiologic differentials for these lesions?
iii. What diagnostic procedure(s) would you do next?

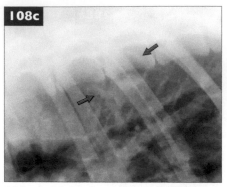

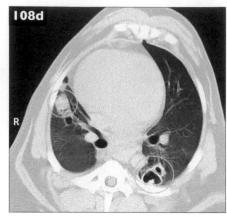

108 i. Multiple cavitary nodules are present. Their walls vary in thickness from uniformly thin, with smooth inner and outer borders, to non-uniform, moderately thick, with mildly irregular inner borders (**108c**, arrows). In some, more than one cavitary lucency is associated, with the soft tissue/fluid rim giving the appearance of a multiloculated cavity. A CT scan done on this patient (**108d**) shows two cavitary lesions, one circled in the dorsal left lung and one in the right ventral lung. PAs adjacent to lobar bronchi are also evident.

ii. Cavitary pulmonary lesions can arise from trauma (bulla, bleb), pneumonia (pneumatocele), bacterial abscess, granuloma, parasitic cysts (*Paragonimus kellicotti*), or neoplasia. The young age of this dog makes neoplasia unlikely. There was no history of trauma and with a normal hemogram and no fever, bacterial infection is unlikely. Paragonimiasis is a strong consideration in endemic regions when access to the crayfish intermediate host is possible. Congenital cavitary lung lesions are also a possibility.

iii. Identification of fluke eggs, which can be recovered from feces, sputum cytology, or tracheal washings, confirms a diagnosis of paragonimiasis.

109 A 7-year-old male Boxer has been losing weight for the past couple of months, but more recently his head and forelimbs have started getting bigger (**109a**). He does not seem painful, but his appetite is poor. Body temperature is normal. The forelimbs, cranial chest, ventral neck, and lips are swollen, cool to the touch, non-painful, and indent with digital pressure. Heart and lung sounds are normal over the mid to caudal thorax, but are muffled over the cranial thorax. The caudal body is quite thin.

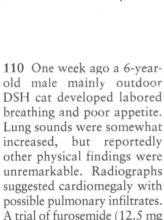

i. Can the location of this dog's disease be identified based on his appearance and physical findings?
ii. What etiologies can cause this condition?
iii. What tests would you recommend next, and why?

110 One week ago a 6-year-old male mainly outdoor DSH cat developed labored breathing and poor appetite. Lung sounds were somewhat increased, but reportedly other physical findings were unremarkable. Radiographs suggested cardiomegaly with possible pulmonary infiltrates. A trial of furosemide (12.5 mg q12h) was prescribed. The owner thinks the cat's signs

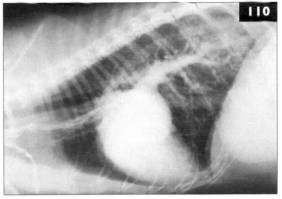

are improved. Cardiac disease of some kind is suspected, but echocardiography is not available. A non-selective angiocardiogram is done (**110**).
i. Does this study suggest a diagnosis of heartworm disease?
ii. Describe the angiographic findings.
iii. What are your recommendations to the owner?

109 i. The swelling is subcutaneous edema. The distribution is typical for the so-called 'cranial caval syndrome', where obstruction of cranial vena caval flow raises venous and capillary hydrostatic pressure in regions that drain into this vessel. Muffled heart and lung sounds over the cranial, but not caudal, thorax suggest a mass lesion pushing the heart and lungs caudally.

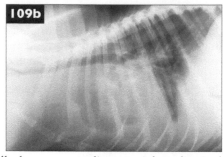

ii. Cranial vena caval compression (usually by an expanding cranial mediastinal lymphoma, thymoma, or other mass) or complete thrombosis leads to this syndrome. Besides bilaterally symmetric cranial edema, as seen here, pleural effusion is common. Caval thrombosis can occur with diseases causing a hypercoagulable state (e.g. immune-mediated thrombocytopenia or hemolytic anemia, sepsis, nephrotic syndrome, and some neoplasia), usually in conjunction with central venous catheter use.

iii. Thoracic radiographs indicated a cranial mediastinal mass (**109b**). Ultrasonography also can identify masses or caval thrombosis, if present. Needle aspirate or biopsy of the mass (lymphoma in this dog), and routine bloodwork and urinalysis, are indicated to guide therapy. Underlying disease process(es) must be sought for caval thrombosis.

110 i. The image was taken after dye passed through the lungs to the left heart, although some residual dye is seen in the cranial vena cava. Dilated and slightly tortuous caudal vessels are seen, but these are pulmonary veins, not arteries. There is no specific indication for heartworm disease here.

ii. There is massive LA enlargement, with dilated pulmonary veins entering caudally. These findings imply chronically high pressure within. The LV is enlarged (note the elevated carina and proximal caudal vena cava) and there appears to be some filling defects within the lumen; possible causes include hypertrophied papillary muscles, irregular mural hypertrophy, and endocardial scarring. Severe hypertrophic or restrictive cardiomyopathy is likely.

iii. Although echocardiography may provide additional information, this study indicates chronic diastolic dysfunction. An increased risk for decompensated heart failure, arterial thromboembolism, and arrhythmias is expected. Furosemide should be continued at the lowest level needed to control pulmonary edema. The owner should monitor the cat's respirations, activity level, and appetite. An angiotensin-converting enzyme inhibitor and therapy to reduce risk of thromboembolism (e.g. aspirin, clopidogrel) are also recommended. Other agents may be helpful for refractory heart failure (e.g. pimobendan, spironolactone) or tachyarrhythmias (e.g. atenolol, diltiazem).

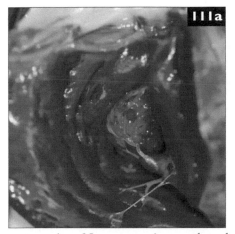

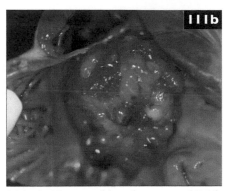

111 A 13-year-old male-neutered Irish Setter is presented for abdominal distension. A palpable fluid wave indicates ascites. No murmur is auscultated, but jugular pulsation and distension are noted. Femoral pulses are normal. Echocardiography shows a serious lesion. The owners elected euthanasia. Postmortem images are shown (**111a**, opened RV with freewall to the right and pulmonary valve at top of image; **111b**, opened RA).
i. Describe the lesion and its location.
ii. Can the dog's clinical signs be attributed to this lesion? Why, or why not?

112 An 18-year-old female spayed DSH cat is presented for episodes of collapse that are becoming more frequent and severe. Over the past few weeks the owner has also noted the cat sometimes has trouble jumping up on the bed. The cat is alert and in good condition. Physical examination is unremarkable. Chest radiographs and BP are normal.

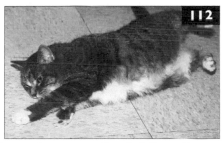

You hospitalize the cat for observation. Later the cat vocalizes briefly, collapses into lateral recumbency, and stiffens her limbs. Several similar episodes occur over the evening. The photograph was taken during one of the episodes (**112**).
i. What are common characteristics of cardiovascular syncope that may help differentiate it from seizure activity?
ii. What differential diagnoses should be considered in this case?
iii. What would you do next in this case?

111 i. In **111a** (viewed from the RV cavity) there is a glistening yellowish mass of tissue protruding through the tricuspid valve orifice. One tricuspid leaflet is seen enveloping the mass (on the left). The mass appears multilobular and gelatinous. In **111b** (from inside the RA looking toward the tricuspid orifice) the mass appears to completely occlude the RV inflow region. This intracardiac tumor was histologically identified as a myxoma. Cardiac myxoma is a benign neoplasm resulting from multipotent mesenchymal cells. It usually arises from the interatrial septum near the fossa ovalis, most commonly in the LA but occasionally from the RA. This tumor type is very rare in dogs.

ii. Jugular pulsation related to atrial contraction can occur with any cause of increased right heart filling pressures. In this case the mass partially obstructed tricuspid inflow and increased resistance to RV filling. Jugular vein distension develops when RA pressure is high. As obstruction to ventricular filling worsens, pulsation of the jugular veins diminishes and may disappear, although venous distension persists. Ascites develops because systemic venous and capillary hydrostatic pressure elevation increases fluid transudation from the capillaries. This mimics right-sided congestive heart failure.

112 i. Syncope is sudden, transient unconsciousness, usually caused by abruptly reduced cerebral perfusion. Collapse into lateral recumbency, limb stiffening, opisthotonic posture, micturition, and vocalization are common. Syncope is often associated with excitement or exertion. Atypical for syncope are facial fits, persistent tonic/clonic motion, defecation, a prodromal aura, (postictal) dementia, and neurologic deficits. Profound hypotension can cause hypoxic seizure-like activity ('convulsive syncope'), but loss of muscle tone usually precedes this. Neurologic seizure activity is usually preceded by atypical limb or facial movement or staring spells before collapse.

ii. Either syncope or seizure activity could be occurring here, although the apparent absence of pre- or postictal mentation change makes cardiovascular syncope more likely. Syncope has many causes, but given this cat's age, absence of cardiac murmur, and normal thoracic radiographs, an intermittent tachy- or bradyarrhythmia would be most likely in this case. Myocardial disease may also be present. Likely differentials for seizure activity include brain tumor, transient cerebrovascular events, and cerebral inflammatory lesion.

iii. An ECG, echocardiogram, neurologic examination, and laboratory database (e.g. CBC, biochemical profile, T_4, urinalysis, heartworm test) are advised. Ambulatory ECG monitoring can help identify or exclude cardiac arrhythmias if resting ECG is normal.

113 The cat in case 112 is being monitored because of frequent collapse events. She collapses during in-hospital ECG monitoring. The heart rhythm just prior to and during the event is shown (113, lead II, 25 mm/s, 1 cm = 1 mV; the top two strips are continuous).

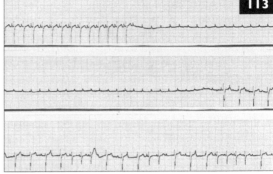

i. What is your ECG interpretation?
ii. Is the underlying problem likely to be within the AV node?
iii. What treatment options are available?

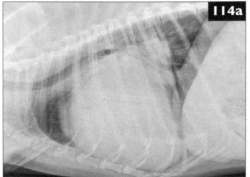

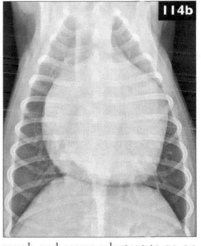

114 A 7-year-old female English Springer Spaniel in good body condition has progressive lethargy and exercise intolerance of several months' duration. Over the past 2 weeks she has developed an occasional soft cough and seems reluctant to go on walks. Examination reveals pink mucous membranes, jugular pulses extending to the laryngeal region, and strong synchronous femoral pulses. Pulse rate is regular at 40 bpm. Holosystolic plateau murmurs are heard over the left and right apex on auscultation. An ejection murmur is also suspected, over the left base region. Lung sounds are normal. Right lateral (114a) and DV (114b) thoracic radiographs are taken.
i. What abnormalities are seen on these chest radiographs?
ii. Identify differential diagnoses for this case based on the information available.
iii. Should a diuretic be administered for congestive heart failure at this time?
iv. What other clinical test(s) are indicated?

113 i. The ECG begins with sinus rhythm at 200 bpm; the QRS complexes have deep and wide S waves typical for right bundle branch block (RBBB). Midway across the top strip, AV conduction fails and only sinus P waves occur. Almost 12 seconds elapse (and syncope occurred) before a ventricular escape rhythm appears (middle strip, right side). Complete AV block with ventricular escape rhythm continues into the bottom strip; after the 5th QRS complex, three sinus P waves are conducted with RBBB, followed by brief alternating periods of AV block with escape rhythm and conduction.

ii. The RBBB apparent during sinus rhythm indicates an intraventricular conduction system abnormality. More widespread intraventricular disease is likely, with intermittent left bundle branch block producing complete heart block. Nevertheless, AV nodal disease may also exist. Most advanced AV block is associated with underlying structural disease (e.g. endocarditis/myocarditis, cardiomyopathy, endocardiosis, fibrosis, trauma).

iii. The intermittent nature of the AV block is problematic. Most cats with persistent third degree AV block are asymptomatic, with ventricular escape rates of 90–120 bpm. The efficacy of medical management is unclear. Artificial pacing can alleviate the syncope. An epicardial approach is now thought to be better in cats as chylothorax commonly develops after transvenous pacing (as in this cat).

114 i. Generalized cardiomegaly is present, with LV and especially LA enlargement being predominant. This is evidenced by the extremely tall (lateral) and elongated (DV) cardiac silhouette. The caudal edge of the enlarged LA overlaps the LV apical region on DV view; the left auricular bulge is seen at the 2 o'clock position. The caudal vena cava is prominent. Pulmonary vessel size and pulmonary parenchyma appear normal.

ii. Differential diagnoses for this case include chronic volume overload dilation secondary to chronic bradycardia, or dilated cardiomyopathy, or chronic AV valve disease with concurrent conduction disturbance. The most likely underlying causes for the regular bradyarrhythmia in this case is complete AV block or, considering the signalment, atrial standstill. Other bradyarrhythmias such as intermittent sinus arrest, sick sinus syndrome, or second degree AV block are classically associated with an irregular heart rhythm.

iii. There is no evidence of pulmonary edema (left-sided heart failure); pulmonary vessels appear normal in size and pulmonary parenchyma appears clear. Diuretics are not needed at this time.

iv. An ECG is indicated for cardiac rhythm diagnosis. An echocardiogram is warranted to evaluate chamber sizes and ventricular systolic function. (See also case **115**.)

115 This ECG (115a, leads I, II, and III at 50 mm/s, 1 cm = 1 mV) is taken from the dog in case 114. An echocardiogram shows severe dilation of the LA and moderate to severe dilation of the LV. LV systolic function is characterized as normal, with a FS of 55%.

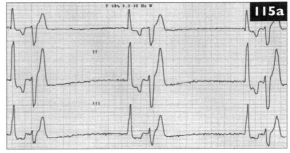

Serum biochemical tests are normal.

i. What is the ECG rhythm diagnosis?

ii. What treatment, if any, would you advise?

iii. What is the long-term prognosis for this patient?

116 An 18-year-old cat is presented for difficulty breathing and weight loss, which began a couple weeks ago. She now shows open-mouth breathing and increased abdominal effort. The cat has long tested positive for feline leukemia and immunodeficiency viruses. On physical examination she appears depressed, thin, and somewhat dehydrated. Respiratory rate is 24 breaths/min and labored; HR is 160 bpm and regular. Wheezes are heard on auscultation. Thoracic radiographs reveal a soft tissue opacity within the distal trachea. Laboratory tests show mild azotemia. Supplemental O_2 and intravenous fluid therapy are instituted prior to anesthesia for bronchoscopy. Images from within the mid (116a) and distal (116b) trachea are shown.

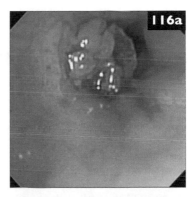

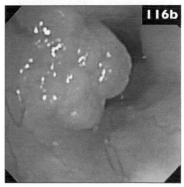

i. What are the bronchoscopic findings?

ii. What would you do now?

iii. What are the most common causes of large airway obstruction in cats?

iv. How would you manage this case after bronchoscopy?

115 i. Atrial standstill with a ventricular escape rhythm and frequent ventricular premature contractions (VPCs). Persistent atrial standstill is characterized by a junctional or idioventricular escape rhythm without detectable P waves. In this ECG a VPC follows every escape complex in a repeatable pattern (ventricular bigeminy), which

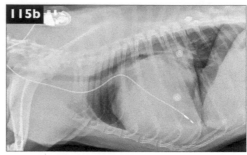

may represent a re-entry path within an area of diseased myocardium. The VPCs occur early enough that an arterial pulse may not be generated. In this dog, serum electrolytes were normal and clinical and radiographic findings indicated severe heart disease.

ii. Medical therapy is usually inadequate for atrial standstill. An atropine challenge test may indicate whether the bradyarrhythmia is responsive to changes in vagal tone. Permanent transvenous pacemaker implantation is the treatment of choice (115b).

iii. Persistent atrial standstill, also called AV muscular dystrophy, has been recognized mainly in Springer Spaniels and Old English Sheepdogs. It has been compared to a type of human muscular dystrophy and involves progressive atrial and ventricular muscle degeneration. Congestive heart failure often results. Even with pacemaker placement, the disorder is usually fatal within 12–18 months of diagnosis.

116 i. An irregular, fleshy mass is attached to the lateral trachea wall near the carina.

ii. Debulk the mass as much as possible with endoscopic biopsy forceps and submit the tissue for histologic examination. A wire snare passed through the bronchoscope's biopsy channel can also be used to remove intratracheal masses in the cat. Incomplete removal may result in regrowth of the mass. However, given the deep intrathoracic location of this mass and the cat's advanced age, surgical resection was deemed too risky.

iii. A neoplastic mass (e.g. lymphoma, adenocarcinoma, squamous cell carcinoma) is most likely, although lymphoplasmocytic inflammatory polyps and lymphoid hyperplasia are also reported. Lymphoid hyperplasia may presage later discovery of neoplasia. Laryngeal masses are more common than tracheal mass lesions. Laryngeal paralysis is another consideration for upper airway obstruction. This mass appeared to be an adenoma or a very well-differentiated carcinoma.

iv. Supplemental O_2 should be continued during anesthetic recovery. Prednisolone (e.g. 1 mg/kg initially then tapering over several days and discontinuing) helps reduce airway inflammation and edema. A broad-spectrum antibiotic may also be used. Long-term prognosis is usually poor because of mass recurrence.

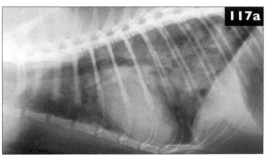

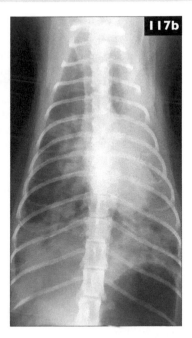

117 A 2-year-old female DLH cat is presented for signs of respiratory distress. She appears anxious and tachypneic. Body temperature, mucous membrane color, pulses, jugular veins, and precordial palpation are normal. HR is 240 bpm. A grade 2/6 systolic murmur and S_4 gallop sound are heard at the left apex. Breath sounds are harsh. Lateral (**117a**) and DV (**117b**) chest radiographs are obtained.
i. Describe the radiographic findings.
ii. What is the most likely diagnosis?
iii. What would you do next?

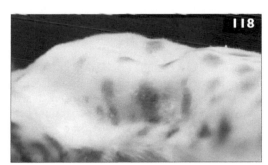

118 A 12-week-old male Bengal kitten is presented for breathing difficulty. The cat is otherwise healthy except for the physical abnormality illustrated (**118**, cat positioned in dorsal recumbency with its head to the left).
i. What is the physical abnormality illustrated?
ii. What is the cause of this condition?
iii. What diagnostic tests are indicated, and why?
iv. What concurrent abnormalities may be found with this condition?

131

117 **i.** The cardiac silhouette is enlarged (VHS ~8.8 v), with moderate tracheal elevation. Diffuse patchy interstitial to alveolar infiltrates are especially prominent in the dorsocaudal lung fields. Pulmonary vessels to the right caudal lobe are seen best and are enlarged (wider than the 10th rib where they cross; **117b**). Aerophagia is consistent with respiratory distress.

ii. Cardiogenic pulmonary edema. This condition in cats usually involves an uneven and patchy distribution of opacities, either extending throughout the lung fields or concentrated in the middle zones. Hypertrophic cardiomyopathy (HCM) most commonly causes an S_4 gallop and congestive heart failure (CHF) in cats, but other cardiomyopathies are other potential causes. Congenital cardiac shunts or mitral dysplasia often cause left-sided CHF. Although enlargement of both veins and arteries often accompanies pulmonary overcirculation, this vascular pattern also occurs with CHF (pulmonary venous congestion and secondary increase in PA pressure). Other differentials for interstitial pulmonary infiltrates include infection, hemorrhage, and neoplasia.

iii. Administer supplemental O_2 and parenteral furosemide. Minimize patient stress and manipulation. When respiration improves, obtain an echocardiogram, along with BP measurement and a complete laboratory database, to guide further therapy. Severe HCM was identified in this cat.

118 **i.** Pectus excavatum. This concave sternal deformity is caused by dorsal deviation of the mid or caudal sternum and associated costal arches.

ii. Pectus excavatum is a congenital deformity of the sternum and costal cartilages that results in dorsoventral narrowing of the thorax. The exact developmental mechanism of this abnormality is not known.

iii. Thoracic radiographs should be obtained to assess the degree of dorsoventral narrowing, as well as to screen for pneumonia and cardiac displacement. These radiographs also provide a baseline for evaluating the effectiveness of treatment. Echocardiography can also be helpful, especially if a heart murmur is heard.

iv. Concurrent abnormalities can include tracheal hypoplasia and congenital heart defects; animals with pectus excavatum are also more susceptible to lower airway infection and pneumonia. However, a cardiac murmur heard in an animal with pectus excavatum may not necessarily indicate a congenital heart defect. Murmurs in affected animals without structural heart disease often disappear after surgical correction of pectus excavatum. Such murmurs are thought to be related to cardiac malpositioning rather than a cardiac defect *per se*.

119 Physical examination of the kitten in case **118** reveals a palpable sternal abnormality. Thoracic radiographs are taken (right lateral view shown [**119**]).

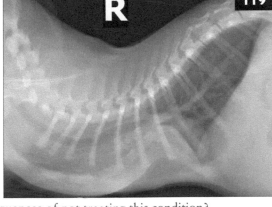

i. What is the physical abnormality illustrated in the radiograph?
ii. What is the recommended treatment for this condition?
iii. How soon should definitive treatment for this condition be performed?
iv. What are the potential consequences of not treating this condition?

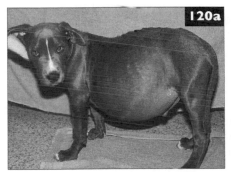

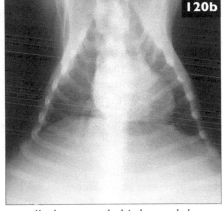

120 A 5-month-old male Pit Bull Terrier is presented for abdominal distension that has developed over the past 2 months (**120a**). He is acting and eating normally, but recently his large abdomen has been slowing him down. The dog is alert and active, with normal mucous membrane color and capillary refill time. Femoral pulses are normal. The jugular veins are not distended or pulsating. HR and rhythm and heart and lung sounds are normal. There is large-volume ascites, which is a modified transudate. Thoracic radiographs show normal heart size and shape, with normal lungs and pulmonary vasculature (DV, **120b**).
i. What are the causes of large-volume modified transudate in the abdomen?
ii. Does this dog have right-sided congestive heart failure (CHF)?
iii. How would you proceed with this puppy?

119 i. The dorsal sternal deviation of pectus excavatum is evident.
ii. Treatment involves fashioning an external frame of lightweight thermoplastic material that is secured with sutures placed around the sternum and through holes in the frame. Sutures are preplaced around the sternum and threaded through holes drilled in strategic locations in the frame. When the sutures are tightened the sternum is pulled toward the frame, reversing the pectus excavatum. The frame is maintained for 3 weeks.
iii. The procedure is ideally performed when the animal is still growing, so that thoracic remodeling will occur quickly and before the animal outgrows the frame.
iv. Respiratory compromise is the most common manifestation of pectus excavatum. The severity of clinical signs relates to the severity of the deformity, thoracic volume reduction, and lung collapse. Secondary pneumonia or cardiac compromise can be complications. Signs can range from mild exercise intolerance to marked respiratory distress and death. Some cases exhibit persistent coughing. Others are asymptomatic except for the physical presence of the defect; however, waiting for clinical signs to develop may not be prudent, because the condition is treated more readily in an actively growing animal than in an adult with a less pliable thorax.

120 i. Ascites usually results from abnormal Starling's forces, often high systemic venous or portal pressure. Increased capillary permeability (e.g. from inflammation), low capillary colloid oncotic pressure (from hypoalbuminemia), and lymphatic obstruction are other mechanisms. Ascites from high venous hydrostatic pressure can be categorized by location of pathology. 'Posthepatic' ('postsinusoidal') ascites occurs from restricted blood flow between the hepatic vein and RV. Excessive fluid formation in hepatic sinusoids then diffuses across the liver capsule to the peritoneal space. Posthepatic ascites is usually secondary to right-sided CHF or cardiac tamponade. Uncommonly, caudal vena caval or RA inflow obstruction or compression are causes. 'Hepatic' ascites, from primary liver disease, usually involves portal hypertension, although other mechanisms are possible. 'Prehepatic' ascites develops from portal vein obstruction; excess fluid transudation from intestinal serosa produces increased lymph formation. Prehepatic ascites is uncommon because collateral portosystemic shunting reduces portal hypertension.
ii. Right-sided CHF should also cause jugular vein distension, as well as other evidence for cardiac enlargement or dysfunction. However, the caudal vena cava appears large on the radiograph.
iii. Recommend echocardiography to examine the proximal caudal vena cava and RA inflow region for obstructive lesions, and possibly abdominal ultrasonography or vena caval angiography.

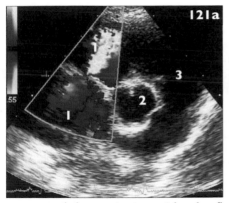

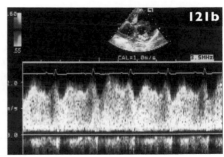

121 An echocardiogram is done on the Pit Bull Terrier puppy described in case 120. A diastolic frame from the right parasternal short axis view with color flow Doppler sector over the RA (121a) and pulsed wave (PW) Doppler with sample volume in the RA above the tricuspid valve (121b) are shown. 1 – RA, 2 – Ao, 3 – RV.
i. Describe the findings in 121a.
ii. What is shown in 121b?
iii. What is your diagnosis?
iv. How can this condition be treated?

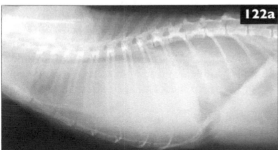

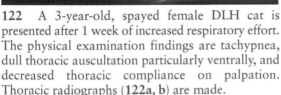

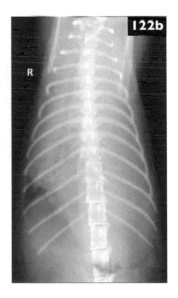

122 A 3-year-old, spayed female DLH cat is presented after 1 week of increased respiratory effort. The physical examination findings are tachypnea, dull thoracic auscultation particularly ventrally, and decreased thoracic compliance on palpation. Thoracic radiographs (122a, b) are made.
i. What are the radiographic abnormalities?
ii. What is the radiographic diagnosis?
iii. What are the etiologic differentials?
iv. Of what value would a CT study be in this patient?

121 i. A perforated membrane bisects the RA. Low velocity flow (coded red) moves through the large caudal RA chamber, accelerating across the membrane's narrow opening into the cranial RA chamber. Tricuspid valve, RV, Ao, and main PA are normal.

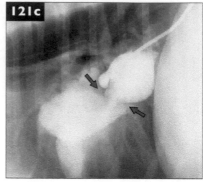

ii. The sample volume is in the cranial RA chamber. Flow velocity is increased (peak >2 m/s) across the intra-atrial membrane, with pressure gradient ~10–20 mmHg throughout the cardiac cycle.

iii. Cor triatriatum dexter. This uncommon malformation occurs when the embryonic right sinus venosus valve fails to regress, creating an abnormal membrane that divides the right (dexter) atrium in two. Caudal vena caval and coronary sinus flows enter the caudal RA chamber. Obstructed flow through the abnormal membrane raises hydrostatic pressure in the caudal vena cava and veins draining into it, causing progressive ascites. Angiography depicts the distended caudal cava and flow restriction at the RA membrane (arrows, 121c).

iv. The abnormal membrane can be surgically excised or the orifice enlarged using balloon dilation catheters.

122 i. Nearly the entire thorax is of soft tissue/fluid opacity. Only the caudal right portion has normal lung lucency. The trachea is markedly displaced dorsally throughout and is shifted to the right. The principal bronchi are also shifted to the right and demonstrate air bronchogram formation. The cardiac shadow is effaced with the exception of a small portion of the apex evident in the DV view that is shifted to the right. The left half of the diaphragm is effaced and the impression is that the right half is displaced caudally. No pleural fissure lines are evident.

ii. Large left-sided thoracic mass, more likely of mediastinal origin than pulmonary or pleural.

iii. Thymic origin neoplasia (lymphoma or thymoma), cranial mediastinal lymphadenomegaly (lymphoma), thymic cyst, and branchial cyst. The diagnosis in this patient was malignant thymoma.

iv. Based on the limited studies in dogs and cats, CT imaging is not likely to provide an etiologic diagnosis for a cranial mediastinal mass. However, it has been found to be useful in the local staging of these masses and thus in the surgical management.

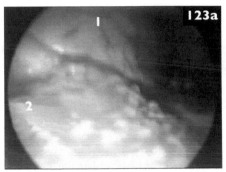
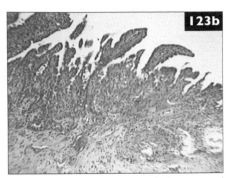

123 A 13-year-old neutered female Beagle presents with a 1-week history of lethargy, followed by cough and respiratory distress that developed 2 days prior to evaluation. The dog appears mildly dyspneic (respiratory rate 45 breaths/min). Physical examination reveals normal body temperature (38.9°C [102°F]), good femoral pulse quality, and no jugular pulsation or distension. The hepatojugular reflux is negative. Chest percussion indicates a bilateral horizontal line of dullness. Other parameters are unremarkable. Thoracic radiographs show increased opacity throughout the ventral aspect of the chest, with retraction and scalloping of lung lobes, consistent with a mild pleural effusion. Echocardiography and abdominal ultrasonography are unremarkable. Thoracocentesis yields 150 ml of serosanguineous fluid: total protein, 50.5 g/l (5.05 g/dl); albumin, 34.1 g/l (3.41 g/dl); globulin, 20.4 g/l (2.04 g/dl); alb/glob ratio, 1.49; pH, 7.4; SG, 1.035; appearance, red turbid fluid; cell preservation, good; cytology, individual small clusters and large rafts of cells with foamy cytoplasm, variable round to oval nuclei and occasional mitoses, cells have a variable nuclear/cytoplasmic ratio, high number of neutrophils in the background; microbiology, negative aerobic and anaerobic cultures.

Thoracoscopy is performed under general anesthesia and an image is obtained (**123a**, 1 – pericardium, 2 – right middle lung lobe). No parenchymal lesions or isolated masses are identified. A pleural biopsy is obtained (**123b**, 25×; H&E).
i. What are the differential diagnoses for this case?
ii. How would you describe the thoracoscopic findings?
iii. What does the biopsy show?

124 What are the effects of, and indications for, pimobendan?

123 i. The effusion is consistent with a pleural exudate. This can occur from inflammation (pleuritis), with increased permeability of the pleural surface to proteinaceous fluid. Causes of pleuritis include bacterial infection, neoplasia (pulmonary, mediastinal, or pleural), thoracic trauma, or even chronic effusion of different causes.

ii. The thoracoscopic image shows several white-gray plaques, a few millimeters in diameter, on the visceral pleural surface. Similar lesions were observed on the pericardium and parietal pleura.

iii. Biopsy and histopathology of the pleural lesions are necessary for definitive diagnosis. In this case, cords of cells, acini, and papillary projections are seen on histologic examination. Some of the larger, bizarre cells observed at the surface in some areas resemble the cells observed in the pleural fluid. In the absence of an obvious primary mass elsewhere, and from the cytologic appearance, these changes are consistent with pleural mesothelioma.

Life expectancy with mesothelioma is often less than a 1 year, although survival time may increase with chemotherapy (and pericardectomy if concurrent pericardial effusion). Intracavitary administration of cisplatin or carboplatin, possibly with piroxicam, may produce clinical remission for several months. The intracavitary route delivers higher drug concentrations to the neoplastic tissue and reduces risk of toxicity.

124 Pimobendan increases cardiac contractility and promotes systemic and pulmonary vasodilation, thereby improving cardiac pump function. It increases contractility by phosphodiesterase-3 (PDE-3) inhibition (enhances adrenergic effects on Ca^{++} fluxes) and by a calcium-sensitizing effect on cardiac contractile proteins. The latter increases contractility without additional myocardial O_2 requirement. PDE-3 inhibition underlies the drug's vasodilating effect. Pimobendan also can modulate neurohormonal and proinflammatory cytokine activation. Pimobendan is indicated for dogs with congestive heart failure (CHF) from chronic valvular disease or dilated cardiomyopathy; it has improved clinical signs and survival when added to conventional CHF therapy. Dogs with other causes of myocardial dysfunction and cats with refractory CHF may also benefit.

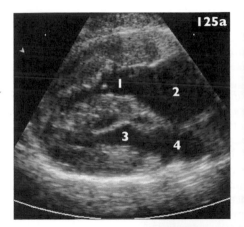

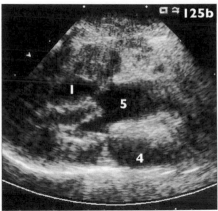

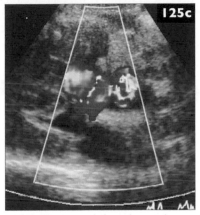

125 A 5-year-old 3 kg (6.5 lb) spayed female cat has episodes of cyanosis and increased respiratory rate and effort, mostly after playing. The referring veterinarian has prescribed enalapril and furosemide, with little improvement. The cat is alert. Respiratory rate is 72 breaths/min, HR is 240 bpm, and temperature is 38.8°C (101.9°F). No cardiac murmur is heard on auscultation, but increased breath sounds are noted. Femoral pulses and jugular veins are normal. After a few minutes of play, slight cyanosis of the oral mucous membranes and increased respiratory effort are evident. An echocardiogram is done; images shown are from the right parasternal long axis position (125a–c). 1 – RV, 2 – RA, 3 – LV, 4 – LA, 5 – Ao.
i. Assess the echo findings.
ii. What is the diagnosis?
iii. Why is no murmur evident?
iv. How should this be managed?

125 i. Moderate RV hypertrophy and RA enlargement are evident (125a). 125b shows a large ventricular septal defect (VSD) with overriding aortic root; flow from both RV (blue) and LV (red) enters into the aorta (125c). The slightly elevated pulmonary outflow velocity is consistent with mild pulmonic stenosis (PS).

ii. Tetralogy of Fallot; component anomalies are VSD, PS, a dextropositioned aorta, and RV hypertrophy. PS can vary from mild (as in this case) to complete PA atresia. The rightward shift of the aortic root facilitates RV-to-aorta shunting. RV hypertrophy develops secondary to systolic pressure overload.

iii. The relatively equilibrated ventricular pressures, along with the mild PS here, explain the lack of murmur. In other cases, hyperviscosity from hypoxia-induced erythrocytosis also reduces turbulence and murmur intensity.

iv. The degree of RV-to-aorta shunting depends on the balance between PS severity (fixed RV outflow resistance) and systemic arterial resistance (variable). Shunting increases with exercise because systemic resistance declines, so exercise restriction is prudent. Hematocrit is periodically monitored. Phlebotomy helps control severe erythrocytosis and hyperviscosity signs. Hydroxyurea and palliative surgery have also been used in dogs. Furosemide and enalapril were discontinued in this case.

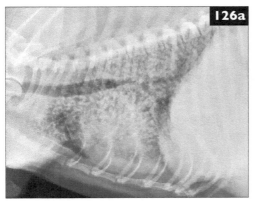

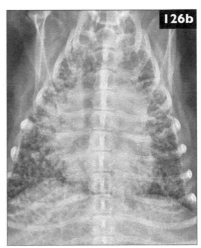

126 An 11-year-old Yorkshire Terrier was recently diagnosed with hyperadreno-corticism (Cushing's disease). At a recheck examination the owner complains that the dog has developed 'breathing problems' and a cough. You hear no cardiac murmur, but there is an occasional soft crackle at the very end of deep inspiration. Lateral (126a) and DV (126b) thoracic radiographs are taken.

i. What radiographic abnormalities are seen?
ii. What is the likely cause?

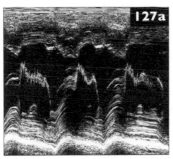

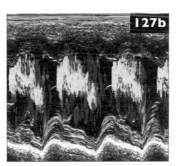

127 A 6-year-old neutered male Pomeranian develops episodic trembling asso-ciated with stiffening of the limbs as well as weakness, vomiting, and panting. An echocardiogram is done (127a, M-mode image at mitral valve level; 127b, color M-mode in same position).

i. What is shown in the figures?
ii. Why does this occur?
iii. What etiologies can cause this?
iv. Are particular physical examination findings likely to result?

126 i. A severe diffuse miliary to nodular coalescing interstitial pattern lung pattern is seen. The pattern is intensely opaque, suggesting pulmonary mineralization/ossification. Moderate RV enlargement and severe RA and main PA enlargement are seen on the DV view, consistent with the 'reverse D' pattern of RV pressure overload. These cardiac changes suggest pulmonary hypertension, likely secondary to the severe interstitial lung condition. Moderate to severe hepatomegaly is also noted.

ii. Cutaneous dystrophic mineralization of the truncal region (calcinosis cutis) is sometimes seen in patients with hyperadrenocorticism. Calcium deposits can also occur elsewhere in the body such as the bronchial or lung tissue. It was suspected that this dog's pulmonary mineralization was related to the endocrinopathy. Mineralization associated with hyperadrenocorticism may be difficult to differentiate from idiopathic pulmonary ossification. Most animals with the latter condition are asymptomatic and the pulmonary lesions are an incidental finding. With hyperadrenocorticism-associated cutaneous mineralization, resolution can occur after weeks to months of endocrine therapy.

127 i. Diastolic flutter of the anterior mitral leaflet is seen (**127a**; arrow, **127c**). Color flow Doppler reveals marked diastolic turbulence within the LV outflow tract, between the septum and the anterior mitral leaflet (**127b**). The mitral E point–septal separation is increased.

ii. A regurgitant jet from aortic valve insufficiency creates diastolic LV outflow turbulence and strikes the mitral leaflet, causing it to vibrate and pushing it away from its fully open position (see case **128**).

iii. Infective aortic valve endocarditis is the most likely acquired cause. Congenital ventricular septal defect with loss of aortic root support, aortic valve malformation, or aortic regurgitation (AR) with subaortic stenosis are other causes.

iv. A diastolic decrescendo murmur is often audible at the left base with moderate to severe AR. A systolic murmur of relative aortic stenosis is also possible because AR imposes a volume overload on the LV, increasing stroke volume. AR causes stronger arterial pulses because diastolic pressure falls more quickly and lower than normal, widening the pulse pressure (difference between systolic and diastolic arterial pressure). Progressive LV dilation, secondary mitral insufficiency, and left-sided heart failure can result from AR.

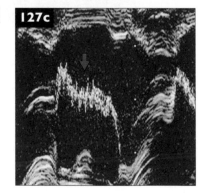

127c

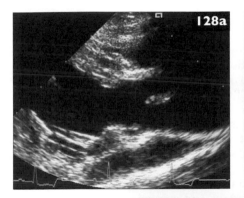

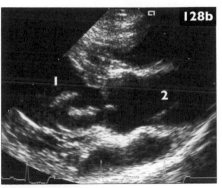

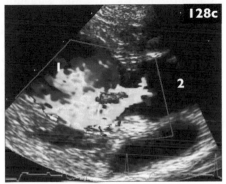

128 A 6-year-old Pomeranian has a history of episodic trembling, stiffening of the limbs, weakness, vomiting, and panting. The dog is lethargic and thin (4.6 kg [10.2 lb]). Body temperature is 40°C (104°F). A grade 4/6 systolic murmur and 2/6 diastolic murmur are heard at the left base. Left femoral pulses are very strong, but no right femoral pulse is palpable. Chest radiographs indicate mild generalized cardiomegaly. Neutrophilia (>25,400/μl) with left shift, mild anemia (PCV 30%), and thrombocytopenia (99,500/μl) are seen on CBC. Echocardiography shows LV volume overload and moderate systolic dysfunction. These images are from the left cranial long axis view (128a, systole; 128b, diastole; 128c, diastole). 1 – LV, 2 – Ao.
i. Describe the echo findings.
ii. What is your assessment of this case?
iii. What is your management plan?

128 **i.** A large, elongated vegetative lesion, attached to the aortic valve, extends into the ascending aorta during systole, then moves back into the LV during diastole. Color flow Doppler (**128c**) reveals marked aortic regurgitation, with turbulent flow surrounding the vegetation.

ii. Infective aortic valve endocarditis is most likely here, based on the large vegetative lesion along with fever, CBC abnormalities, evidence for arterial thromboembolism (absent right femoral pulse), and other findings. In general, presumptive diagnosis of endocarditis is based on positive blood cultures with either echocardiographic evidence of vegetations or valve destruction (e.g. ruptured chordae, flail leaflet tip) or documented recent onset of a regurgitant murmur.

iii. Goals include identifying the organism and source of infection, choosing appropriate bactericidal antibiotic therapy, and managing complications (e.g. cardiac, thromboembolic). *Enterococcus faecalis* was cultured here; however, negative blood and urine cultures do not rule out infective endocarditis.

Aggressive antibiotic therapy is begun immediately after obtaining culture samples, modified if necessary based on results, and continued for at least 6–8 weeks. A combination of cephalosporin, penicillin, or synthetic penicillin derivative with an aminoglycoside or fluoroquinolone is commonly used. Clindamycin or metronidazole adds anaerobic efficacy.

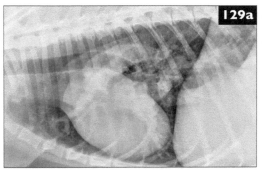

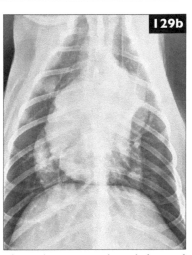

129 A 10-year-old spayed female English Setter is presented for progressive exercise intolerance, excessive panting, and, recently, collapse with minimal exertion. The dog is in poor body condition. Cardiovascular examin-ation indicates pale pink mucous membranes, jugular pulsations, and weak femoral pulses that are correlated with the cardiac apex beat. Thoracic auscultation reveals a holosystolic murmur heard best over the right apex and a 'snappy' second heart sound, but no other auscultatory abnormalities. Right lateral (**129a**) and DV (**129b**) thoracic radiographs are obtained.

i. What abnormalities are seen on the thoracic radiographs?
ii. What differential diagnoses should be considered?
iii. What additional clinical tests would be indicated?

130 A 4-month-old male DSH kitten is presented for cardiac evaluation because of occa-sional collapse episodes. Physical examination is unre-markable. An ECG is recorded (**130a**, leads as marked, 25 mm/s except lower right segment of lead II at 50 mm/s, 1 cm = 1 mV).

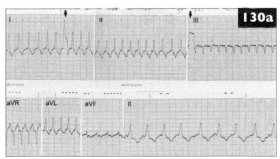

i. What do the arrows point to?
ii. What is your ECG interpretation?
iii. Describe the conduction abnormality present.
iv. Could this be associated with the collapse episodes? If so, how?

129 i. The main PA and major branches (especially the right) are severely enlarged, but become markedly truncated peripherally. The mildly rounded right heart (**129b**) and main PA bulge (1–2 o'clock position) create a 'reverse D' cardiac appearance. The rounded RV also lifts the LV apex dorsally off the sternum (**129a**).

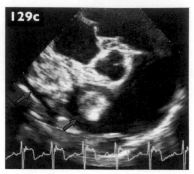

ii. The 'reverse D' appearance suggests RV pressure overload. Common causes are congenital pulmonic stenosis (PS) and PA hypertension (PAH). PS is unlikely as the murmur in this older dog is not characteristic of PS. However, the tricuspid regurgitation (TR) murmur and loud second heart sound are typical for severe PAH, although not always heard. PAH can develop with chronic airway disease, infiltrative lung disease, and pulmonary vascular disease, including heartworm disease and pulmonary thromboembolism (PTE), as well as chronic left-sided heart failure.

iii. Echocardiography can confirm PAH and suggest severity. Classic findings include RV hypertrophy, right heart and PA dilation, and TR. Peak TR jet velocity is used to estimate RV and (when PS is absent) PA systolic pressures. Vascular abnormalities are sometimes identified, including the chronic in-situ PTE seen here (**129c**); two hyperechoic thrombi (arrows) are within the dilated right PA.

130 i. Calibration marks (with QRS complex superimposed in lead I).

ii. HR 220–240 bpm, with sinus rhythm. Mean electrical axis (0°) is normal. PR interval is short (~0.03 second), QRS duration is increased (~0.06 second), and in lead I, R wave amplitude (maximum QRS excursion) is greater than normal at 1.3 mV.

iii. Ventricular pre-excitation. PR intervals are shortened because an accessory conduction pathway bypasses the normal slow-conducting AV node. With extranodal (outside the AV node) accessory pathways, the early ventricular depolarization causes a widened and slurred QRS upstroke or 'delta' wave (arrows, **130b**). This is typical for Wolff–Parkinson–White type pre-excitation. The increased QRS amplitude here is probably secondary to abnormal ventricular activation.

iv. Yes. Re-entrant supraventricular tachycardia can occur via a macro-re-entry circuit involving the accessory pathway and AV node (AV reciprocating tachycardia). Usually, a ventricular impulse is conducted backwards through the accessory pathway to the atrium, then down the AV node in the normal ('antegrade' or 'orthodromic') direction to re-enter the ventricles. Rapid AV reciprocating tachycardia can cause weakness, syncope, congestive heart failure, and death. Atenolol therapy controlled this cat's collapse episodes.

131 A young female Cocker Spaniel has poor exercise ability (**131**). The owners have become quite concerned over the past 5 months because she has had increasingly frequent episodes of weakness or paralysis in her hindlimbs when outside playing. At other times she seems normal. Oral mucous membranes are pink; femoral pulses are normal. The

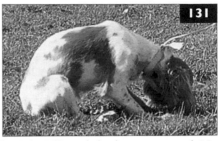

precordial impulse is strong, especially on the right. HR and rhythm are normal. No cardiac murmur is heard, but the second heart sound is quite prominent. Respirations are normal. You take the dog outside and walk her; after a short time, she becomes weak in the rear and resists walking further. The dog remains alert with a normally pink tongue and oral membranes.

i. What are your initial differential diagnoses?

ii. Is the absence of a murmur surprising in this dog?

iii. Is evaluation of tongue/oral membrane color adequate to detect cyanosis with exercise in this dog?

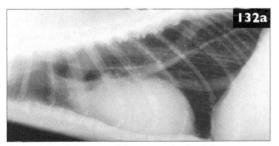

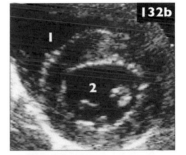

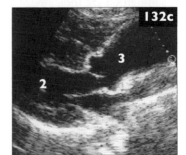

132 A 16-year-old spayed female cat was previously diagnosed with hyperthyroidism and is receiving methimazole. HR is 200 bpm. Respirations are normal. An S_4 gallop sound, but no murmur, is heard. BP is 220 mmHg, systolic. A lateral thoracic radiograph is obtained (**132a**) and echocardiography is undertaken (**132b, c**). 1 – RV, 2 – LV, 3 – Ao.

i. What are the radiographic abnormalities?

ii. Describe the echocardiographic findings.

iii. How would you manage this cat's hypertension?

131 i. Most likely a right-to-left shunting (reversed) patent ductus arteriosus (PDA). The observed hindlimb weakness and 'apparent paralysis' with exercise are typical with reversed PDA because the caudal body receives relatively unoxygenated blood through the shunt. The strong right precordial impulse suggests RV hypertrophy (secondary to severe pulmonary hypertension). A loud, snapping (and sometimes split) S_2 sound on auscultation suggests pulmonary hypertension. Other considerations could be arterial thromboembolic or other vascular disease affecting the hindlimbs (although the normal femoral pulses contradict this) or a neuro-muscular disorder. The abnormal precordial and auscultatory findings would not be expected with these conditions.

ii. There is often no murmur or only a soft systolic murmur with reversed PDA; a continuous murmur is not heard. Factors contributing to this include the reduced pressure gradient between PA and aorta and an increase in blood viscosity as secondary polycythemia develops.

iii. No. Reversed PDA causes cyanosis of the caudal mucous membranes alone (differential cyanosis). The cranial body receives normally oxygenated blood via the brachycephalic trunk and left subclavian artery, which arise from the aortic arch upstream from the ductus. Intracardiac shunts cause equally intense cyanosis throughout the body.

132 i. The horizontal cardiac orientation is common in geriatric cats. Mild cardiomegaly (VHS ~8.5 v) is consistent with chronic hypertension. The thoracic aorta appears undulant (wavy). Aortic root enlargement and undulant thoracic aorta are reported in hypertensive cats.

ii. Mild interventricular septal (7 mm, **132b**) and LV free wall (6 mm) hypertrophy are seen. Chronic systemic hypertension can stimulate mild to moderate LV hypertrophy. This cat's gallop sound likely reflects increased ventricular stiffness despite minimal hypertrophy. The ascending aorta is dilated (**132c**). Correlation between ascending aortic diameter and systolic BP (SBP) has been shown in cats, although aortic valve annulus diameter typically is normal. A proximal ascending aortic diameter:aortic annulus diameter ratio ≥1.25 is reported in hypertensive cats.

iii. Hemogram, serum biochemistries (including T_4), urinalysis, and ocular examination are indicated. Underlying or concurrent disease is treated if possible. Antihypertensive therapy is especially indicated when hypertension is severe (e.g. >200/110 mmHg); SBP below (160–)170 mmHg is the usual therapeutic goal. Amlodipine is the first-line therapy for most hypertensive cats. However, a beta blocker is advocated for hyperthyroid-induced hypertension, so T_4 measurement is particularly important in this cat. Combination of benazepril with amlodipine may be advantageous if there is underlying renal disease.

133 A 16-year-old male Miniature Poodle is presented for respiratory distress (**133**). He has a history of coughing for the past month, with lethargy and poor appetite developing recently. Although the dog has coughed when excited or nervous for a 'long time', this seems different. One week ago, another veterinarian prescribed furosemide and torbutrol, believing the lungs to be 'very congested and the HR irregular and slow'. The clinical signs

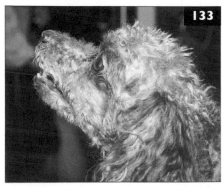

may have improved initially, but then worsened. Amoxicillin was also prescribed for dental disease. The dog is orthopneic with marked inspiratory effort. Mucous membranes are slightly cyanotic. Vital signs are temperature 38.9°C (102°F), respirations 24 breaths/min, HR 130 bpm. A grade 2–3/6 systolic murmur over the mitral area and increased breath sounds during inspiration are heard.
i. Is cardiogenic pulmonary edema likely in this dog? Why, or why not?
ii. What does this respiratory pattern usually signify?
iii. Besides providing supplemental O_2, what would you do next?

134 A 3.5-year-old intact male Pomeranian is presented for respiratory distress associated with recurrent pneumothorax. Thoracic radiographs reveal the lesion seen in these two intraoperative photographs (**134a, b**, the animal's head is to the left). The surgical approach is via median sternotomy.
i. What lesion has caused recurrent pneumothorax in this dog?
ii. Why is median sternotomy a better surgical approach than lateral thoracotomy for this condition?
iii. What intraoperative disadvantage is encountered with median sternotomy versus lateral thoracotomy for treatment of this condition?
iv. What is the reported advantage of surgical treatment versus conservative management for this condition?

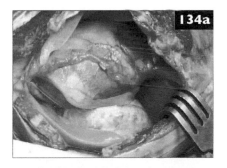

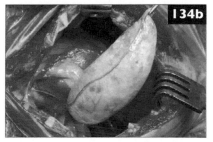

133 i. No. Although the murmur is consistent with chronic mitral regurgitation, which would be the most common cause of cardiogenic pulmonary edema in this case, the relatively slow respiratory rate with labored inspiration is atypical, especially with edema severe enough to cause cyanosis.

ii. Slow and labored inspiration is most often associated with upper airway obstruction. Causes include laryngeal paralysis, severe cervical tracheal collapse, laryngeal or tracheal foreign body, granuloma, tumor, or other mass lesion.

iii. It is important to maintain a patent airway and support oxygenation. If patient stability allows, radiographs of the laryngeal, cervical, and thoracic regions may help localize the obstructive lesion. However, immediate sedation for laryngeal examination and tracheal intubation (or, if necessary, tracheostomy under general anesthesia) may be required. In this dog, one lateral radiograph permitted localization of the obstructive lesion (see case 9), which was then surgically removed.

134 i. A large pulmonary bulla encompasses nearly the entire right cranial lung lobe. A pulmonary bulla is an air-filled space in the lung parenchyma formed when adjacent alveoli become confluent. The cause of this confluence in most cases is idiopathic. Spontaneous rupture of a bulla results in pneumothorax.

ii. Median sternotomy is performed when pulmonary bullae are diagnosed or suspected, because multiple bullae and blebs may be present, and because lateral thoracotomy does not allow exploration of all lung lobes.

iii. The disadvantage of median sternotomy is that lung lobectomy is technically more difficult than when lateral thoracotomy is performed, because the lobar bronchus, PA, and pulmonary vein are located deep in the dorsal aspect of the pleural cavity.

iv. Surgical treatment is preferred instead of conservative management because recurrence rates are lower with surgical intervention. Often, the bulla that has ruptured has already sealed at the time of surgery, but the remaining lesion and additional bullae can be excised, usually via partial lung lobectomy, to prevent future episodes of spontaneous pneumothorax. Also, small blebs can be ruptured intraoperatively and allowed to seal in a controlled, monitored situation to prevent them from causing recurrent spontaneous pneumothorax.

135 A 15-year-old female Schipperke has sinus node dysfunction with prolonged periods of sinus arrest and syncope. A transvenous pacemaker system is implanted via the right jugular vein using a pulse generator in VVIR mode. The following day this ECG is recorded (135a, leads as marked, 25 mm/s, 1 cm = 1 mV).

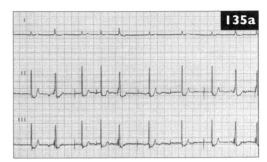

i. What does VVIR mean?
ii. Does the ECG show a normal paced rhythm?
iii. What is your ECG interpretation?
iv. How can this happen?

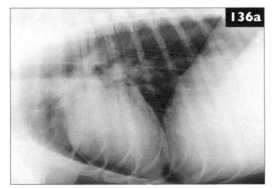

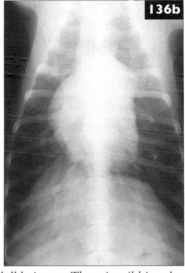

136 A 7-year-old spayed female mixed breed dog is presented for reduced exercise tolerance, a mild cough, and weight loss over the past several weeks. Her vaccination status is uncertain. She is on no medications. Another dog in the household was recently diagnosed with heartworm disease. The dog is thin, with a dull haircoat. There is mild jugular distension and pulsation, a loud S₂ sound heard best at the left base, and a grade 3/6 systolic murmur at the right apex. Lung sounds are harsh, but no crackles or wheezes are heard. You obtain lateral (136a) and DV (136b) chest radiographs.

i. What is your radiographic interpretation?
ii. Do the dog's physical findings suggest heartworm (HW) disease?
iii. What test(s) would confirm a diagnosis of HW disease?

135 i. This pacemaker nomenclature code indicates: chamber paced, Ventricle; chamber where spontaneous electrical activity is sensed, Ventricle; pacemaker response to sensed event, Inhibited (i.e. pacemaker does not discharge when spontaneous cardiac activation is detected within preset timing cycle); and, pacemaker is Rate responsive (i.e. rate of pacing changes with activity).

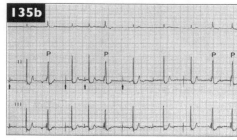

ii. No.

iii. HR is 80 bpm. Only occasional QRS complexes are pacemaker stimulated ('P', 135b); the others are junctional escape complexes. Six pacing artifacts that fail to stimulate a QRS are seen (arrows denote some), indicating pacemaker 'exit block'. Also, occasional failure to sense spontaneous cardiac activity ('entrance block') is evident (3rd arrow from left). Spontaneous (non-paced) cardiac activation should be sensed and pacemaker output inhibited for a preset interval to avoid triggering tachyarrhythmias. Sinus node activity is not evident, but occasional abnormal negative P' waves appear.

iv. Pacing and sensing failure can result from electrode dislodgement, cardiac perforation, lead fracture or insulation break, loose connector pin, and increased pacing threshold from tissue inflammation or fibrosis. Reprogramming of pulse generator output and sensing parameters may restore normal function in the latter case. Chest radiographs may depict lead dislodgement or fracture.

136 i. The overall heart size is normal (VHS ~10.5 v), but there is right heart prominence especially on the DV view. The main PA segment is enlarged and caudal PAs are slightly larger than the 9th ribs, where they cross (136b); the cranial PA (136a) is larger than the accompanying vein. Pulmonary hypertension is likely. The lung fields are normal.

ii. The jugular distension and pulsation indicate high right heart filling pressure and, in view of the right apical murmur, tricuspid insufficiency. The loud S_2 sound is consistent with an underlying cause of pulmonary hypertension, which often causes a loud and 'snapping' or split S_2. Given the history, HW disease is the likely etiology.

iii. An adult HW antigen test. Circulating microfilariae are naturally absent in some ('occult') HW infections and monthly HW preventive drugs also eventually eliminate microfilariae by impairing worm reproduction. Because this dog is not on monthly HW preventive, a test for circulating microfilariae may yield the diagnosis (as it did in this dog). Microfilaria concentrations tests (e.g. millipore filter or modified Knott technique) are more accurate than fresh wet blood smear examination.

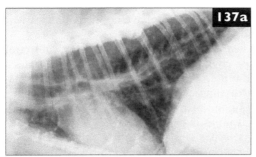

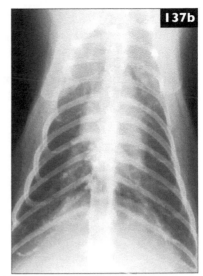

137 A 13-year-old spayed female DSH cat from the USA midwest has been coughing intermittently for 2 years. She appears in good physical condition, but is slightly tachypneic. Physical findings include moderate dental disease and mild lenticular sclerosis. Auscultation indicates normal HR and rhythm, with no obvious cardiac murmur; however, soft pulmonary crackles are heard over the ventral lung fields. Lateral (137a) and DV (137b) radiographs are taken.
i. Is heart failure likely in this cat?
ii. What are the main causes of coughing in cats?
iii. Describe the radiographic findings.
iv. What additional testing is recommended?

138 A Maine Coon cat is presented for acute onset of tachypnea and respiratory distress. The cat is open-mouthed breathing and the oral mucous membranes appear dark red. The owners mention that the cat tends to be very curious and raided one of the kitchen cabinets yesterday, spilling its contents onto the floor. Thoracic radiographs are interpreted as normal. Blood is submitted for routine CBC and bio-

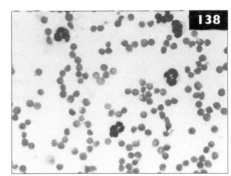

chemistry tests. This blood smear (138) is stained with new methylene blue (100×, oil immersion).
i. Is an abnormality seen on this blood smear?
ii. How is this related to the cat's clinical signs?
iii. How would you manage this case?

153

137 i. No. Although some cats with cardiomyopathy have no murmur, cats with congestive heart failure rarely cough.

ii. Reactive airway disease (asthma), heartworm disease, and lungworm infection are the most common diseases causing coughing in cats within this geographical region. Lack of cough receptors in the pulmonary alveolar regions of cats may explain an absence of coughing with lung parenchymal disease. Pharyngeal irritation, nasopharyngeal polyp, drainage of nasal/pharyngeal secretions, and hairballs also cause coughing/gagging sounds in cats.

iii. The heart size is normal. The PAs, especially those to the caudal lobes, are markedly enlarged, but not tortuous. Bronchointerstitial lung infiltrates are present, especially in the caudal lobes. There is a small amount of air in the cranial thoracic esophagus; other findings include spondylosis, mild sternal deformity, healed rib fractures (right caudal two ribs), and mild hepatomegaly.

iv. Heartworm serologic tests are indicated, as the pulmonary infiltrates and arterial enlargement are typical of this disease. Echocardiography can identify heartworm disease when an adult worm is visualized in the PA or right heart. Airway washings and fecal examination can be used to screen for lungworms. Serologic heartworm tests were negative in this cat, but one adult worm was found at necropsy.

138 i. Heinz bodies are seen as pale blue bodies protruding from the surface of red cells. Heinz bodies represent aggregates of precipitated, oxidized hemoglobin. Oxidative damage to the red cell can occur as a result of ingestion of acetaminophen, onions, zinc, methylene blue, phenazopyridine, benzocaine, vitamin K_3, DL-methionine, propylene glycol, and phenolic compounds.

ii. Oxidation of heme iron results in methemoglobin formation, which cannot bind O_2. Clinical hypoxia and cyanosis result.

iii. The only known compound to which the cat could have been exposed was acetaminophen (in the kitchen cabinet). Treatment involves supportive care, removal of the oxidative substance if possible, and administering N-acetylcysteine (140 mg/kg PO or IV loading dose, followed by 70 mg/kg q6h for 7 treatments) to provide an alternate substrate for conjugation with the reactive acetaminophen metabolites. The prognosis in acetaminophen toxicity is variable and depends on the dose ingested, identification (or suspicion) of the toxin, and treatment promptness. This cat responded well to therapy and was discharged from the hospital 4 days later.

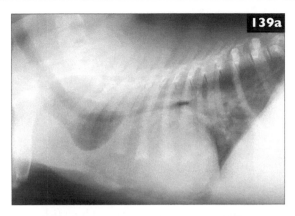

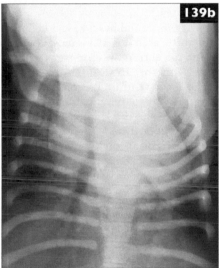

139 A 7-week-old female Chow Chow cross is presented for her first examination and vaccinations. The owners note that she regurgitates her food frequently. The puppy is thin, but otherwise appears healthy. Auscultation reveals a continuous murmur heard high at the left base and a systolic murmur that is loudest at the right sternal border. Lateral (**139a**) and DV (**139b**) chest radiographs are obtained.
i. Describe the radiographic findings.
ii. Is the cause for the dog's regurgitation evident?
iii. What additional radiographic test is commonly done to verify this?
iv. Are the auscultatory findings typical for this problem?

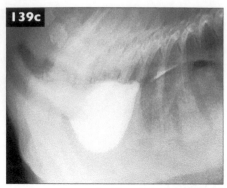

139 i. The cranial thoracic esophagus is dilated and air filled. The cardiac silhouette is enlarged. An interstitial infiltrate is in the caudal lung fields. Dilated pulmonary vessels are seen on the DV view.

ii. Esophageal distension at the cranial heart base is characteristic for vascular ring anomaly. Persistent right aortic arch (PRAA) is most common, but other embryonic aortic arch malformations can entrap the esophagus within a vascular ring. PRAA encircles the esophagus with the aortic arch (right and dorsal), ligamentum arteriosum (left), and heart base (ventral). Because solid food cannot pass normally, regurgitation and stunted growth commonly develop within 6 months of weaning. Food and air can accumulate in the dilated esophageal segment. Aspiration pneumonia is a common complication. Other radiographic signs of PRAA can include leftward tracheal deviation near the cranial heart border (not seen well here), focal tracheal narrowing and ventral displacement cranial to the heart, and cranial mediastinal widening.

iii. A barium esophagram depicts the esophageal stricture and cranial dilation (**139c**).

iv. Vascular ring anomalies do not cause murmurs. Concurrent patent ductus arteriosus and ventricular septal defect caused the murmurs, cardiomegaly, pulmonary overcirculation, and early pulmonary edema in this dog.

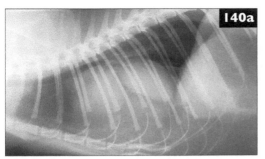

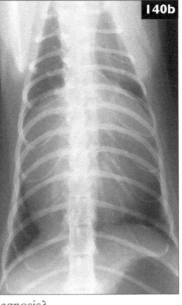

140 A 3-year-old female spayed DSH cat is presented for lethargy and vomiting over the past 2 days. The abdomen is non-painful and thin. Heart sounds are normal on the left, but hard to hear on the right. The physical examination is otherwise unremarkable. Extended thoracic radiographs (**140a, b**) are taken.
i. Describe the radiographic findings.
ii. What is the most likely diagnosis?
iii. How does this occur?
iv. What other tests can be used to confirm the diagnosis?

141 A 7-year-old castrated male DSH cat is presented for lethargy of 3-week duration and intermittent respiratory difficulty over the past week. The cat appears depressed. Heart sounds are muffled, although a grade 2–3/6 systolic murmur is heard at the left sternal border. Pleural effusion is identified on thoracic radiographs; the cardiac silhouette is enlarged and globoid in appearance. Echocardiography reveals the presence of pericardial effusion. Samples of pericardial fluid are prepared for cytologic examination. A cytospin preparation is shown (**141**, Wright's stain, 50× oil).
i. What is the most likely diagnosis?
ii. What additional tests would be useful?

140 i. The cardiac silhouette is extremely enlarged and not clearly separated from the diaphragmatic border. The trachea is displaced dorsally. Fat and soft tissue opacities are seen within the silhouette. A pleural fold (**140c**, arrow) is evident between the silhouette and diaphragm.

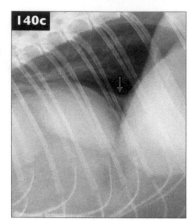

ii. Peritoneopericardial diaphragmatic hernia (PPDH).

iii. Abnormal embryonic development, probably of the septum transversum, allows persistent communication between the pericardial and peritoneal cavities at the ventral midline. The pleural space is not involved. Although the peritoneal–pericardial communication is not trauma induced, trauma can facilitate movement of abdominal contents through a pre-existing defect. PPDH is the most common pericardial malformation in dogs and cats.

iv. Plain radiography is often diagnostic or highly suggestive of PPDH. Other findings can include gas-filled bowel loops within the pericardial sac, a small liver, few organs in the abdominal cavity, and sternal or other thoracic deformity. Echocardiography can show liver, fat, or bowel within the pericardium. A gastrointestinal barium series is diagnostic if stomach or intestines are in the pericardium. Non-selective angiography (especially if only falciform fat or liver has herniated), positive contrast peritoneography, or CT are also useful.

141 i. Lymphoblasts are the predominant cell type in this sample, therefore a cytologic diagnosis of lymphoma was made. This diagnosis was confirmed at necropsy. Multiple thoracic organs were involved (heart, mediastinal lymph node, parathyroid). Neoplastic pericardial effusion is much less common in cats compared with dogs. In cats, congestive heart failure and feline infectious peritonitis are more common causes of pericardial effusion.

ii. A CBC, chemistry panel, urinalysis, and FeLV testing would be useful to help determine other organ involvement and prognosis. Abdominal imaging and bone marrow sampling could also be performed for lymphoma staging. Additionally, although a diagnosis of lymphoma can be confirmed with cytology alone, immunophenotyping of cytologic samples is only available from certain laboratories at this time. In this case, B cell lymphoma was confirmed with immuno-histochemistry from histopathology samples taken at necropsy.

142 A 3-year-old spayed female German Shorthair Pointer is presented for lethargy, fever, stiff gait, and swollen limbs. Radiographs of the distal forelimb (142a) and pelvis (142b) are shown.
i. What are the radiographic findings?
ii. Why would thoracic radiographs be indicated for this patient?

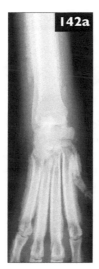
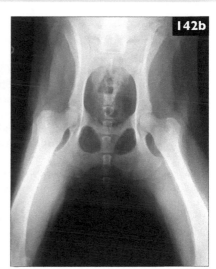

143 A 12-year-old English Cocker Spaniel was diagnosed with a heart condition 2 weeks ago at another clinic. At that time, digoxin, furosemide, and aspirin were prescribed. For the past week the dog has been lethargic and sleeps excessively. His appetite is now poor. The dog is quiet, but alert. Vital signs are normal. There is a grade 5/6 systolic murmur at the left apex; lung sounds are normal. CBC is normal; mildly

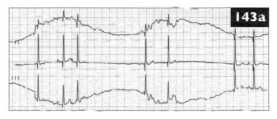
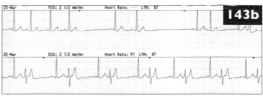

elevated alkaline phosphatase and cholesterol are the only biochemical abnormalities. Radiographs show marked cardiomegaly with LA enlargement; pulmonary vessels and lungs are normal. An ECG is recorded at admission (143a, leads as marked, 25 mm/s, 0.5 cm = 1 mV) and 6 hours later in hospital (143b, non-continuous lead II, 25 mm/s, 0.5 cm = 1 mV).
i. Describe the ECG findings.
ii. Are other tests indicated at this time?
iii. What are your recommendations for this case?

142 **i.** Each femur shows smooth solid periosteal new bone along the medial and lateral length of the diaphysis. The metacarpals, radius, and ulna show a palisade pattern of diaphyseal periosteal new bone. Similar, but more faintly evident, periosteal new bone is visible on the diaphyses of the first phalanges. No cortical lysis is evident.

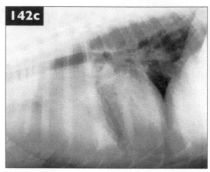

ii. The character and distribution (particularly on metacarpals 2 and 5) of the periosteal new bone is classic for hypertrophic osteopathy (HO). HO is a systemic condition most commonly precipitated by concurrent thoracic cavity disease. A wide variety of thoracic diseases, including pulmonary, cardiac, and esophageal abnormalities, have been associated with HO. Many dogs are presented for lameness caused by the HO rather than the underlying thoracic disease. Thus, recognition of the lesions of HO should prompt radiographic investigation for thoracic disease. The lateral thoracic radiograph (**142c**) of this dog showed a large cranial thoracic mass determined to be a malignant sarcoma.

143 **i.** HR is 50 bpm (**143a**). The rhythm is sinus bradyarrhythmia with periods of sinus arrest. One junctional escape complex is seen (1st QRS from left). Increased R wave voltage (3.8 mV) suggests LV dilation. Intermittent first degree AV block occurs (3rd complex from the left). Baseline artifact is present. Later, sinus bradyarrhythmia with variable PR intervals continues (**143b**) and multiform ventricular premature complexes appear (last complex on top and in bigeminal pattern on bottom).
ii. The ECG abnormalities and clinical signs suggest digoxin toxicity. Serum digoxin concentration should be measured and the digoxin dose closely evaluated. This 15 kg (33 lb) older dog was receiving 0.25 mg digoxin PO q12h (2–3 times the recommended dose). Serum digoxin concentration was 6.5 ng/ml in this dog (therapeutic range 0.5–2.0 ng/ml). Echocardiography and BP measurement are also indicated. Besides the arrhythmias here, digoxin toxicity can also cause more serious ventricular as well as supraventricular tachyarrhythmias, junctional rhythms, and second degree AV block.
iii. Discontinue digoxin immediately; monitor cardiac rhythm, serum electrolytes, and pulmonary status. Cautious fluid administration with supplemental potassium will promote digoxin excretion and reduce myocardial binding. If necessary, use atropine or glycopyrrolate for excessive bradycardia. For severe digoxin-induced ventricular tachyarrhythmia, use lidocaine first (or, if ineffective, diphenylhydantoin). For critical digoxin overdose cases, digoxin-specific antigen-binding fragment (digoxin-immune Fab) therapy is available.

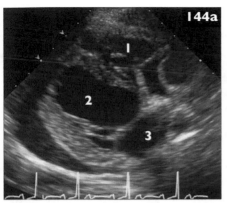

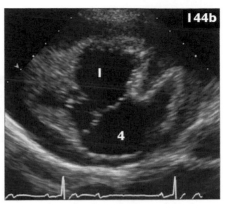

144 A 10-year-old neutered male Golden Retriever has developed signs of weakness and abdominal fluid accumulation. On physical examination, his mucous membranes are pale pink, femoral pulses are slightly weak, and jugular veins are prominent. The precordial impulse is difficult to palpate. Heart sounds are very soft, but lung sounds are normal. Chest radiographs show generalized cardiomegaly with a large caudal vena cava. An echocardiogram is done: 2-D images from right parasternal (144a) and left cranial (144b) long axis views are shown. 1 – RV, 2 – LV, 3 – LA, 4 – RA.
i. Describe the echocardiographic findings.
ii. What is cardiac tamponade?
iii. What echo views are of particular importance in a case such as this?

145 A 9-year-old female German Shepherd Dog is presented for lethargy, abdominal distension, and a gagging-type cough. Her HR is rapid. Breath sounds are prominent and occasional pulmonary crackles are heard. An ECG is recorded (145, leads as marked, 50 mm/s, with a segment of lead aVF at 25 mm/s (bottom); 1 cm = 1 mV).
i. What is your ECG diagnosis?
ii. Is IV lidocaine therapy indicated?
iii. How would you manage this case?

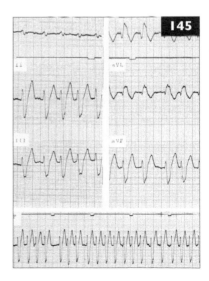

144 i. The echo-free space between the bright parietal pericardium and epicardium is pericardial effusion (**144c**, 5). Collapse of the right atrial wall in diastole and early systole (**144c**, arrows) indicates cardiac tamponade. LA size appears compromised. No mass lesion is evident in these images.

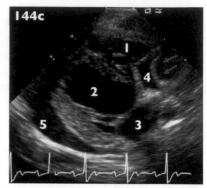

ii. Cardiac tamponade occurs when pericardial effusion increases intrapericardial pressure above normal cardiac diastolic pressure. This external cardiac compression progressively limits RV then LV filling; systemic venous pressure increases and cardiac output falls. Weakness, exercise intolerance, collapse, jugular vein distension, ascites, pleural effusion, and weak femoral pulses are common sequelae.

iii. Pericardial effusion in older dogs is usually of neoplastic origin. Most cardiac tumors involve the right heart, especially the right atrial appendage (hemangiosarcoma), or the aortic root region (chemodectoma and others). Mesothelioma is another consideration and may have no discrete mass lesion. Although a complete echo examination is important to visualize all possible structures, the best view of the right auricle (**144b**) is obtained from the left cranial long axis position.

145 i. HR is 240 bpm. The rhythm is atrial fibrillation (AF); there are no identifiable P waves and the rhythm is irregular as well as rapid. QRS complexes are wide (~0.10 second) and abnormal; the mean electrical axis is shifted right and cranial (between -150 and -90°). Right bundle branch block is likely, as the latter part of the QRS is especially wide. Causes of right ventricular enlargement should be considered.

ii. IV lidocaine is only occasionally effective against AF, although a standard initial bolus is unlikely to be harmful.

iii. IV diltiazem can rapidly reduce heart (ventricular response) rate in AF. Auscultation after the HR is slowed may reveal abnormal heart sounds. Chest radiographs and an echocardiogram are indicated to evaluate cardiopulmonary status. This dog had dilated cardiomyopathy with congestive heart failure.

Conversion to sinus rhythm is unlikely with severe cardiac disease. The usual goal is to control HR (by slowing AV conduction) as well as manage underlying disease and signs of heart failure (see also cases **38, 95, 124, 157, 187, 189, 190, 216**). In-hospital HRs <150 bpm are desirable. Long-term AF therapy in dogs with heart failure usually includes digoxin combined with PO diltiazem or a beta blocker.

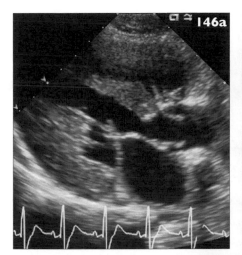

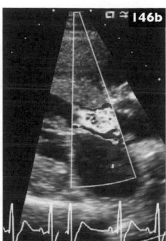

146 A 1-year-old female Newfoundland developed progressive exercise intolerance and episodic collapse over the past 2 weeks. Her body condition, mentation, respirations, membrane color, and jugular veins are normal. Femoral pulses are hypokinetic. A grade 4/6 systolic heart murmur is heard over the low left base, with radiation to the right base. Lung sounds are normal. CBC and serum chemistries are unremarkable. The cardiac silhouette appears mildly enlarged (VHS 10.6 v), with left heart prominence. Pulmonary vessels and

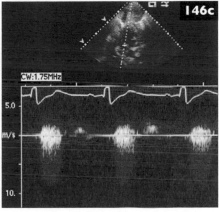

parenchyma are normal. Systolic BP is 110 mmHg. Echocardiography is done; images are from right parasternal long axis view in systole (146a, 2-D; 146b, color flow Doppler) and subcostal view, LV outflow (146c, continuous wave Doppler).

i. Describe the echocardiographic findings.
ii. What is the diagnosis?
iii. Does this explain the dog's clinical signs?
iv. How would you manage this case?

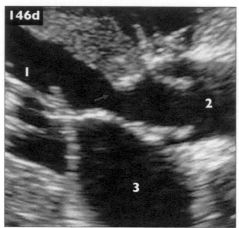

146 **i.** An area of increased echogenicity protrudes from the interventricular septum (**146a, d,** arrow), narrowing the LV outflow region. Marked systolic turbulence occurs here (**146b**). Peak LV outflow velocity is greatly increased at 8.4 m/s (284 mmHg estimated pressure gradient, **146c**). LV free wall and papillary muscle hypertrophy is seen (**146a**). (**146d,** 1 – LV, 2 – Ao, 3 – LA.)

ii. Severe congenital subaortic stenosis (SAS).

iii. Yes. Severe SAS may prevent sufficient increase in cardiac output to sustain normal exercise. Paroxysmal tachyarrhythmias or reflex bradycardia also can cause syncope. Severe SAS causes hypokinetic pulses because of slower rise to systolic arterial pressure. The systolic ejection murmur of SAS is heard best at the low left base (near the stenosis) and at the right base (radiating to the ascending aorta and aortic arch).

iv. Exercise restriction and beta blocker therapy may reduce ischemia-induced arrhythmia. The dog should not be bred; SAS is known to be inherited in Newfoundlands. Risk for aortic valve endocarditis is increased with SAS, so prophylactic antibiotic therapy is used for dental and other 'dirty' procedures. Sudden death and congestive heart failure are common with severe SAS. Surgical procedures have not convincingly improved prognosis.

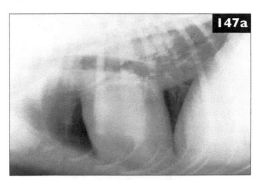

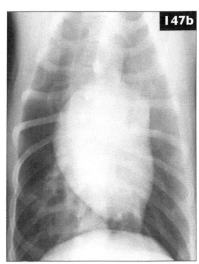

147 An 11-month-old male mixed breed dog weighing 31.8 kg (70 lb) was hit by a grain truck 2 days ago. He was treated for shock and then referred for evaluation of pelvic injuries. On physical examination, the lung and heart sounds are muffled and the heart rhythm is irregular. Thoracic radiographs are made (147a, b).

i. What potential thoracic abnormalities should be suspected based on the physical examination?

ii. What radiographic abnormalities are present?

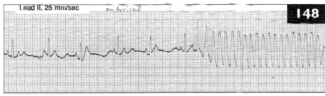

148 An 8-year-old male Dobermann has become progressively less active over the past month. Two brief collapse episodes occurred recently. He now has a soft persistent cough and a poor appetite but mildly increased thirst. The dog's body condition is good. Temperature is 37.8°C (100°F), pulse 170 bpm, and respiratory rate 75 breaths/min with labored effort. Membranes are pale with 2.5 seconds capillary refill time. The heart rhythm is occasionally irregular. A grade 1/6 systolic murmur and a low-pitched soft diastolic sound are heard over the left apex. Inspiratory pulmonary crackles and some wheezes are heard over all lung fields. An ECG is recorded (148, lead II, 25 mm/s, 0.5 cm = 1 mV).

i. What is your ECG interpretation?

ii. What is your assessment of this dog?

iii. What is the most likely cause for the diastolic sound heard on auscultation?

iv. How would you proceed with this case?

147 i. Pneumothorax, pleural effusion (hemorrhage), rib fracture, pulmonary hemorrhage (contusion), traumatic bullae, and diaphragmatic rupture should all be considered as possible thoracic sequelae of vehicular trauma. The physical examination findings can vary widely with these lesions. Although less common, trauma to cardiac structures could cause pericardial bleeding/effusion.

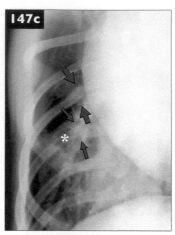

ii. Single fractures in the proximal region of right ribs 7 and 8 are present (147c, arrows). The distal segment of each rib is moderately displaced cranioproximally. Rib fractures, particularly in the proximal third, are difficult to detect radiographically. Careful tracing of the borders of each rib and comparing intercostal space width can improve detection of these fractures. The lung in the region of the fractures has a moderate interstitial pattern consistent with pulmonary hemorrhage. Within this region of soft tissue opacity is a thin-walled circular lucency (asterisk in the center) consistent with a traumatic bulla.

The dog was successfully anesthetized the following day for replacement of a right coxofemoral luxation and stabilization of a right femoral fracture.

148 i. Normal sinus rhythm is seen at the beginning of the strip (some baseline artifact is present), but a rapid paroxysm of ventricular tachycardia (VT; at 390 bpm) develops soon after. Sinus complex measurements are normal.
ii. Signalment, history, and clinical findings are consistent with dilated cardiomyopathy (DCM) and left-sided congestive heart failure. Paroxysmal VT is common in Dobermanns with DCM and often leads to syncope or even sudden death.
iii. The timing, location, and low-pitch indicate a gallop sound, most likely the S_3 (ventricular) gallop. This is associated with ventricular dilation and failure, typically from DCM.
iv. Most urgent initially is to improve oxygenation (resolve pulmonary edema) and suppress rapid VT. Supplemental O_2, furosemide, and lidocaine should be used to effect (or maximum recommended dose). Chest radiographs, echocardiogram, and laboratory database are obtained as soon as patient stability allows. In addition, pimobendan and angiotensin-converting enzyme inhibitor therapy is started. Monitoring of heart rhythm, respirations, BP (IV inotropic support may be needed), metabolic status, and general supportive care are important. If lidocaine does not control the VT, other antiarrhythmic therapy (e.g. amiodarone or sotolol) should be tried and continued PO if effective. Spironolactone can be added for long-term therapy.

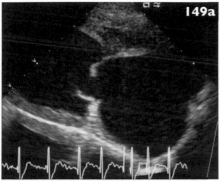

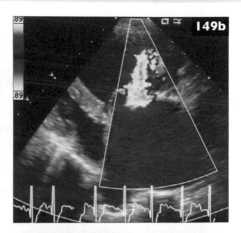

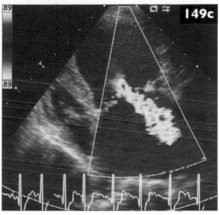

149 A 9-month-old female black Labrador Retriever is presented for evaluation of exercise intolerance and increased panting. The referring veterinarian has prescribed furosemide and amoxicillin; the owner reports this has helped her breathing. The dog is alert and excited. She is small in stature. Respirations are 48 breaths/min with slightly increased effort. HR is >180 bpm. Mucous membranes are pink, femoral pulses are of variable intensity and irregular, and jugular veins are normal. There is a grade 5/6 systolic murmur loudest at the left apex, but heard all over the precordium. Blood pressure is 120 mmHg, systolic. Chest radiographs show marked cardiomegaly (VHS 12.5 v) with LA and LV prominence. Mild pulmonary interstitial infiltrates are seen in the dorsal/hilar region. An echocardiogram is done (149a, 2-D right parasternal long axis in diastole; 149b, left apical color flow in diastole; 149c, left apical color flow in systole)

i. Describe the echocardiographic findings shown.
ii. What is your assessment of this dog's problem(s)?
iii. How would you manage this case?

150 What general guidelines are important when treating bacterial pneumonia?

149 i. Findings include markedly dilated LA and LV, atrial fibrillation, and thickened and deformed mitral leaflets with restricted opening (**149a**). Diastolic flow acceleration (with aliasing) near the mitral valve orifice indicates mitral stenosis (**149b**). Mitral regurgitation occurs in systole (**149c**).

ii. Mitral valve dysplasia, with regurgitation and stenosis, is the underlying problem. Atrial fibrillation with uncontrolled ventricular rate contributes to early congestive heart failure. Mitral dysplasia occurs mostly in large-breed dogs. Malformations include shortened or overly elongated chordae, direct valve–papillary attachments, thickened or cleft leaflets, and malformed papillary muscles. Valve regurgitation ranges from mild to severe. Mitral stenosis is relatively uncommon, but further raises LA pressure. Medical management for congestive failure is used as needed; surgical valve reconstruction or replacement could be an option. Prognosis is poor with severe malformations.

iii. The HR must be controlled (conversion to sinus rhythm is unlikely here); diltiazem (with or without digoxin) is recommended. Furosemide is prescribed for pulmonary edema, along with an angiotensin-converting enzyme inhibitor and pimobendan for initial chronic heart failure management.

150 Antibiotic therapy and supportive care are fundamental. Airway secretion culture and sensitivity testing should guide antibiotic selection whenever possible. Amoxicillin–clavulanate (20–25 mg/kg PO q8h) or cephalexin (20–40 mg/kg PO q8h) is often used while awaiting culture results. More aggressive or intravenous antibiotic therapy is warranted if clinical signs are severe. Appropriate antibiotic therapy is continued for a week or longer after signs disappear. Supportive care includes supplemental O_2, if needed, and good airway hydration to facilitate secretion clearance. Fluid therapy and sterile saline nebulization (several times daily) are helpful. Physiotherapy, by inducing deeper breaths and coughing, promotes airway secretion/exudate mobilization. Chest coupage and/or mild exercise can be used, and ideally follows nebulization. A bronchodilator may help some animals, but can also promote ventilation/perfusion mismatching. Individual patient monitoring is important. In general, cough suppressants, glucocorticoids, and diuretics are avoided with bacterial pneumonia.

151 A 13-year-old female Cocker Spaniel is presented for a 4-month history of coughing, which has worsened over the past month. She now often produces mucus at the end of a coughing fit. Therapy with amoxicillin–clavulanate, butorphanol, and prednisone has been tried, but the cough persists. Physical examination reveals harsh lung sounds, but no cardiac murmur. Radiographs show a moderate bronchial pattern. CBC shows mild thrombocytosis, mild lympho-penia, and mild eosinophilia. Serum chemistry tests are normal. Heartworm antigen test is negative. Bronchoscopy (151a, b) with BAL is performed. BAL cytology reveals low to moderate cellularity, consisting of 31% neutrophils, 6% macrophages, and 63% eosinophils, with mucus and cellular debris. No obvious etiologic agents or neoplastic cells are observed.

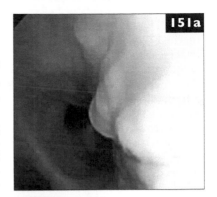

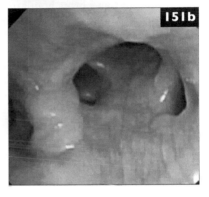

i. What is your assessment of the broncho-scopic findings?
ii. What etiologies should be considered?
iii. How would you manage this case?

152 A 14-year-old DSH cat is euthyroid and clinically well. A grade 2/6 systolic murmur is heard at the left sternal border. Echocardio-graphy shows mild septal hypertrophy and mild mitral systolic anterior motion. An ECG is recorded (leads I and II, 25 mm/s, 1 cm = 1 mV) (152).

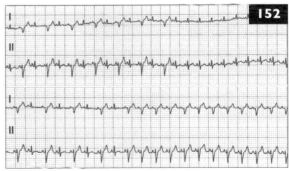

i. What is your ECG interpretation?
ii. How does this abnormality occur?
iii. What could happen if it worsens?
iv. Is cardiac drug therapy indicated at this time?

151 i. The airway mucosa is diffusely thickened and irregular. BAL cytology shows marked eosinophilic and moderate neutrophilic inflammation, suggesting hypersensitivity response.

ii. Allergic bronchitis, lungworm or heartworm infection, and eosinophilic lung disease should be strongly considered. Bacterial bronchitis is less likely, but routine microbiologic culture of BAL samples is recommended. The negative heartworm antigen test and radiographic pattern make this disease unlikely. Fecal tests for lungworms are indicated in endemic areas even though BAL samples were negative for parasites; fecal tests were negative in this dog.

iii. Allergic bronchitis can result from hypersensitivity to inhaled or, possibly, ingested allergens. Definitive identification of specific allergens is rare. Management involves eliminating potential allergens and palliative gluocorticoid (e.g. 1–2 mg/kg q12h initially) and bronchodilator therapy. Environmental allergens can include smoke, dust, and mold/mildew. Food allergy may affect some cases; dietary trials using novel protein and carbohydrate sources may help. Hypersensitivity to insects that contaminate dry food during storage is possible; a canned-only diet can be tried. Allergic bronchitis in dogs typically causes coughing without respiratory distress, unless there is more widespread eosinophilic lung disease (pulmonary infiltrates with eosinophils or eosinophilic granulomatosis). Peripheral eosinophilia occurs inconsistently. Long-standing allergic bronchitis can cause airway pathology similar to chronic bronchitis.

152 i. HR is 240 bpm, with regular sinus rhythm. Intermittent right bundle branch block (RBBB) is seen, sometimes alternating with normal QRS conduction and sometimes affecting multiple complexes in succession. Other measurements and intervals are normal.

ii. Slowed or blocked conduction within any of the major branches of the intraventricular conduction system (aberrant conduction) causes the region of ventricular muscle served by the affected bundle branch to be activated late and slowly. This widens the QRS complex and shifts orientation of the terminal QRS forces toward the area of delayed activation, in this case the right ventricle. RBBB can result from right ventricular disease or distension, but sometimes it occurs in otherwise normal cats and dogs. In contrast, left bundle branch block is usually related to clinically relevant LV disease. The left anterior fascicular block pattern is common in cats with hypertrophic cardiomyopathy

iii. The major intraventricular conduction pathways (the right bundle branch and the left anterior or posterior fascicles of the left bundle branch) can be affected singly or in combination. If conduction were to fail in all three major branches, third degree (complete) heart block would result.

iv. No, RBBB alone does not cause hemodynamic impairment.

153 A 7-year-old female Miniature Pinscher is presented for coughing of 2-week duration. The cough has worsened; it occurs during both day and night, but is more intense with excitement. Exercise tolerance and appetite are now poor. The dog appears slightly depressed. HR and rhythm are normal. Respiratory rate is moderately increased. Lung sounds are harsh, with increased effort and occasional expiratory wheezes. A dry cough is easily elicited by tracheal palpation. Other physical findings are unremarkable. Thoracic radiographs show a 3 cm mass in the right caudal or middle lung lobe region. A hemogram reveals marked eosinophilia (>7 × 10³/µl), with a mild increase in band neutrophils. Bronchoscopy and a fine needle aspiration (FNA) of the lung mass are performed. FNA cytology shows many eosinophils with both non-degenerate and degenerate neutrophils, macrophages, cellular debris, and occasional ciliated epithelial cells. Some macrophages contain phagocytized red blood cells and eosinophil granules. Broncho-scopic images of the distal trachea (153a) and proximal right bronchus (153b) are shown.

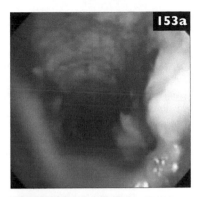

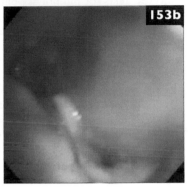

i. What do the bronchoscopic images show?
ii. What differential diagnoses should be considered?
iii. How would you manage this case?

154 What treatments are used for angiostrongylosis in dogs?

153   i. A thick, mucopurulent exudate. The mucosa appears inflamed and edematous.

ii. Eosinophilic inflammation indicates a hypersensitivity response. Common causes in endemic regions include pulmonary parasites and heartworm disease. Occasionally, fungal or neoplastic disease can induce an eosinophilic response; inhaled allergens or allergic drug response are other considerations. However, in the absence of such causes, this dog's pulmonary mass, FNA findings, and peripheral eosinophilia are consistent with eosinophilic pulmonary granulomatosis. Pulmonary nodule formation characterizes this severe form of eosinophilic lung disease in dogs. Hilar lymphadenopathy, eosinophilic bronchitis, and peripheral eosinophilia also variably occur. An underlying etiology is often not found. Bronchoscopic samples in this dog showed a purulent eosinophilic exudate, with no bacterial growth on cultures. Tests for pulmonary parasites and heartworms were negative.

iii. If definitive diagnosis is still unclear after searching for identifiable causes of eosinophilic pulmonary disease, lung mass biopsy can be helpful. Cure is more likely if the triggering antigen can be identified and eliminated. Anti-inflammatory glucocorticoid therapy (e.g. prednisone, 1–2 mg/kg PO q12h initially) is indicated, especially if an inciting cause is not found. Addition of more aggressive immunosuppressive therapy (e.g. cyclophosphamide, 50 mg/m^2 PO q48h) is usually necessary for dogs with large pulmonary nodules.

154   Drugs used to kill *Angiostrongylus vasorum* include: fenbendazole (20–50 mg/kg for [5–]21 days); the combination of imidacloprid with moxidectin (10[–25] mg/kg imidacloprid plus 2.5[–6.25] mg/kg moxidectin as a single dose topical [0.1 ml/kg]); or milbemycin oxime (0.5 mg/kg PO once weekly for 4 weeks).

Supportive therapy should be given according to individual case need. This can include supplemental O_2, blood transfusion, antibiotics, and possibly a corticosteroid. An angiotensin-converting enzyme inhibitor and diuretic are used for congestive heart failure signs. Baermann fecal testing for 3 consecutive days at 3–6 weeks after anthelmintic treatment is advocated to assess treatment efficacy.

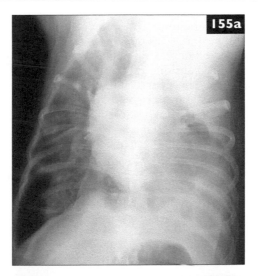

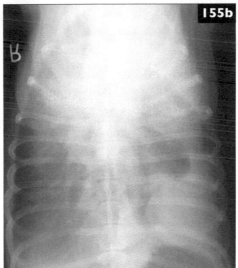

155 A 7-year-old male Boxer is presented for anorexia, weight loss, and more recently, increased panting. On physical examination, the dog is tachycardic (180 bpm) and has labored respirations. An ECG reveals sinus tachycardia; other parameters are normal. VD (155a) and DV (155b) thoracic radiographs are available.
i. What radiographic findings are useful in assessing the cause of pleural effusion?
ii. What radiographic features in this case are suggestive of a thoracic mass versus pleural effusion?

155 i. Although radiography cannot differentiate between pleural effusion types, thoracic structural changes can provide clues to the cause. For example, cardiomegaly with concurrent abdominal enlargement and effusion in dogs suggests a transudate from right-sided congestive heart failure. Rib fracture(s) strongly suggests hemorrhage. Aggressive bone lesions may indicate neoplastic transudate, hemorrhage, or exudate. Nevertheless, a fluid sample should be obtained for analysis.

This patient has active periosteal new bone formation on the caudal borders of left ribs 9 and 10 at the curvature of the chest wall (155c).

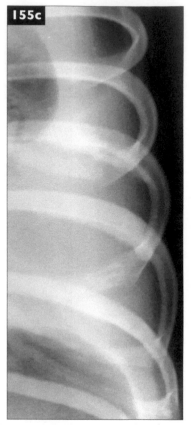

155c

ii. Pleural fluid redistribution depends on fluid type; transudates redistribute more evenly within the thorax than exudates. A mass tends not to move with positional changes. A fluid opacity that cannot be moved from a thoracic region by positional change indicates either trapped or loculated fluid or a mass.

Another finding that suggests a mass is altered shape or position of adjacent organ(s). This is easier to evaluate when the adjacent organ provides contrast with the mass, as in this dog's DV view. A concave shape change in the left caudal lung lobe's lateral border from the 9th to 11th ribs, along with adjacent rib changes, strongly suggests a mass near or involving the thoracic wall. Biopsy indicated a fibrosarcoma.

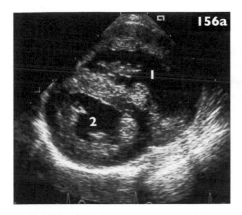

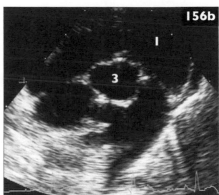

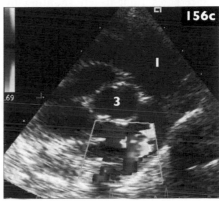

156 A 4-month-old male Sheltie puppy is presented for cardiac examination because of a heart murmur and declining exercise tolerance. The puppy is alert but quiet. Mucous membranes are pink. Heart sounds are clearly heard, as well as a grade 2/6, ill-defined systolic murmur at the left base. Lung sounds are normal. A prominent right apical impulse is noticed, but other examination parameters are unremarkable. Hematocrit is 0.47 l/l (47%). An echocardiogram, among other tests, is done (right parasternal short axis views; **156a**, ventricular level, diastole; **156b**, heartbase; **156c**, color flow Doppler, systole). 1 – RV, 2 – LV, 3 – Ao.

i. What is the significance of a prominent right apical impulse on chest palpation?
ii. Describe the findings shown in the figures.
iii. What recommendations would you give this owner?

157 List important general guidelines for re-evaluating patients with chronic heart failure.

156 i. The precordial impulse is normally strongest over the left cardiac apex. A stronger impulse on the right can occur with RV hypertrophy or cardiac displacement to the right, as from a mass lesion, lung atelectasis, or chest deformity.
ii. There is RV hypertrophy and dilation (**156a**) consistent with systolic pressure overload. The mildly dilated main PA appears to divide into three branches (**156b**), rather than only right and left PAs; the third vessel, oriented downward, is a large patent ductus arteriosus (PDA). Flow within this vessel moves away from the transducer (coded blue, **156c**), from PA towards aorta. This dog has severe pulmonary hypertension with a right-to-left shunting (reversed) PDA.
iii. Pulmonary hypertension associated with congenital shunts is usually irreversible. Reversed shunts cause hypoxemia and exercise intolerance. Reversed PDA causes greater hindlimb weakness and differential (caudal but not cranial) cyanosis because unoxygenated blood enters into the descending aorta (see case **131**). Exercise exacerbates right-to-left shunting by reducing peripheral vascular resistance; exercise restriction is advised. Secondary erythrocytosis can compromise tissue perfusion; hematocrit should be periodically monitored.

Sildenafil citrate may reduce pulmonary resistance and right-to-left shunting, thereby improving clinical signs; 're-reversal' to left-to-right ductal flow is rare.

157 Periodic re-evaluation is important because heart disease is progressive and complications often occur:
- Review medications and dosage schedules with the owner at each visit.
- Ask about any problems with drug administration (and compliance) and possible adverse effects.
- Ask about the pet's diet, appetite, resting breathing rate (which the owner should be routinely monitoring at home), activity level, and any other concerns.
- Do a thorough physical examination.
- Check BP.
- Depending on patient status, other appropriate tests might include a resting ECG or ambulatory monitoring, thoracic radiographs, hemogram, serum biochemical tests (especially renal function and electrolytes), echocardiogram, or serum digoxin concentration.
- For patients with early and stable heart failure, recheck examinations every 4–6 months may suffice. More frequent visits are needed for advanced disease.

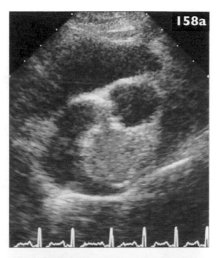

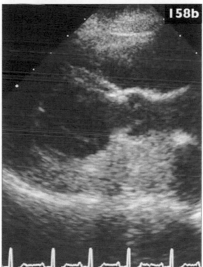

158 A 7-year-old spayed female Boxer is presented for cardiac screening prior to anesthesia for removal of a skin mass. She has normal exercise tolerance and cardiovascular examination findings. Echocardiography reveals an occasional ventricular premature complex, but normal cardiac chamber size and function; right parasternal short axis (158a) and long axis outflow (158b) images are shown.

i. What abnormality is seen on these images?
ii. What dogs are more likely to be affected by this?
iii. What is the usual natural history?
iv. Is treatment usually effective?

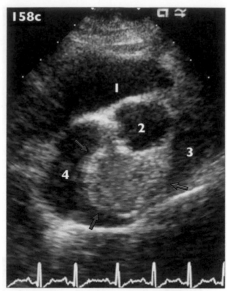

158 i. Note the (~3 cm) mass (arrows, **158c**, 1 – RV, 2 – Ao, 3 – PA, 4 – LA) at the aortic root between LA and PA. An aortic body tumor (ABT) is most likely, although ectopic thyroid or parathyroid tumors occasionally occur at the heart base.

ii. The majority of canine ABTs are reported in brachycephalic breeds, particularly Boxers, Boston Terriers, and Bulldogs, but other breeds can be affected.

iii. ABT (chemodectoma) is the second-most common cardiac tumor. ABTs arise from clusters of chemoreceptor cells near the aortic root (aortic bodies) that sense blood O_2 and CO_2 tension. About half of affected dogs are between 10 and 15 years and about a third are 7–10 years old when diagnosed. ABTs are usually slow growing and locally invasive, but sometimes metastasize. They can be an incidental finding, as in this dog, unless or until they cause pericardial effusion and cardiac tamponade or dysfunction of surrounding structures.

iv. If cardiac tamponade develops, partial pericardiectomy or balloon pericardiotomy may prolong survival for months to years, depending on tumor growth rate. Surgical resection is rarely possible because of local invasion. ABTs are fairly unresponsive to chemotherapy.

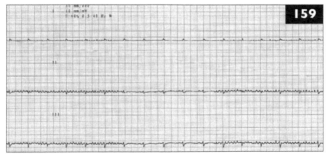

159 An 8-year-old neutered DLH cat with sneezing and serous nasal discharge is referred for cardiopulmonary examination. Physical examination is unremarkable. Although cardiac disease is not expected in this case, the owner requests additional assurance regarding cardiac status. Thoracic radiographs and an ECG are done (159; simultaneous leads I, II, and III at 50 mm/s; 1 cm = 1 mV). Radiographs are normal.

i. What is the ECG interpretation?
ii. Is there an abnormal heart rhythm? If so, what is it?

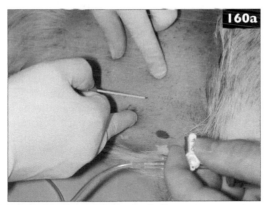

160 A 9-year-old dog develops abdominal distension, weakness, and increased panting. Poor pulses, jugular distension, ascites, and muffled heart sounds are found on examination. Chest radiographs enhance your suspicion of pericardial effusion with tamponade. You perform pericardiocentesis (160a).

i. What equipment is used for pericardiocentesis?
ii. How is the patient positioned and prepared?
iii. Describe how to perform pericardiocentesis.

159 i. The HR is 200 bpm. The rhythm is normal sinus rhythm. The mean electrical axis is thought to be normal. Complex measurements are also normal.

ii. No. The saw tooth appearance seen in the baseline at the beginning and near the end of the strip is an artifact, created by purring. With close evaluation, one can identify underlying sinus complexes that occur at the same intervals as the sinus complexes seen clearly in the middle of the strip. The underlying sinus complexes are seen best in leads I and III.

160 i. An over-the-needle catheter system, with gauge and length determined by patient size (some small side holes can be cut near the tip of large [12–16 g] catheters for faster fluid removal); sterile extension tubing attached to a three-way stopcock and a collection syringe; a collection bowl; sterile clot and EDTA tubes for fluid samples; an ECG monitor.

ii. Manually restrain the patient in left lateral or sternal recumbency. Alternatively, use an elevated echocardiography table with a large cut-out, restrain the patient in right lateral recumbency, and tap from underneath (**160b**). Echo guidance is not usually necessary. Prepare the skin surgically from right 3rd–7th intercostal spaces and sternum to costochondral junction. Using sterile gloves and aseptic technique, palpate for the cardiac impulse at the puncture site (usually between 4th and 6th rib), then infiltrate 2% lidocaine into the skin, underlying intercostal muscle, and pleura.

iii. Attach the prepared extension tube assembly to the needle stylet within the catheter. Advance the needle/catheter through a small stab incision, avoiding intercostal vessels caudal to the rib. An assistant applies gentle suction to the collection syringe as you slowly advance the needle towards the heart; aim the needle towards the patient's opposite shoulder. Pleural fluid may be aspirated first. Pericardial contact causes increased resistance to needle advancement and a subtle scratching sensation. Gently press through the pericardium; you may feel a loss of resistance as pericardial fluid, usually dark red, appears in the tubing. Advance the stylet/catheter unit slightly into the pericardial space before removing the stylet. Attach the extension tubing to the catheter itself. Save samples for analysis then drain as much fluid as possible.

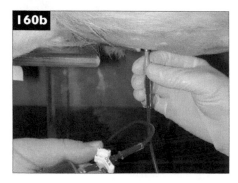

161 You are performing pericardiocentesis on the dog from case **160** and obtain this hemorrhagic fluid (**161a**).
i. How do you know that you are withdrawing pericardial fluid and not intracardiac blood?
ii. What complications can occur from pericardiocentesis?

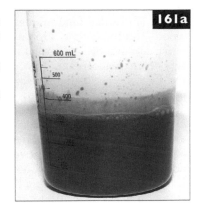

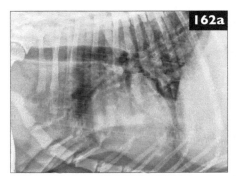

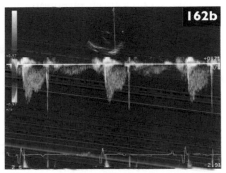

162 A 6-year-old female Labrador Retriever from southern England is presented for coughing and respiratory difficulty, which began 3 weeks ago and has worsened considerably. Initial treatment with antibiotics and corticosteroids has not been helpful. The owner notes frequent coughing and labored breathing now, and mentions that recently a small wound on the dog's tongue bled for a long time. Hemoptysis has not been observed. The dog is bright and alert, but quickly becomes tachypneic when walking around the room. Thoracic auscultation reveals pulmonary crackles over all lung fields and a grade 3/6 holosystolic heart murmur, loudest over the right parasternal region. Other physical findings are unremarkable. Thoracic radiographs (**162a**) and an echocardiogram are obtained. Echocardiography shows RV enlargement, diastolic interventricular septal flattening, moderate tricuspid regurgitation (TR), with peak systolic velocity of 4.8 m/s, and an abnormal PA flow profile (**162b**).
i. What is your radiographic interpretation?
ii. How would you interpret the echocardiographic findings?
iii. What additional tests might be helpful?

161 i. Pericardial fluid in dogs is usually dark red like venous blood. To differentiate, drop a small amount onto the table or into a serum tube. Pericardial fluid does not clot unless there is very recent hemorrhage. Also, spin some in a hematocrit tube; the PCV of pericardial fluid is usually lower than that of peripheral blood, with yellow-tinged (xanthochromic) super-natant (161b, left). As pericardial fluid is removed, the patient's ECG complex amplitude usually increases, tachycardia diminishes, and the animal often appears more comfortable.

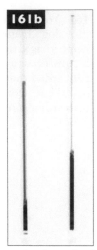

ii. Pericardiocentesis is a relatively safe procedure when carefully done and extraneous needle movement within the chest avoided. If the needle/catheter contacts the heart, a scratching or tapping sensation is felt or the device moves with the heart beat; retract slightly to avoid cardiac trauma. Direct myocardial injury or puncture commonly causes ventricular premature beats, which usually cease when the needle is withdrawn. Lung laceration is a potential complication; pneumothorax and/or hemorrhage can result. Spread of infection or neoplastic cells into the pleural space occurs in some cases. Coronary artery laceration can occur and cause myocardial infarction or further intrapericardial bleeding, but this is rare, especially with a right-sided approach to pericardiocentesis.

162 i. Overall cardiac size is normal (VHS 10.5 v), although there is mild RV prominence. Bronchointerstitial pulmonary infiltrates, with areas of alveolar pattern, are seen ventrally and cranially.

ii. Whenever septal flattening occurs, RV pressure exceeds LV pressure, during diastole in this case. The high peak TR velocity indicates a systolic pressure overload on the RV. Estimated RV systolic pressure is ~95–100 mmHg (Bernoulli pressure gradient = 4 × peak velocity^2 plus assumed RA pressure of 3–8 mmHg). The normal PA peak systolic velocity indicates pulmonary hypertension (PH) as the cause of the RV pressure overload. The late systolic notching of the pulmonary flow signal is abnormal and consistent with severe PH. RV enlargement and TR are common sequelae. PH can result from severe lung or pulmonary vascular disease.

iii. Routine laboratory and coagulation tests help screen for systemic disease and possible bleeding disorder. Persistent cough indicates airway involvement. Bronchoscopy and airway lavage for cytology and culture are indicated. Thoracic CT could further characterize the pulmonary infiltrates or reveal other abnormalities. *Angiostrongylus vasorum* can sometimes cause PH and is of growing concern in the UK and northern Europe. Baermann fecal tests may detect its larvae. Heartworm disease (*Dirofilaria immitis*) is generally not expected in this geographic region, although its worldwide occurrence is spreading.

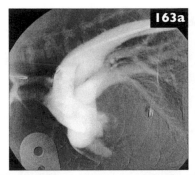
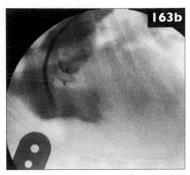

163 Routine physical examination of a 10-month-old Collie reveals a loud murmur at the high left heart base. Additional diagnostic tests are done and cardiac catheterization procedures are pursued (163a, initial aortic angiogram; 163b, postprocedure aortic angiogram).
i. What is shown on the initial angiogram, and what is your clinical diagnosis?
ii. Has the procedure been successful?

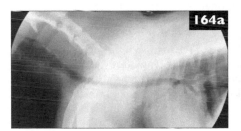
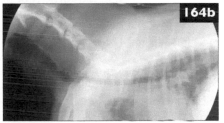

164 An 11-year-old spayed female Chihuahua-mix weighing 6.4 kg (14 lbs) is presented for an intermittent dry and occasionally 'honking' cough. She was diagnosed previously with degenerative mitral valve disease and pulmonary hypertension, and has moderate mitral and tricuspid valve regurgitation.

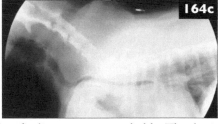

Besides the murmur, the physical examination findings are unremarkable. The dog's trachea is evaluated fluoroscopically during resting respiration and an induced cough (164a is at peak inspiration; 164b at end expiration; 164c during the cough).
i. What is your diagnosis based on these images?
ii. What other conditions are commonly associated with this radiographic diagnosis?

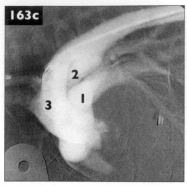 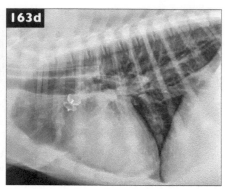

163 i. A bolus of radiopaque contrast has been delivered to the aortic root via a catheter ascending from the femoral artery. Contrast material is also present in the main PA and its branches because of a left-to-right shunting patent ductus arteriosus (PDA) (see **163c**: 1 – PA, 2 – ductus, 3 – Ao).
ii. Yes. A self-expanding device (Amplatz® Canine Duct Occluder) has been successfully deployed. The narrow waist of the device straddles the junction between PA and ductal ostium; the larger (top) portion is inside the ductal ampulla. The dense nitinol mesh of the device occludes ductal flow. Contrast (appears dark in **163b**) delivered to the aortic root no longer passes through the ductus into the PA. **163d** shows the appropriately positioned duct occluder.

164 i. **164b** and **164c** show complete collapse of the mainstem bronchi. **164c** shows partial collapse of the intrathoracic trachea during the cough. This image also shows extrathoracic movement and a striking curvature of the trachea during the cough. However, there is no collapse of the portion showing pronounced ventral curvature. Mild to moderate LA enlargement associated with mitral valve disease is also seen (**164a**). Although marked LA enlargement can compress the main bronchi and contribute to collapse, in this case echocardiographic examination indicated that the LA enlargement was only mild.

This dog's signalment is typical for dogs with collapsing trachea. Standard radiography may be successful at demonstrating either extra- or intrathoracic tracheal collapse particularly if comparative lateral images are acquired; one at the peak of the inspiratory breath and one at end expiration. Some dogs only demonstrate collapse during coughing. In such patients, dynamic evaluation by fluoroscopy is needed. Fluoroscopic assessment usually shows a greater degree of collapse than plain radiographs.
ii. These patients are often obese, but may be thin. They may have concurrent acquired valve disease and chronic bronchitis.

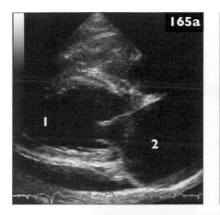 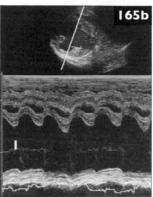

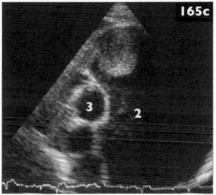

165 An 11-year-old male neutered cat is presented after 2 weeks of respiratory difficulty. The cat is in good body condition, alert, and responsive, but appears slightly uncomfortable. Respirations are rapid and shallow, with increased abdominal effort. Femoral pulses are weak but regular. Thoracic auscultation reveals sinus tachycardia (250 bpm), with an intermittent gallop rhythm. Pulmonary crackles are heard over the caudal lung fields. Systolic BP is slightly low (100 mmHg). Hematology, serum biochemistry, and thyroid test results are normal. Thoracic radiographs show cardiomegaly, pulmonary venous engorgement, patchy alveolar infiltrates, and mild pleural effusion. An echocardiogram is done; images from the right parasternal position are shown (**165a**, 2-D long axis LV inflow; **165b**, M-mode at ventricular level; **165c**, 2-D short axis at heart base). 1 – LV, 2 – LA, 3 – Ao

i. What is the clinical significance of an audible gallop rhythm?
ii. What is your diagnosis based on the clinical and echocardiographic findings?
iii. What therapeutic strategy would you advise for this patient?

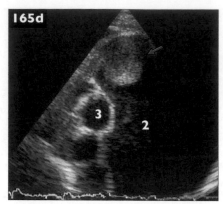

165 i. 'Gallop rhythm' refers to audible S_3 and/or S_4 sounds. These diastolic sounds are not heard in normal cats and dogs. They can become audible when myocardial compliance is reduced (e.g. by myocardial hypertrophy or fibrosis) and ventricular filling pressure is increased. The S_4 gallop is most common in cats.

ii. Findings indicate congestive heart failure (CHF). Echo images show LA and LV enlargement with mild pericardial effusion, ascribed to CHF (**165a, c**). LV free wall motion is markedly hypokinetic (**165b**, bottom). A thrombus (arrow, **165d**) is evident within the left auricular appendage. Restrictive cardiomyopathy (RCM) was diagnosed. RCM is characterized by a restrictive filling pattern, minimal or no LV hypertrophy, and severe LA enlargement. Myocardial fibrosis is common. Myocardial infarction may explain the regional LV hypokinesis.

iii. Furosemide is indicated for congestive signs. Pimobendan may improve systolic function. Efficacy of other agents (e.g. angiotensin-converting enzyme inhibitor or beta blocker) is unclear; some cats with RCM may benefit. However, with marked systolic dysfunction (as in this cat), beta blockers are generally avoided or used only cautiously because of their negative inotropic effect. The LA thrombus indicates increased risk for arterial thromboembolism; low-dose aspirin, clopidogrel, or possibly both, is advised, although prophylactic efficacy remains unclear. The prognosis is guarded.

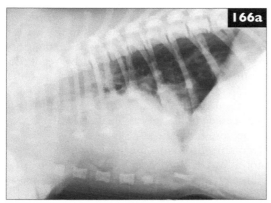
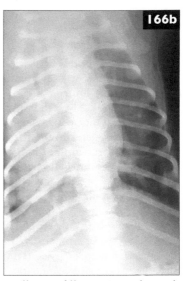

166 A 2-month-old male Bichon Frise developed a paroxysmal, nonproductive ('honking') cough 1 week ago. Two days ago, respiratory distress also developed. The puppy appears lethargic, with increased respiratory effort. Mucous membranes are slightly dry and capillary refill time is prolonged. Rectal temperature is 39.8°C (103.6°F). CBC shows moderate leukocytosis (19.7 × 10⁹/l, normal 6.0–15.0) with neutrophilia (15.7 × 10⁹/l; normal 3.0–11.5). Serum biochemistry tests are normal. Thoracic radiographs are shown (**166a, b**).

i. What is your radiographic interpretation?
ii. What additional tests may be useful for this case?
iii. What empirical treatment would be indicated pending these test results?

167 A 4-year-old spayed female mixed breed dog is presented for acute onset of respiratory distress after eating a rawhide chew. A lateral radiograph of the neck is taken (**167**).
i. Is the rawhide chew evident in this image?
ii. If not, what views will you add to the evaluation?

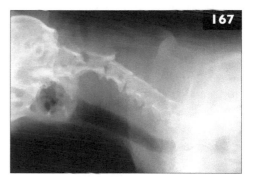

166 i. There are diffuse interstitial and alveolar pulmonary infiltrates, most severe throughout the right lung. Several air bronchograms are visible. Infiltrates are less severe in the left lung. Cardiac size is normal. Considering this dog's age and history, canine infectious tracheobronchitis ('kennel cough') complicated by secondary pneumonia is most likely. Canine influenza is another differential for the initial cough and lung injury.

ii. BAL or tracheal wash is indicated to obtain samples for bacterial culture and cytologic evaluation. Tests to rule out canine influenza can include PCR for viral RNA, antigen detection, virus isolation, and serologic testing.

iii. A wide-spectrum antibiotic is recommended while awaiting bacterial culture results or if additional testing is not allowed. *Bordetella* spp. infection is often susceptible to potentiated amoxicillin (e.g. amoxicillin–clavulanate 20–25 mg/kg q8h), fluoroquinolones (e.g. enrofloxacin 10–20 mg/kg q24h), and tetracyclines (e.g. doxycycline 5–10 mg/kg q12h). Patient hydration should be optimized. Oxygen supplementation and cage rest are advised in severe cases. Mild sedation can help reduce anxiety in particularly distressed patients. Nebulization and coupage can help loosen and mobilize secretions. Gentamicin nebulization has been helpful against *Bordetella* spp. in some cases. Some animals may need parenteral nutritional support.

167 i. An irregular, gas and soft tissue-mixed opacity is evident in the pharyngeal region, overlapping with the larynx. Although this odd appearance could raise suspicion of a foreign body, there are two findings that suggest this is unlikely. Note the oblique positioning of the head and neck. This is evident by the excellent definition of the dens of C2 and separation of the tympanic bullae. The ability radiographically to evaluate the pharyngeal and laryngeal regions is markedly compromised when positioning is oblique because of the summation of soft tissue, bone, and gas-filled structures. The complex opacity in this case is the summation of the ear pinna with the oropharynx. When producing radiographic images, it is important to think about the placement of body parts, such as the pinna and skin folds, as well as other objects external to the animal, such as collars, leashes, and fluid administration tubing. At the caudal end of this image, the trachea deviates more ventrally than normal at the thoracic inlet. This suggests an abnormal thoracic esophagus.

ii. Lateral and DV or VD views of the thorax are indicated.

168 A 13-year-old female Labrador Retriever is presented for coughing of 1-month duration. Chest radiographs reveal a diffuse interstitial lung pattern and a mass-like opacity in the right caudal thorax. Bronchoscopy (168a, b, right lobar bronchi), with BAL and biopsy, is done to further evaluate the lungs before surgical removal of the pulmonary mass is attempted. BAL fluid is only moderately cellular; cytospin preparation shows basophilic cell clumps scattered among numerous foamy macrophages, with occasional neutrophils and eosinophils. Clumped cells have basophilic cytoplasm, one or more prominent nucleoli, and marked anisocytosis and anisokaryosis; some are multinucleated. Biopsy specimens show neoplastic cuboidal epithelial cells aligned in tubular or papillary formations separated by dense fibrous connective tissue.

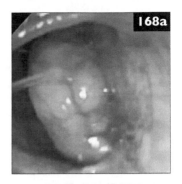

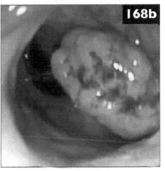

i. What is seen in the bronchoscopic images?
ii. What is your assessment of this case?
iii. What are the most common tumor types in the lung?

169 An 11-year-old spayed female Shih Tzu is presented for chronic cough, weight loss, and a mass on the right forelimb 4th digit. The dog has always lived in the midwest region of the USA. In addition to the mass, hyperemia of the associated foot pad, tachypnea, and an enlarged right prescapular lymph node are noted on physical examination. A stress leukogram and mild hypoalbuminemia are the only abnormal findings on

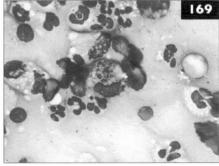

CBC and chemistry panel. Thoracic radiographs show a diffuse alveolar pattern. BAL is performed and samples submitted for cytologic evaluation and microbiological culture. Shown is a direct preparation from the endotracheal tube following BAL procedure (169, Wright's stain, 50× oil).
i. Identify the etiologic agent present in the figure.
ii. What is the preferred treatment?
iii. What is the prognosis?

168 i. Irregular soft tissue masses protrude into the bronchial lumen in each figure. **ii.** The biopsy findings are consistent with pulmonary adenoma or well-differentiated pulmonary adenocarcinoma (bronchioloalveolar carcinoma). Although malignancy is not clear based only on the biopsy specimens, the presence of more than one bronchial nodule, along with the radiographically evident pulmonary mass and the atypical, neoplastic cells found on BAL cytology, indicate this dog has metastatic bronchioloalveolar carcinoma. **iii.** Lung tumors can be primary, multicentric, or metastatic. Primary lung tumors are usually malignant. Carcinomas are most common, especially adenocarcinoma, bronchoalveolar carcinoma, and squamous cell carcinoma. Multicentric tumors involving the lung include lymphoma, malignant histiocytosis, and mastocytoma. Pulmonary metastases are common and can originate from primary pulmonary tumors as well as distant neoplasms. Pulmonary neoplasia causes variable clinical signs depending on the structures involved and the extent of respiratory compromise. In this case the cough presumably was triggered by metastases in the airways. Prognosis for patients with pulmonary neoplasia not only relates to the tumor's histology, but also to whether metastasis has occurred. Surgical resection can be effective for solitary pulmonary masses. Metastatic disease is often minimally responsive to chemotherapy, with relentless progression and death from hypoxemia.

169 i. In the middle of the figure is a macrophage containing oval bodies that have a thin clear halo surrounding a purple center. These are intracellular yeast, morphologically consistent with *Histoplasma capsulatum*. There are also increased numbers of neutrophils in the sample. **ii.** Itraconazole is the preferred treatment for histoplasmosis in small animals. Fluconazole may also be used and may be a better choice than itraconazole if the central nervous system (CNS) and/or eyes are involved. Ketoconazole is less efficacious against *Histoplasma* spp. infection, and therefore is generally not recommended. Some cases of pulmonary histoplasmosis may be self-limiting; however, antifungal therapy is still recommended to prevent dissemination of the organism. **iii.** The prognosis for appropriately treated disseminated histoplasmosis ranges from fair to good, depending on which organ systems are involved. Infections involving the eye, CNS, epididymis, and bone are more difficult to treat and therefore carry a poorer prognosis.

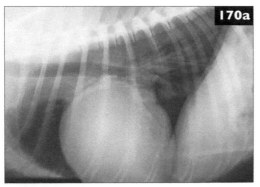

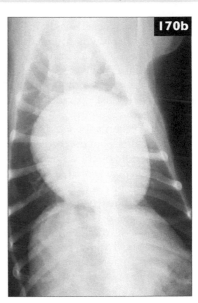

170 A 7-year-old male American Cocker Spaniel is presented for presurgical evaluation. Lateral (170a) and DV (170b) chest radiographs are obtained.
i. Describe the radiographic findings.
ii. What are your likely differential diagnoses?
iii. What do you recommend?

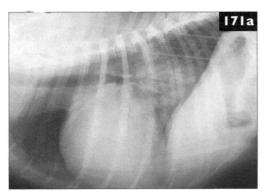

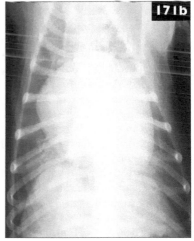

171 The dog in case 170 returns 2 weeks later. He has been breathing harder and coughing recently. No medications have been given. Lateral (171a) and DV (171b) radiographs are shown. Echocardiography shows dilation of all cardiac chambers, poor ventricular wall motion, and moderate AV valve regurgitation.
i. Describe the radiographic findings.
ii. What is the underlying disease process?
iii. How would you manage this case?

170 i. There is generalized cardiomegaly (VHS ~12.7 v). The heart shadow is rounded, yet the contours of the enlarged LA (**170a**) and LV apex (**170b**) are seen. A cranial lobar pulmonary vein (large arrow, **170c**) is distended compared with the accompanying artery (small arrow). Pulmonary parenchyma is normal.

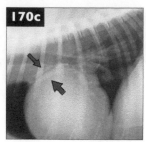

ii. Dilated cardiomyopathy or chronic mitral and tricuspid regurgitation are most likely. Pericardial effusion is also possible, but the cardiac silhouette is not truly globoid and pulmonary venous distension would be unexpected. Tricuspid regurgitation alone (either congenital or acquired) would not cause this pulmonary vascular pattern.

iii. Careful physical examination and auscultation may provide additional clues about the underlying cardiac disease. Echocardiography will depict abnormal cardiac structure and function. Dilated pulmonary veins imply high pulmonary venous pressure and incipient left-sided congestive heart failure. Resting respiratory rate and activity level should be closely monitored and a reduced salt diet instituted. Initiating angiotensin-converting enzyme inhibitor (or pimobendan) therapy now is reasonable. Low-dose furosemide can also be considered. Follow-up examination within 1–2 weeks is advised.

171 i. In addition to the cardiomegaly and pulmonary venous congestion seen in previous radiographs (see **170a, b**), pulmonary interstitial and alveolar infiltrates in the hilar and caudal regions indicate cardiac decompensation with fulminant pulmonary edema.

ii. Echocardiographic findings are consistent with dilated cardiomyopathy (DCM). Although DCM is most common in large dog breeds, Cocker Spaniels are also known to develop DCM. Low plasma taurine, and sometimes carnitine, concentrations have been found in American Cocker Spaniels with DCM. Concurrent degenerative AV valve disease is common in Cocker Spaniels and likely contributes to valve regurgitation in this case.

iii. Therapy for congestive heart failure includes furosemide, pimodendan, an angiotensin-converting enzyme inhibitor, supplemental O_2, and other supportive care as needed. Plasma or whole blood taurine concentration measurement is recommended; plasma concentrations <25(–40) nmol/ml and blood concentrations <200 (or 150) nmol/ml are considered deficient. Plasma carnitine concentration is not a sensitive indicator of myocardial carnitine deficiency. Oral taurine and L-carnitine supplementation (see Drugs used for cardiac and respiratory diseases, pp. 255–261) can improve LV function and reduce heart failure medication requirement in Cocker Spaniels. Taurine alone is useful in some but not all Cockers with DCM. Three to 4 months is allowed to determine if echocardiographic improvement will occur.

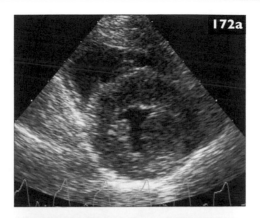

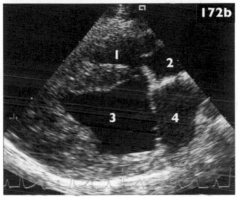

172 A 17-year-old spayed female Keeshond is presented late at night after two episodes of collapse that day. She is otherwise well and has no previous history of collapse. She is alert, with slight tachypnea and tachycardia. No cardiac murmur is heard and lung sounds are normal. An ECG shows sustained ventricular tachycardia, which converts to normal sinus rhythm after a lidocaine bolus. Constant rate lidocaine infusion is given through the night. Chest radiographs the following morning are unremarkable. An echocardiogram is done; right parasternal views are shown (172a, short axis at ventricular level; 172b, long axis 4-chamber). 1 – RV, 2 – RA, 3 – LV, 4 – LA.

i. Describe the echo findings.
ii. What are your differential diagnoses?
iii. Are other tests or therapy indicated?

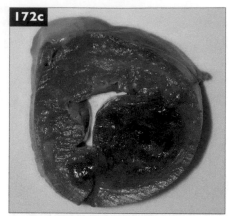

172 i. The anteromedial papillary muscle and LV apical area are thickened and slightly hypoechoic compared with the surrounding myocardium (**172a**).
ii. The asymmetric thickening and altered echogenicity suggest infiltrative disease. Myocardial lymphoma or other neoplasm, including hemangiosarcoma (HSA) or metastatic tumor, should be considered. Other unusual differentials include granulomatous inflammatory lesions or asymmetrical hypertrophic cardiomyopathy (although hypoechogenicity would not be expected).
iii. Careful peripheral lymph node and abdominal palpation, thoracic and abdominal radiographs, routine laboratory database, and abdominal ultrasonography to look for evidence of neoplastic or inflammatory disease elsewhere. Cardiac troponin assay may indicate ongoing myocardial damage (suggested by ventricular tachyarrhythmia). Ventricular antiarrhythmic therapy is indicated.

Several splenic masses were identified ultrasonographically. Postmortem examination confirmed HSA in the LV (**172c**), spleen, and other organs. The LV location is unusual; most cases of cardiac HSA involve right heart structures, especially the right auricle. Also unusual is the dog's advanced age. Although cardiac tumor occurrence increases with age, prevalence drops in dogs older than 15 years.

173 A 9-year-old female mixed breed dog is referred for repair of a fractured femur. The dog has been healthy and active until she was hit by a car 2 days ago. Her heart rhythm is irregular. Pulses are strong; mucous membrane color, capillary refill time, and

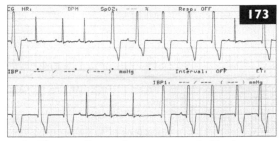

hydration are normal. BP is normal. Chest radiographs are normal. She is on no medication. An ECG is recorded (173, lead II, 25 mm/s, 0.5 cm = 1 mV).
i. What is the ECG rhythm diagnosis?
ii. Should lidocaine or another antiarrhythmic drug be given?
iii. How would you manage this case?

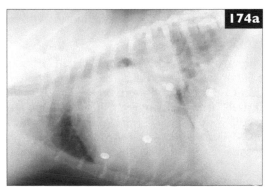

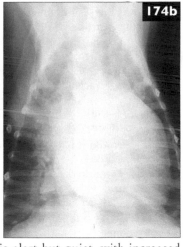

174 A 4-year-old female Labrador Retriever is referred for evaluation of an arrhythmia. Two months ago she began coughing. One week ago she had an episode of respiratory distress that improved after furosemide administration. She is alert but quiet, with increased respiratory rate and effort. Mucous membranes are pale pink, with a 2–3 seconds capillary refill time. HR is ~220 bpm and irregular. Harsh lung sounds and soft crackles are ausculted; a murmur is suspected, but tachycardia and increased lung sounds make it difficult to characterize. The ECG rhythm is atrial fibrillation. Lateral (174a) and DV (174b) chest radiographs are shown (ECG electrodes are visible).
i. What are the radiographic findings?
ii. What are your differential diagnoses?
iii. What would you do next?

173 i. Sinus arrhythmia with an intermittent accelerated idioventricular rhythm at approximately the same HR as the sinus rhythm (90–100 bpm). The ventricular rhythm appears as the sinus rate slows. First degree AV block with variable PR intervals is also present and may reflect high vagal tone or AV nodal injury/disease. PR prolongation is greatest as the increasing sinus rate interrupts the idioventricular rhythm, suggesting partial retrograde AV conduction.
ii. No. The dog's physical condition and normal chest radiographs indicate good hemodynamic status.
iii. Continued monitoring of HR, rhythm, AV conduction, and hemodynamic status is important. If the idioventricular rate increases markedly (e.g. >140–150/min), or multiform or irregular ventricular tachycardia develops, antiarrhythmic therapy may become necessary. Fracture repair and continued supportive care are indicated. Post-traumatic cardiac arrhythmias usually appear within 1–2 days after trauma. Possible causes of myocardial injury and arrhythmias could include acceleration–deceleration forces, autonomic imbalance, ischemia, or electrolyte and acid–base disturbance. Ventricular premature complexes, ventricular tachycardia, and accelerated idioventricular rhythm (usually 60–100 bpm) are common. Accelerated idioventricular rhythm is usually benign, often evident only when the sinus rate slows, and generally disappears within 1–2 weeks in animals without underlying heart disease.

174 i. Cardiomegaly (VHS >15 v) with marked LV and LA enlargement (**174a**) is present, with increased hilar interstitial opacity suggesting cardiogenic pulmonary edema. A left auricular bulge is evident (2–3 o'clock position) on DV view. Caudal pulmonary vessels and aorta are not well visualized, but cranial lobar pulmonary vessels look slightly dilated. In dogs, the width of the cranial lobar vessels, where they cross the 4th rib, is normally 0.5–1.0 times the width of the proximal 1/3 of that rib. Caudal lobar vessels are normally 0.5–1.0 times the width of the 9th rib where they cross.
ii. Causes of marked left heart enlargement include dilated cardiomyopathy, chronic severe mitral valve insufficiency (either acquired or congenital), and certain congenital left-to-right cardiac shunts; all of these can cause pulmonary edema. Enlarged lobar pulmonary vessels can occur from pulmonary overcirculation or venous congestion with pulmonary hypertension secondary to left-sided heart failure.
iii. Additional furosemide (for pulmonary edema) and diltiazem (to reduce HR from atrial fibrillation) are indicated immediately. As respiration improves and HR becomes more controlled, auscultatory findings should be reassessed. Echocardiography is warranted to evaluate cardiac structure and function, and further direct therapy.

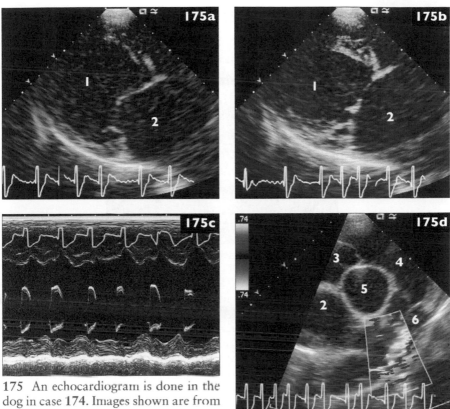

175 An echocardiogram is done in the dog in case 174. Images shown are from the right parasternal position (175a, long axis in diastole; 175b, long axis in systole; 175c, M-mode at mitral valve level; 175d, short axis color flow in diastole). 1 – LV, 2 – LA, 3 – RA, 4 – RV, 5 – Ao, 6 – PA.

i. Describe the echo abnormalities seen.
ii. Does this dog have idiopathic dilated cardiomyopathy?
iii. How would you manage this case?

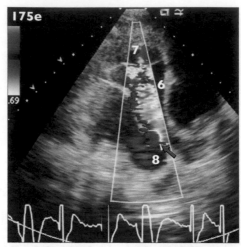

175 i. There is severe LA and LV dilation, with little change from diastolic to systolic chamber size, and wide mitral E-point–septal separation (>10 mm, **175c**) consistent with marked LV dysfunction. Restricted mitral motion from congenital valve stenosis or aortic regurgitation are other causes of wide E-point–septal separation, but were not found here. Atrial fibrillation caused irregular mitral opening with 'A' point loss (**175c**). **175d** shows diastolic flow disturbance into the dilated left PA from a left-to-right shunting patent ductus arteriosus (PDA), which led to severe LV and LA volume overload, myocardial dysfunction, atrial fibrillation, and congestive heart failure. A left cranial long-axis image (**175e**, 6 – PA, 7 – RV outflow tract, 8 – descending Ao) shows the PDA jet (arrow) from the descending aorta into the PA.

ii. No. Cardiac failure is secondary to chronic PDA.

iii. First, treat the congestive signs and uncontrolled heart rate using standard therapies (pimobendan, furosemide, angiotensin-converting enzyme inhibitor, diltiazem +/- digoxin, and dietary salt and exercise restriction). After the patient is stable, PDA closure is recommended to reduce hemodynamic load. Medical management for heart failure and heart rate control is continued as needed.

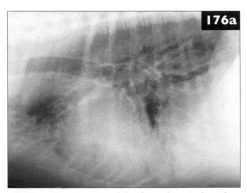

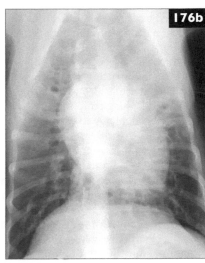

176 A 6-year-old female Labrador Retriever is presented for chronic coughing. She appears to be doing well otherwise. Thoracic radiographs (**176a, b**) are obtained.

i. What is the abnormal radiographic pattern present?

ii. What is the significance of this pattern?

177 The 2-month-old Bichon Frise puppy in **166** is evaluated. Chest radiographs reveal diffuse pulmonary interstitial and alveolar infiltrates, especially throughout the right lung. Bronchoscopy shows edema and inflammation of the bronchial mucosa, with fluid and mucus partially obstructing the bronchial lumen. A cytologic specimen from BAL fluid is shown (**177**).

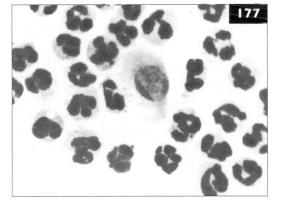

i. What is the predominant feature of the BAL cytology?

ii. What other assessment should be done?

iii. Based on the information available, how would you manage this case?

176 i. The ventral lung regions show dilated bronchi extending to the lung periphery (176c). Some of these bronchi have a beaded contour and some show saccular terminal dilations. This is a bronchial pattern with bronchiectasis. An alveolar pattern is also present in the periphery of the middle lung region.

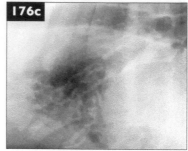

ii. This bronchial pattern generally indicates chronic airway disease, involving either the bronchial wall or supporting connective tissue surrounding it. Bronchiectasis is an irreversible dilation of the bronchial lumen; it usually is associated with chronic bronchial inflammation/infection, with consequent mural weakening and accumulation of secretions.

Several types of bronchiectasis are described: (1) cylindrical, characterized by dilated bronchi without peripheral tapering (the most commonly reported type in dogs); (2) varicose, where the wall assumes a beaded appearance; (3) saccular, with single or multifocal bulbous (saccular) dilations at the distal bronchus; and (4) cystic, where strings or clusters of rounded cavities occur along the dilated bronchus ('balloons on a stick'). The usual presenting complaint with bronchiectasis is coughing. Dogs older than 10 years, as well as American Cocker Spaniels, West Highland White Terriers, Miniature Poodles, Siberian Huskies, and English Springer Spaniels, may be at increased risk.

177 i. The BAL fluid cytology indicates septic neutrophilic inflammation. There is a mild amount of mucus and some extracellular material resembling bacterial rods. These findings are consistent with infectious bronchopneumonia.

ii. Bacterial culture and sensitivity testing is indicated to identify the etiologic agent and the most appropriate antibiotic treatment. In this case, *Bordetella bronchiseptica*, which was sensitive to amoxicillin–clavulanate, enrofloxacin, gentamicin, streptomycin, and tetracycline, was isolated from the BAL culture. *B. bronchiseptica* is a small gram-negative bacterium that commonly causes canine infectious tracheobronchitis (kennel cough). Other infectious agents that can be involved include canine adenovirus-2, parainfluenza virus, and canine respiratory coronavirus. The disease is usually self-limiting unless complicated by bronchopneumonia, which may develop in unvaccinated puppies or immunocompromised adults.

iii. Antibiotic therapy should be provided based on the culture results. Supportive care is also important. Depending on patient status, this can include hospitalization, supplemental O_2, and parenteral antibiotic and fluid administration (to maintain good hydration). Physiotherapy (coupage) and airway nebulization can help mobilize airway secretions. Cough suppressants are avoided with bacterial pneumonia.

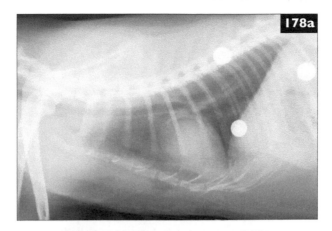

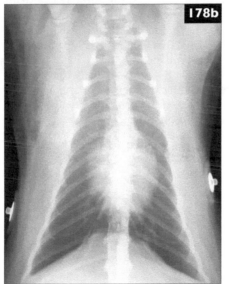

178 A 5-year-old spayed female DSH cat is presented for suspected trauma after being found in the neighbor's yard breathing with difficulty. The cat is laterally recumbent, with open-mouth breathing and in apparent shock. After initial stabilization, physical examination reveals a chin abrasion and small holes with bruising on the ventral thorax. Thoracic auscultation is normal. Palpation of the limbs and abdomen is normal. Despite a return to closed-mouth breathing, the respiratory rate remains elevated. Thoracic radiographs (178a, b) are taken.
i. Are thoracic wall abnormalities present?
ii. Are intrathoracic abnormalities present?

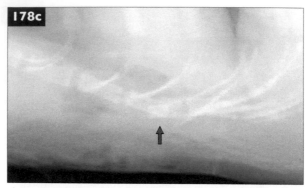

178 i. Three electrocardiographic electrodes have been applied to the skin of the thoracic wall. There are small subcutaneous gas shadows present along the sternum, particularly between sternebrae 3 and 6. Similar gas shadows are present in the right thoracic wall from the axilla to the 5th rib. There is increased bone opacity at the caudal half of the 6th sternebra due to cranial luxation (overlapping) of the 6th intersternal joint (**178c**, arrow). There is also detachment of the sternocostal joint as noted by the ventral positioning of the distal ends of the 7th costal cartilages. The small holes in the skin are likely due to bite wounds.

ii. There is no radiographic evidence of pleural space, lung, or cardiac abnormalities. The absence of radiographic pneumothorax does not exclude the potential for a bite wound to enter the thoracic cavity. Careful evaluation of the bite wounds, including probing, is needed. Respiratory rate can increase as a response to pain, no doubt associated with the sternal luxation.

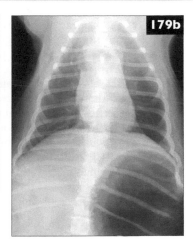

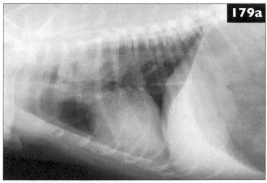

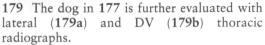

179 The dog in **177** is further evaluated with lateral (**179a**) and DV (**179b**) thoracic radiographs.

i. What is the location of the rawhide chew?

ii. What is the explanation for the gastric shadow size?

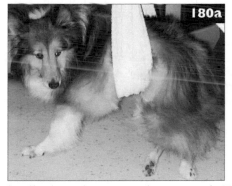

180 A 10-year-old neutered male Sheltie is presented for progressively worsening hindlimb weakness over the past week. There has been no known trauma. The dog is alert, but unable to support weight with his hindlimbs (**180a**), which are slightly cool to the touch and show abnormal conscious proprioception (**180b**). Femoral pulses are non-palpable. Body temperature is 37.7°C (99.9°F), HR is 132 bpm; respirations are labored at 76 breaths/min. Other physical findings are unremarkable. Chest and abdominal radiographs show no abnormalities.

i. What is the most likely cause of this dog's hindlimb weakness?

ii. What tests would be useful to confirm this?

iii. What underlying conditions can predispose to this?

iv. What are the general management goals in cases such as this?

179 i. The thoracic images show moderate ventral and sharp rightward deviation of the trachea at the level of the 3rd rib. In the DV view (enlargement, **179c**), a circular radiolucency with a soft tissue border summated (superimposed) with T3 is seen on the left side of the tracheal deviation. This feature has about the same diameter as the width of T3. Thin, parallel soft tissue opacity lines course through the mid and caudal thorax at the expected location of a thoracic esophagus that appears moderately dilated. The

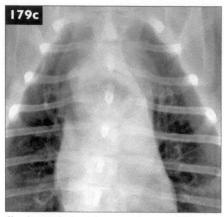

stomach is in a normal position, but markedly distended with gas. The combination of findings indicates that the foreign material is in the cranial thoracic esophagus at approximately the level of the 3rd rib.

ii. Patients in acute respiratory distress are often aerophagic. This can cause dilation of all parts of the alimentary tract with air.

180 i. Caudal aortic thromboembolism (TE). Dogs with arterial TE usually show clinical signs for days to weeks, in contrast to the peracute paralysis typical in cats. Signs include pain, hindlimb paresis, lameness or weakness (often progressive or intermittent), and chewing or hypersensitivity of affected areas. Physical findings are similar to those in cats with aortic TE: absent or weak femoral pulses, cool extremities, hindlimb pain, loss of sensation in affected digits, hyperesthesia, cyanotic nailbeds, and neuromuscular dysfunction.

ii. Aortic TE usually can be visualized with abdominal ultrasonography or other imaging modalities. TE elevates circulating D-dimer concentration, although a modest increase can accompany neoplasia, liver disease, immune-mediated and other diseases. Skeletal muscle ischemia and necrosis from arterial TE also elevates muscle enzyme concentrations.

iii. Diseases causing vascular endothelial damage, blood stasis, or hypercoagulability promote TE. Arterial TE in dogs has occurred with protein-losing nephropathies, neoplasia, hyperadrenocorticism, chronic interstitial nephritis, gastric dilatation–volvulus, pancreatitis, sepsis, endocarditis, vasculitis, and other conditions.

iv. Management goals are to stabilize the patient (fluids and other supportive care as needed), prevent additional TE (antiplatelet and anticoagulant therapy), and identify underlying disease(s) and treat as possible. Thrombolytic therapy is sometimes given, but there are dosage uncertainties, intensive monitoring requirements, and potentially serious or fatal complications.

181 A 14-year-old female Schnauzer/Poodle-cross develops coughing and recent exercise intolerance. She was previously diagnosed with chronic mitral and tricuspid regurgitation and mild pulmonary edema, for which furosemide, aminophylline, and digoxin were prescribed. Chest radiographs today indicate cardiomegaly but no pulmonary edema. You hear an arrhythmia and record this ECG (181a, b, leads as marked, 25 mm/s, 1 cm = 1 mV).

i. What is your ECG interpretation?
ii. What does the arrow in 181b indicate?
iii. How would you adjust this dog's medication?

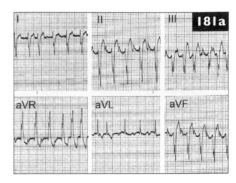

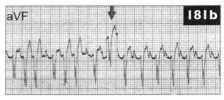

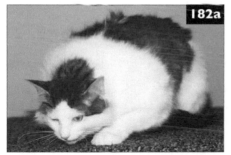

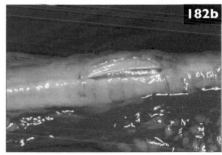

182 A 14-month-old spayed female mixed breed cat (182a) is presented for emergency treatment of acute-onset respiratory distress and whole body 'bloating'. Ten days prior to this an ovariohysterectomy was performed; incisional dehiscence occurred but was subsequently repaired. The cat's respiratory distress resolves with supplemental O_2 and she remains stable overnight. Nevertheless, the owners request euthanasia. A lesion is discovered at postmortem examination (182b).

i. What is the medical term for the whole body 'bloating' in this cat?
ii. What is the cause of this cat's respiratory distress and 'bloating'?
iii. Does the cat's previous surgery relate to this condition? If so, how?
iv. What other procedure is commonly associated with this condition in cats, and why?
v. Does surgical or non-surgical management yield better results in this condition?
vi. What can be done to prevent this condition from occurring?

181 i. HR is 180 bpm. The rhythm is sinus tachycardia with frequent atrial premature complexes (singles and pairs; asterisks, **181c**). The mean electrical axis is shifted rightward (to -150°). The widened terminal portion of the QRS

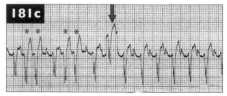

suggests right bundle branch block, although marked right ventricular enlargement is possible. The P waves, seen more easily as HR slows (**181b**), are widened at 0.06 second, consistent with LA enlargement. PR intervals are upper normal to slightly prolonged (0.13–0.16 second), which could be a digoxin-induced effect or indicate more widespread conduction system disease.

ii. Calibration signal superimposed on a sinus QRS complex.

iii. More frequent atrial tachyarrhythmias could underlie these clinical signs. Aminophylline's sympathomimetic effects can exacerbate arrhythmias; reducing the dose or discontinuing aminophylline may help. Ambulatory ECG monitoring can detect intermittently worse arrhythmias. Alternatively, diltiazem or atenolol can be added as a clinical trial. Digoxin suppresses some atrial tachyarrhythmias, but its serum concentration should be verified. Serum chemistries should also be measured. Pimobendan and an angiotensin-converting enzyme inhibitor are recommended for chronic heart failure management.

182 i. Subcutaneous emphysema is the accumulation of air in the subcutaneous tissues.

ii. The cause of subcutaneous emphysema and respiratory distress in this cat was a tracheal tear.

iii. The tracheal tear probably occurred during either the ovariohysterectomy or hernia repair as a result of endotracheal tube trauma.

iv. Dentistry procedures are frequently implicated in tracheal tears. The repeated repositioning of the animal during such procedures causes rotation of the endotracheal tube, which can strain and tear tracheal tissue.

v. Surgical treatment involves tracheal suturing or resection of the damaged trachea and anatomosis. However, conservative management of a simple tracheal tear, like the one shown in **182b**, is often as effective as surgical repair.

vi. Careful endotracheal tube selection and insertion can prevent tracheal tearing. Endotracheal tubes with high-volume, low-pressure cuffs are preferred over those with low-volume, high-pressure cuffs because they minimize tracheal injury. However, the main preventive measure during anesthesia is to disconnect the endotracheal tube from the anesthetic tubing whenever the animal must be repositioned. The torque on the trachea at the inflated cuff as the tube is twisted is the most likely cause of the tear.

183 A 14-year-old spayed female German Shepherd Dog is presented for evaluation of a large abdominal mass. The owners mention that over the last 6 months she has seemed slower and pants more, but otherwise has no clinical signs. The dog is alert and pants constantly. Body temperature is 39.2°C (102.6°F), mucous membranes are pink, and capillary refill time is <2 seconds.

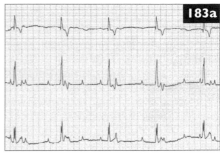

The heart is difficult to hear on auscultation, but the rate seems slow; a systolic murmur is suspected on the left. Lung sounds are normal. A large, firm mid-abdominal mass is palpated. Mild cardiomegaly is seen on radiographs. An ECG is recorded (183a, leads as marked, 25 mm/s, 1 cm = 1 mV).

i. What is your ECG diagnosis?
ii. What additional tests do you recommend at this time?
iii. The owner wishes to pursue abdominal exploratory surgery and mass removal. What do you advise?

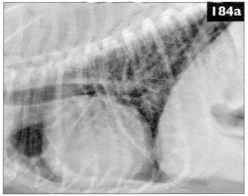
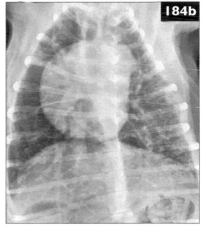
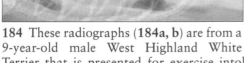

184 These radiographs (184a, b) are from a 9-year-old male West Highland White Terrier that is presented for exercise intolerance of several month's duration. Recently, an occasional cough has been noted. The dog has had no other past medical problems and is current on routine vaccinations and heartworm preventive.

i. What is the likely disease process(es)?
ii. What other diagnostic tests are indicated?
iii. How would you manage this case?

183 i. Heart rate is 40 bpm. P waves are evident, but none appear to be conducted (complete AV block). A regular ventricular escape rhythm is present. The upright configuration of these ventricular complexes is less common than the wide, negative QRS of many idioventricular rhythms. P waves are

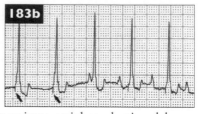

wide (0.06 second), suggesting LA enlargement or intra-atrial conduction delay.

ii. An atropine challenge (see case 37) will test for vagal influence on AV conduction; most dogs with complete AV block show no response. Echocardiography is indicated to evaluate cardiac structure and function. Other tests include BP measurement, routine laboratory database, and abdominal imaging to identify the source and extent of the mass.

iii. Considering this dog's age, large abdominal mass, and complete AV block, prospects for a positive outcome seem slim. Nevertheless, if a fully-informed owner wants to pursue abdominal exploratory, pacemaker implantation is recommended first. A transvenous pacemaker was implanted; postoperative ECG shows pacing artifacts (arrows, 183b) at the QRS onset. Two weeks later a 20 cm mass (necrotic omental lipoma) was surgically removed. The dog thrived for another 1.5 years.

184 i. These radiographs would support the diagnosis of idiopathic pulmonary fibrosis, sometimes called 'Westie lung disease'. This condition was first described in West Highland White Terriers, but recent reports suggest that other breeds of dogs may be affected, particularly Staffordshire Bull Terriers. Note the right heart enlargement, main PA and right PA enlargement, and the diffuse bronchointerstitial lung pattern creating a coarse honeycomb-like appearance. A very small amount of pleural fluid is also seen.

ii. A lung aspirate and/or BAL may be helpful to identify pathologic organisms and rule out other causes of parenchymal infiltration. In many cases these tests reveal only mild to moderate inflammation. A lung biopsy is often needed to obtain a definitive diagnosis. An echocardiogram can document PA hypertension and may be used to monitor pulmonary pressures during therapy.

iii. The principal therapy for idiopathic pulmonary fibrosis is a corticosteroid (e.g. low-dose prednisone). Bronchodilators and azathioprine may benefit some cases. Sildenafil may decrease pulmonary hypertension, which can improve symptoms; however, systemic hypotension is a potential side-effect. The prognosis for pulmonary fibrosis is often poor because the disease is progressive and tends to be advanced at the time of diagnosis.

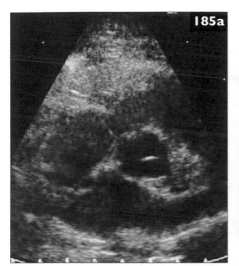

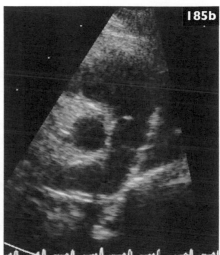

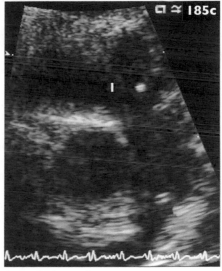

185 A 6-year-old neutered male DSH cat is presented for vomiting a reddish brown material last night. He frequently goes outdoors during the day and lives in the American midwest. In the past he has ingested various foreign objects such as rubber bands and flower stems. The cat is tachypneic (60 breaths/min) and slightly hypothermic (36.9°C [98.5°F]). Lung sounds are increased; no heart murmur is heard. BP and abdominal radiographs are normal. Chest radiographs show increased right lung opacities and enlarged caudal lobar arteries. Right parasternal short axis echocardiographic images of the Ao/LA (185a) and main PA (185b) and a left cranial short axis view of the Ao and PA (185c, enlarged, 1 – PA) are shown.

i. What are the echo findings?
ii. Are the clinical findings consistent with this diagnosis?
iii. How would you manage this case?

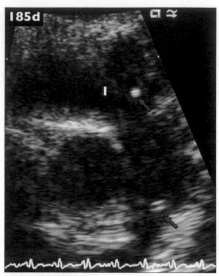

185 i. LA, Ao, and PA sizes are normal. Characteristic parallel echos of an adult heartworm are inside the PA (185c, d, arrows).

ii. Yes. Feline heartworm disease has variable signs. Tachypnea, dyspnea, or paroxysmal cough can mimic feline asthma. Vomiting is common. Lethargy, anorexia, syncope, neurologic signs (especially with aberrant larval migration), and sudden death can also occur.

iii. An adulticide is not recommended for cats; acute worm death can cause severe complications. Respiratory signs usually respond to prednisone (e.g. 2 mg/kg q24h, reduced gradually over 2 weeks to 0.5 mg/kg q48h, then discontinued after 2 more weeks). This is repeated if necessary. Monthly heartworm prophylaxis and restricted activity are also recommended. Severe respiratory distress and death can occur any time, especially after worm death. Signs of pulmonary thromboembolism (PTE) include fever, cough, dyspnea, hemoptysis, pallor, pulmonary crackles, tachycardia, and hypotension. Supportive care includes an IV glucocorticoid (e.g. 100–250 mg prednisone sodium succinate), fluid therapy, a bronchodilator, and supplemental O$_2$. Diuretics are not indicated for PTE. Pleural effusion from right-sided heart failure is managed with thoracocentesis, furosemide, and an angiotensin-converting enzyme inhibitor.

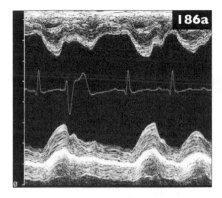

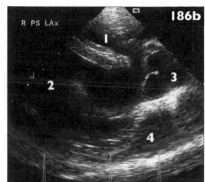

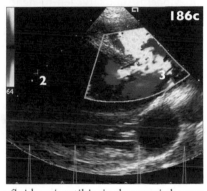

186 An 8-month-old mixed breed dog is presented for vomiting, bloody diarrhea, and weight loss (body condition score 2/5). A grade 6/6 systolic heart murmur, loudest at the right sternal border, is discovered on physical examination. A grade 1/6 diastolic murmur is also heard at the left heart base. Mucous membranes are pink, but capillary refill time is prolonged. Body temperature is normal. Ventricular premature complexes are seen on ECG. Blood work indicates marked neutropenia, mild hypoalbuminemia, and a positive parvovirus test. Supportive fluid and antibiotic therapy is begun and an echocardiogram is obtained. M-mode at ventricular level (186a) and right parasternal long axis (186b, in diastole; 186c, color flow in systole) images are shown.
1 – RV, 2 – LV, 3 – Ao, 4 – LA.

i. What abnormalities are seen on the echo images?
ii. Are the auscultatory findings consistent with this?
iii. Do these findings influence your therapy?

187 What strategies can be helpful for managing chronic refractory (stage D) congestive heart failure?

186 i. Marked LV dilation is evident. There is a 6–7 mm ventricular septal defect (VSD) just below the aortic valve (**186b**), with left-to-right systolic flow (**186c**). VSDs volume overload the lungs, left heart, and RV outflow tract. However, the degree of LV dilation here seems disproportionate and probably reflects additional LV volume loading from concurrent aortic valve insufficiency, as well as mild LV dysfunction. Although LV FS is within normal range (~35%), more vigorous LV motion is expected with the reduced LV afterload afforded by shunt flow into the relatively low-pressure RV. Occasional ventricular premature beats are also present.
ii. A holosystolic murmur heard best at the right sternal border is typical for VSD. The soft, left basilar diastolic murmur is consistent with aortic valve regurgitation. This sometimes occurs with VSD, presumably because the deformed septum provides inadequate support for the aortic root.
iii. Moderate and large left-to-right shunting VSDs can lead to left-sided congestive failure. This is of great concern in this dog because aggressive fluid therapy may be needed to manage parvovirus infection. Careful monitoring of respiratory rate and effort (and, ideally, pulmonary capillary wedge pressure) is recommended.

187 First, verify dosage and frequency of all drugs and supplements being administered. The following strategies can be used sequentially or in combinations, depending on individual needs:
• Increase dose and/or frequency of furosemide.
• Add pimobendan, if not being used (INBU).
• Add an angiotensin-converting enzyme inhibitor (ACEI), INBU.
• Add spironolactone, INBU.
• Increase ACEI to q12h and maximal recommended dose.
• Identify and manage arrhythmias, if present.
• Add arteriolar vasodilator to further reduce afterload (e.g. amlodipine or hydralazine). (**Note:** Not recommended for patients with hypertrophic cardiomyopathy or fixed ventricular outflow obstruction [e.g. subaortic stenosis]).
• Add sildenafil, if moderate/severe pulmonary hypertension.
• Add digoxin, INBU.
• Add thiazide diuretic (closely monitor renal function!).
• Further restrict dietary salt intake and exercise.

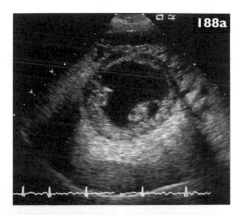

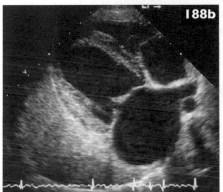
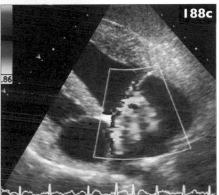

188 A 7-year-old male Brittany is presented for recent lethargy, vomiting, and inappetence. A couple days ago he ingested a mouse toy. One week ago he had successful surgical repair of a ruptured anterior cruciate ligament. On examination the dog is alert but quiet. Body temperature is normal, HR is 140 bpm and irregular, respiratory rate is increased, pulse deficits are noted, and heart sounds are muffled. Systolic BP is 130 mmHg. Recent chest radiographs forwarded by the referring veterinarian show a large, globoid cardiac silhouette (VHS 15 v) that almost fills the thoracic cavity and abuts the diaphragm; visible lung fields are normal. An echocardiogram is done; images are from right parasternal short axis (**188a**) and long axis (**188b**) and left apical (**188c**) positions.

i. What abnormalities are seen in the figures?

ii. What is your assessment of this case?

iii. What are your recommendations?

188 i. Marked LA and mild LV dilation are seen. Mitral valve thickening (**188b**) and insufficiency (**188b**) are evident. The pericardial space is greatly distended with soft-tissue opacities (pericardial echos near ECG trace in **188a, b**). The ECG rhythm is atrial fibrillation (AF).

ii. Differentials for soft tissue within the pericardial space include abdominal organs displaced through a congenital peritoneopericardial diaphragmatic hernia (PPDH) or neoplastic mass lesion(s). The mitral valve thickening suggests degenerative valve disease. Based on LA size, significant mitral regurgitation has existed for quite some time. AF is common with chronic atrial enlargement.

iii. Further imaging is warranted to search for diaphragmatic discontinuity and abdominal organ displacement (from PPDH) or for other causes of the intrapericardial soft tissue and clinical signs. Also recommended are diltiazem (possibly with digoxin) to control HR, echocardiographic evaluation of LV systolic function, and close monitoring for early signs of cardiac decompensation. In this case, PPDH was confirmed with abdominal ultrasonography and surgically repaired; displaced tissues included gallbladder and portions of atrophied liver, spleen, small intestine, and pancreas. An immature pyloric-to-diaphragm adhesion was also found; this was thought to have precipitated the recent vomiting and inappetence.

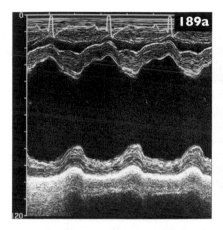

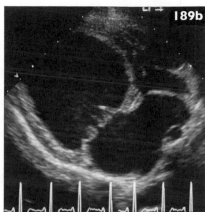

189 An 18.6 kg (41 lb) 9-year-old female English Pointer has a history of chronic mitral valve disease (endocardiosis) with congestive heart failure (CHF) and, possibly, small airway disease. Current medications are: furosemide, 12.5 mg q12h; enalapril, 10 mg q24h; digoxin, ½ a 0.125 mg tab q24h; theophylline, 100 mg q12h; and a heartworm preventive. Some coughing and increase in resting respiratory rate have recently developed. The dog is alert and active during examination. HR is 140 bpm and somewhat irregular. A grade 5/6 mitral

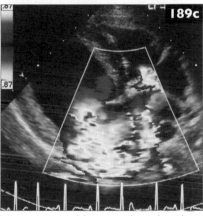

regurgitation (MR) murmur and soft pulmonary crackles are heard. Chest radiographs show cardiomegaly with dorsohilar pulmonary infiltrates. An ECG reveals sinus rhythm with frequent supraventricular premature complexes. Renal function and serum electrolytes are normal; heartworm test is negative. An echocardiogram is done. Right parasternal M-mode at ventricular level (189a), and systolic long axis 4-chamber (189b, c) images are shown.

i. What are the echo findings?

ii. What do you recommend at this time?

iii. What complications might be anticipated in cases like this?

190 What are the important principles for treating acute heart failure in dogs?

189 i. Marked LV and LA dilation, mitral valve thickening, and severe MR (**189c**) are evident. LV FS is 32%. FS provides an afterload-dependent estimate of contractility. Consequently, with well preserved contractility but severe MR, an increased FS is expected. The 'normal' (range 27–40%) FS in this dog therefore suggests some myocardial dysfunction.

ii. For decompensated CHF add pimobendan, increase furosemide dose, and increase enalapril to q12h. Try reducing the dose of or discontinuing theophylline, as it may be exacerbating the tachyarrhythmia. Measure trough serum digoxin concentration; if low, consider increasing to q12h dosing as an antiarrhythmic measure. Verify reduced dietary salt intake and restrict exercise. Closely monitor renal function, serum electrolytes, BP, heart rhythm, resting respiratory rate, appetite and activity. Low-dose carvedilol therapy and an omega-3 fatty acid (fish oil) supplement may be helpful.

iii. Complications could include: more severe arrhythmias, including atrial tachycardia or fibrillation and ventricular tachyarrhythmias; recurrent, refractory pulmonary edema; persistent dry cough from bronchial compression; pulmonary hypertension; and biventricular failure with body cavity effusions. Intensified CHF therapy can promote azotemia, electrolyte disturbances including hypo- or hyper-kalemia, hypotension, inappetence, and other adverse drug effects or toxicity.

190
- Severe cardiogenic pulmonary edema requires urgent therapy, but it is important to minimize patient stress. Cart (or carry) if patient needs to be moved. No exercise should be allowed.
- Provide supplemental O_2, but avoid increasing the patient's anxiety level.
- Induce diuresis with parenteral furosemide – dose aggressively as needed (can give IM initially until IV catheter can be safely placed).
- Monitor respiratory rate (RR) and effort frequently; adjust diuretic dosing accordingly.
- Promote vasodilation (hydralazine or angiotensin-converting enzyme inhibitor with or wthout nitroglycerine, or alternatively, nitroprusside if fulminant pulmonary edema).
- Support myocardial function (pimobendan).
- Minimize anxiety (butorphanol or morphine).
- If moderate to large pleural effusion is present, remove by thoracocentesis.
- For hypotension or myocardial failure, add dobutamine or other positive inotrope as needed to support BP.
- Monitor BP, HR and rhythm, as well as RR; treat arrhythmias as indicated.
- Evaluate serum chemistries and perform other tests to clarify underlying cardiac and other abnormalities as soon as patient stability allows.

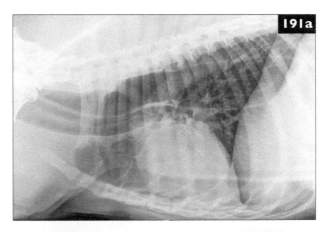

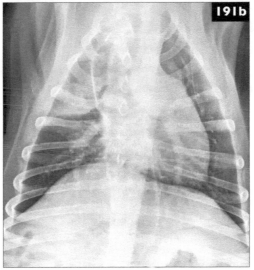

191 A 9-year-old neutered male Labrador Retriever is presented for 2 days of vomiting after being given a linear dental chew. He appears weak and lethargic. Physical examination findings include a body temperature of 39.8°C (103.7°F), HR of 152 bpm, respiratory rate of 36 breaths/min, and normal mucous membrane color and capillary refill time. Heart sounds are normal, but pulmonary crackles are heard over the right mid-lung field. Right lateral (191a) and DV (191b) thoracic radiographs are made.

i. What is your radiographic assessment?

ii. What etiologic differentials should be considered in this patient?

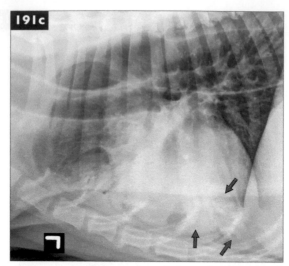

191 **i.** There is diffuse caudal cervical and thoracic megaesophagus with right cranial and right middle lung lobe consolidation most consistent with aspiration pneumonia.

Aspiration pneumonia is a common consequence of megaesophagus, as well as impaired swallowing reflexes. The right middle lobe is the most commonly affected single lobe, followed by the right cranial lobe. Variable infiltrate distribution occurs when multiple lobes are affected. Using both lateral radiographic projections better reveals the extent of lung involvement. In this dog, the left lateral view (**191c**) shows air bronchograms in the right cranial and middle lobes (arrows). Although right cranial lobe changes are evident on the DV view, right middle lobe abnormalities are only clear on the left lateral view (arrows), summated (superimposed) with the cardiac apex.

ii. Megaesophagus is described radiographically as focal or segmental versus diffuse. General causes of megaesophagus include neuromuscular diseases, mechanical causes, and idiopathic. Diffuse esophageal dilation is more likely with neuro-muscular diseases, including myasthenia gravis, endocrinopathies (hypoadreno-corticism, hypothyroidism), immune-mediated disease, and toxins. Mechanical causes include intraluminal foreign objects, mural masses, and strictures (as from esophagitis or vascular ring anomalies). Focal megaesophagus is more likely with mechanical causes, although diffuse dilation can accompany obstructions near the lower esophageal sphincter. Aerophagia associated with excitement, respiratory distress, and anesthesia should be differentiated.

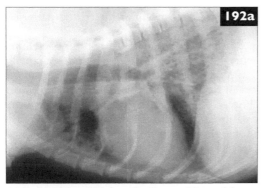

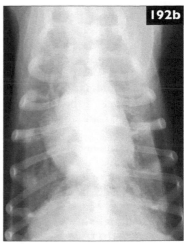

192 A 6-year-old female Basset Hound has a 3-week history of coughing and rapid respiration. Enlarged peripheral lymph nodes are found on physical examination; other parameters are unremarkable. On auscultation, lung sounds are found to be harsh. Right lateral (192a) and DV (192b) thoracic radiographs are shown.

i. What radiographic changes are present?
ii. Does this patient have concurrent pneumothorax?
iii. What will be your next diagnostic procedures?

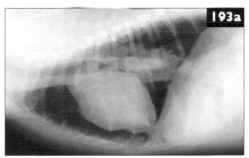

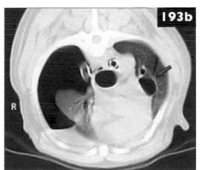

193 An 11-year-old male Scottish Terrier is presented with a history of two episodes of spontaneous pneumothorax. The dog has a chronic cough not associated with any particular activity or event. On presentation his breathing is labored and harsh lung sounds are heard. A right lateral thoracic radiograph (193a) and a CT scan image (193b) are shown.

i. What is evident radiographically?
ii. Is a cause for the pneumothorax evident in the CT image and if so, what and where is it?
iii. What are the causes of and diagnostic options for spontaneous pneumothorax?

192 i. A diffuse pulmonary unstructured to small nodular interstitial pattern is evident. There is incidental T4/5 spondylosis deformans.
ii. No. In the DV view there is a distinct lucent-soft tissue interface positioned in the lateral portion of each hemithorax extending from ribs 4–10. Note that cranially the interface is at the thoracic wall and at the caudal level the interface curves medially. Pulmonary shadows are evident in the left 8th intercostal space between the interface and the thoracic wall border. The lucent-soft tissue interface is the effect of skin folds and/or the conformation of the thoracic cavity. The influence of the latter is particularly prominent in some chondrodystrophic breeds. Both of these effects can simulate pneumothorax. However, there is no evidence of pneumothorax seen in the lateral view of this dog.
iii. Fine needle aspiration of the enlarged lymph nodes and cytologic examination should be done. In this dog, lymphoma was diagnosed.

There is a broad list of etiologic differential diagnoses consistent with the interstitial pattern. Besides lymphoma, these include mycotic pneumonia, diffuse pulmonary metastasis, eosinophilic bronchopneumopathy, and hemorrhage. Pulmonary histopathology from necropsy in this patient showed neoplastic lymphocytes in cuffs around blood vessels and airways, as well as in lymphatic vessels.

193 i. The heart is markedly displaced from the sternum. There is a large radiolucent space with no pulmonary vascular shadows in the dorsocaudal thorax. The caudal lung lobes are markedly collapsed.
ii. Yes. The patient is in sternal recumbency for the CT scan and the image is immediately cranial to the tracheal bifurcation. A segment of chest tube is seen dorsally, adjacent to the right side of the mediastinum. A large-volume pneumothorax is present in the right hemithorax causing right lung collapse and shifting of the heart to the left. There is minimal pleural air between the left cranial and caudal lobes dorsally. An air attenuating cavity (arrow), of diameter equal to the trachea, is seen ventral to a left lobar bronchus and adjacent to the left border of the pulmonary trunk. This is consistent with a large superficial bulla.
iii. Spontaneous pneumothorax is a closed pneumothorax that occurs without traumatic or iatrogenic cause. Pneumonia, abscesses, neoplasia, bullous emphysema, heartworm disease, and pulmonary bullae and blebs are the reported causes. Although radiography clearly indicates the pneumothorax, it has poor sensitivity for blebs and bullae when pneumothorax is present. CT is more sensitive for detecting blebs and bullae, and assessing their extent prior to surgical treatment.

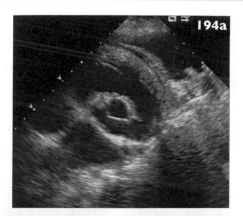

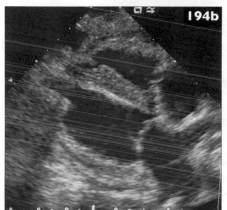
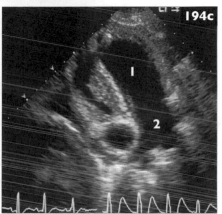

194 A 6-year-old male Labrador Retriever is brought to the Emergency Service with a several hour history of lethargy, inappropriate defecation, and weakness. The dog runs outside, but there was no known trauma or toxin exposure. On presentation, he is lethargic and weak. Mucous membranes appear 'muddy' and his tongue is bluish. He is panting, HR is 140 bpm, and temperature is 37.8°C (100°F). A small wound is seen on the left thorax. Systolic BP is 75 mmHg. IV fluid and O$_2$ are administered. An ECG shows paroxysmal ventricular tachycardia. Subsequent bloodwork shows a PCV of 0.23 l/l (23%), thrombocytopenia, hypokalemia, and increased creatinine. Pleural effusion consistent with hemorrhage is detected. An echocardiogram is done; right parasternal short axis (194a) and long axis (194b) and left apical (194c) views are shown. 1 – LV, 2 – LA.

i. Describe the echo findings.

ii. What is the likely etiology?

iii. How would you manage this case?

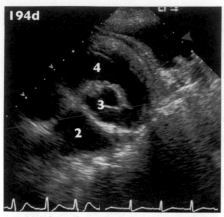

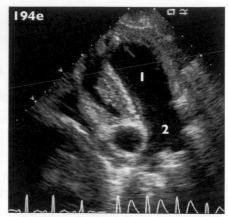

194 i. Pleural (arrowhead) and small pericardial (arrow) effusions are seen (**194d**); atrial size is normal. There is a focal, markedly hyperechoic area near the LV apex (arrow, **194e**) that appears to protrude into the lumen and casts an acoustic shadow deep to this area. 1 – LV, 2 – LA, 3 – Ao, 4 – RV. The monitor ECG shows ventricular tachycardia.

ii. A bullet or other metallic projectile is the likely cause (documented radiographically). The difference in acoustic impedance between tissue and metal (also air) is so great that most of the ultrasound energy is reflected and deeper structures cannot be seen. Antemortem identification of penetrating cardiac wounds is rare because most rapidly cause death from uncontrolled bleeding, cardiac dysfunction, and arrhythmias. This dog recovered without residual cardiovascular signs.

iii. Initial goals are to stabilize BP, control ventricular tachycardia, improve oxygenation (including blood transfusion and thoracocentesis, if needed), correct metabolic abnormalities, and control infection.

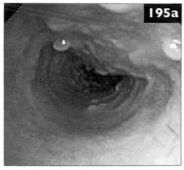
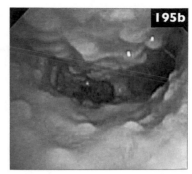

195 A 12-year-old spayed female Miniature Pinscher is presented with a 9-month history of coughing and wheezing that worsens with excitement and exercise. Currently she is on no medications. A moist, hacking cough is noted during the examination. Thoracic radiographs show normal lung fields, slightly thickened bronchial walls, and mild cardiomegaly. CBC, serum chemistry, and urinalysis tests are unremarkable. Tracheobronchoscopy is done; images from the thoracic inlet region (195a) and just cranial to the carina (195b) are shown.
i. What abnormalities are seen on the images?
ii. What other tests should be done?
iii. What is your assessment?
iv. What are the management principles for this condition?

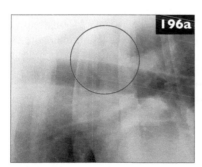
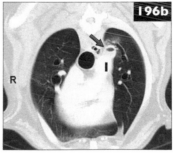

196 A 7-year-old neutered male mixed breed dog weighing 43.6 kg (96 lb) is referred for possible surgical treatment of spontaneous pneumothorax. Thoracic drainage tubes had been used to remove free air from the pleural space. Thoracic radiographs at presentation show no pneumothorax and no abnormalities other than the subtle lesion shown in the left lateral view (196a). A CT study is done to further define this region (transverse post-contrast CT image shown in 196b, 1 – aorta).
i. What is the subtle lesion (circled) shown in 196a?
ii. What additional information is provided by the CT study?

195 i. Small mucosal nodules are present and especially numerous near the carina, along with mucosal edema and inflammation (195b). The sagging dorsal tracheal membrane indicates tracheal collapse.

ii. Besides visual airway inspection, tracheobronchial muscosal brushings and BAL fluid should be collected for cytologic examination and bacterial culture/sensitivity testing.

iii. Chronic bronchitis (CB) is likely. CB is defined as coughing occurring on most days for 2 or more consecutive months, in the absence of other causative disease. Airway inflammation with excessive mucus production, epithelial hyperplasia, fibrosis, and sometimes polypoid mucosal proliferation (as here) occurs, along with small airway obstruction. Infection, allergy, or inhaled irritants can trigger CB. Complications can include bacterial bronchitis and pneumonia, airway collapse, pulmonary hypertension, and bronchiectasis. In this dog, cytology showed intense inflammation (neutrophils and eosinophils), but no organisms. However, cultures were positive for *Pseudomonas* and *Citrobacter* spp. An uncommon cause of reactive nodules within the carina and main bronchi is *Oslerus osleri* parasitic infection.

iv. Avoid potential inhaled irritants and other cough triggers; be alert for complications. Bronchodilators, glucocorticoids, and cough suppressants can help control signs. Antibiotic therapy for bacterial infection is ideally based on culture/sensitivity results. Saline nebulization and coupage help mobilize secretions.

196 i. There is a focal circular lucency, ventral to T4, which partially overlaps the trachea just proximal to the carina.

ii. The CT scan confirms a cavitary lesion in the left dorsal medial edge of the left cranial lung (arrow, 196b). The ovoid shape of the gas in the cavity suggests the presence of fluid in the ventral portion, although the average Hounsfield unit (HU) of 40 is more typical of tissue or blood. However, higher HU numbers are associated with fluid of high protein content. The CT scan also shows the proximity of the lesion to the aorta. The advantage of CT in this patient is that it provides improved localization of the lesion for surgical planning. The lesion was adhered to the lateral aspect of the aorta; however, successful surgical dissection and removal was accomplished. Microbial culture of the lesion was negative and histopathology showed it was an inflammatory lesion.

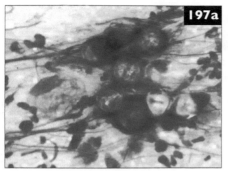
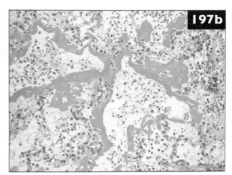

197 A 4-year-old castrated male Saint Bernard from the American midwest is presented for a cough and purulent nasal discharge. Two week earlier he was referred to an ophthalmologist for unilateral uveitis. At that time, panophthalmitis was identified. Vitreal fluid cytology revealed prior hemorrhage; a presumptive diagnosis of rickettsial disease was made. Thoracic radiographs were normal. The dog was sent home on doxycycline and prednisone while awaiting definitive test results.

Physical examination reveals panophthalmitis, purulent nasal discharge, and tachypnea with increased respiratory effort. The patient also has a harsh, productive cough. Thoracic radiographs show a diffuse nodular interstitial pulmonary pattern, with an additional ventrally-distributed alveolar component. Cardiovascular structures are normal. A sputum sample is submitted for cytologic examination (**197a**, Wright's stain, 100× oil). Despite aggressive therapy, severe acute respiratory distress develops and the dog dies. A photomicrograph of a lung section taken at necropsy is shown (**197b**, H&E stain, 20×).

i. What is seen in **197a**?
ii. What was the likely cause for the patient's rapid deterioration and death?
iii. Are the histologic findings in **197b** consistent with the patient's clinical course?

198 Normal breath sounds, caused by turbulent air flow in larger airways, are similar to the sound of wind gently blowing through trees. Describe the different types of abnormal lung sounds and their general associations.

197 i. The basophilic round, thick-walled structures (**197c**, arrow) are yeast organisms, morphologically consistent with *Blastomyces dermatitidis*. Yeast are approximately 7–15 microns in diameter and exhibit broad-based budding.

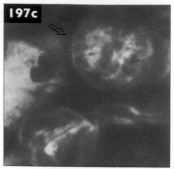

ii. The dog's progressive respiratory signs, diffuse interstitial pulmonary infiltrates, and sudden onset of severe respiratory distress are consistent with acute respiratory distress syndrome (ARDS), in this case secondary to pulmonary blastomycosis. ARDS is a clinicopathologic condition in which diffuse lung injury, often triggered by a systemic inflammatory response, leads to sudden and severe respiratory distress. ARDS has been associated with a variety of conditions, including bacterial pneumonia, aspiration pneumonia, and sepsis. In people, ARDS is a common complication in critical care patients and generally carries a poor prognosis; the prognosis for ARDS associated with pulmonary blastomycosis is grave.

iii. The lung section shows lesions characteristic of the exudative phase of ARDS. Note the diffuse alveolar damage, characterized by loss of type I pneumocytes and hyaline membrane formation. Alveolar lumens contain cellular debris, erythrocytes, and fibrin. These histopathologic lesions represent a severe, acute process that would markedly impair respiration if widespread, as they were in this case. The rapid clinical deterioration of this patient is consistent with these changes.

198 Although some disagreement about the classification of respiratory sounds exists, the terms crackles, rhonchi, and wheezes are recognized in the international classification system as abnormal respiratory sounds.

Crackles (previously known as râles) are fine, popping, crackling, discontinuous, non-musical sounds. They are usually heard during inspiration, resulting from explosive opening of small, previously-collapsed airways. Fine crackles are more common over ventral lung fields, but may be heard elsewhere over peripheral lung fields. Causes include small airway disease and pulmonary edema.

Rhonchi (or coarse crackles) sound similar to crackles, but tend to be associated with larger airways (rather than peripheral regions). Rhonchi have a more 'liquid' sound than crackles and usually involve secretions moving in large bronchioles and bronchi (e.g. with chronic bronchitis).

Wheezes are high-pitched, squeaking or musical, continuous sounds that are heard mainly during expiration, although they can occur throughout the respiratory cycle. Wheezes stem from airway wall vibrations caused by lower airway narrowing, constriction, or spasm. Causes include asthma, congestive heart failure, fibrosis, and pneumonia.

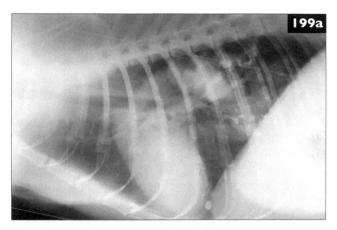

199a

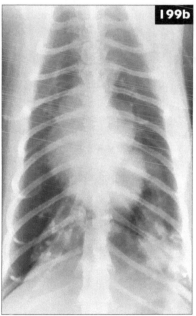

199b

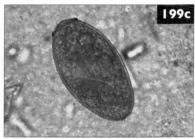

199c

199 A 9-year-old spayed female DSH cat is presented for coughing, which has occurred since the cat was found as a stray 8 years ago when the owner was living in the mid-west USA. The cat has been housed indoors only since adoption. Recently, she has intermittently shown respiratory distress. The owner has given prednisone off and on over the years, but it does not seem to be helping lately. Chest radiographs (lateral, **199a, b**), tracheal wash, heartworm test, and a fecal examination (**199c**) are done.

i. What radiographic abnormalities are seen?
ii. What does the fecal test show?
iii. What is your diagnosis?
iv. How would you treat this case?

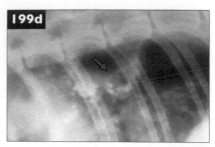

199 i. Multiple soft tissue opacities in the dorsal and caudal lung fields, with several smaller areas of randomly distributed calcification. Some of the opacities contain cystic areas (**199d**, arrow) suggestive of parasitic lung disease, abcesses, or granulomas.

ii. A *Paragonimus kellicotti* egg (note single operculum at top). Multiple eggs were found in the feces and tracheal wash cytology.

iii. Chronic paragonimiasis. *P. kellicotti* is a parasitic lung fluke found in North America usually, although sometimes elsewhere. It requires two intermediate hosts (snail, then crayfish or crab). After the host ingests an infected intermediate, larvae migrate to the lungs. Eggs produced by adult flukes are coughed up, swallowed, and passed in the feces. Diagnosis is by identification of eggs on fecal examination (sedimentation technique is best) or airway washings. Adult flukes can live for many years. Host pulmonary changes include granulomatous reaction around adults or generalized inflammatory reaction to fluke eggs. Signs often mimic those of allergic bronchitis. Spontaneous pneumothorax occurs when cystic lesions rupture. Some animals are asymptomatic. *P. kellicotti* infection is more common in cats, but dogs and other species can be affected.

iv. Fenbendazole (50 mg/kg PO q4h for 14 days) or praziquantel (23 mg/kg PO q8h for 3 days).

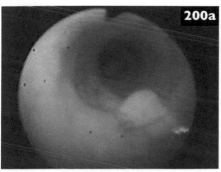

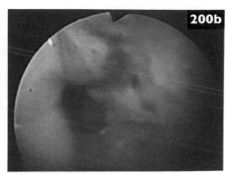

200 A 9.5-year-old neutered female Staffordshire Bull Terrier is referred because of a chronic cough that has worsened over the previous 2 months. The cough is described as productive and is accompanied by a 'gurgling noise'. Retching and spasmodic abdominal contractions also occur during coughing. The dog has been treated with a variety of medications, including wide-spectrum antibiotics, without notable improvement. Yesterday she coughed up a frothy white fluid tinged with fresh blood.

The dog is alert, responsive and in excellent body condition. Physical examination is unremarkable. A cough can be elicited by moderately strong tracheal palpation, but sounds different from the dog's chronic cough. Hematology and serum biochemistry test results are unremarkable. Thoracic radiographs show a mild bronchial pattern, thought to be age related. Abdominal sonography is unremarkable. Laryngeal anatomy and function appear normal during anesthesia induction for bronchoscopic examination, which reveals only a small amount of mucus in the distal trachea and main bronchi (200a). BAL fluid contains low cell numbers, with no cytologic abnormalities or bacterial growth.

Because of the retching and gagging history, upper gastrointestinal endoscopy is also performed. An image of the distal esophagus is shown (200b). Several wood fragments are found in the stomach; most are removed with endoscopic forceps. Multiple duodenal and gastric biopsies indicate histopathologically normal gastrointestinal mucosa.

i. What abnormalities are observed in the endoscopic images?
ii. What is the most likely cause of coughing and retching in this dog?
iii. How would you manage this case?

201 What is amlodipine, and when is it indicated?

200 i. The images show moderate inflammation of the distal esophageal lining, characterized by mucosal hyperemia and ulcerations.

ii. Esophageal reflux is the likely cause of coughing and retching in this dog, thought to be similar to gastroesophageal reflux disease in people. Coughing can occur when gastric contents reflux up to the hypopharynx and are aspirated, stimulating the laryngeal cough receptors. An esophageal–bronchial reflex may also be stimulated when gastric acid refluxes onto the distal esophageal mucosa. Although definitive diagnosis would require invasive long-term pH monitoring, the history and clinical signs accompanied by esophageal erosions strongly suggest gastroesophageal reflux disease.

iii. A change in diet or feeding frequency and antacid therapy may help minimize esophageal reflux and control the related cough. This dog was successfully treated with sucralfate, ranitidine, and frequent small meals (4–5 small meals per day instead of larger meals given twice daily).

201 Amlodipine besylate is a dihydropyridine L-type Ca^{++} channel blocker. It causes vasodilation without appreciable cardiac effects. Amlodipine is the initial drug of choice for hypertensive cats, including those with chronic renal failure. It can be useful for hypertensive dogs that respond inadequately to an angiotensin-converting enzyme inhibitor. Amlodipine is also used for additional afterload reduction in dogs with refractory congestive heart failure. Amlodipine is usually administered q24h, but it can be dosed q12h if needed. Several days are required to achieve maximal effect, so low initial doses and weekly BP monitoring during slow up-titration are recommended.

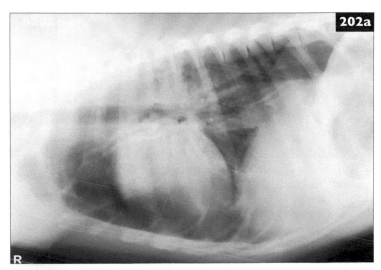

202 A 1-year-old female Chesapeake Bay Retriever is presented after being in an accident with a farm machine. The dog is reluctant to stand or walk, is non-weight bearing on the left hindlimb, has puncture wounds on the left side of the chest and lumbar area, and has a mild increase in respiratory effort. Right lateral (202a) and VD (202b) thoracic radiographs are taken to assess thoracic trauma.

i. What findings indicate that substantial thoracic trauma has occurred?

ii. Based on the findings in the thoracic radiographs, what other body system needs to be more thoroughly assessed?

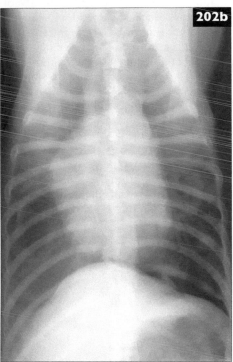

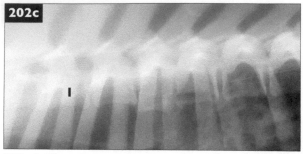

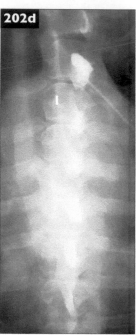

202 i. There is partial to complete effacement of the ventral cardiac border, caudal vena cava, and ventral and right half of the diaphragm. Several thin pleural fissure lines are visible (both views). There is a well defined gas–soft tissue border in the caudodorsal thorax, with a decrease in lung vascular markings between this border, the spine, and the left crus of the diaphragm. A mild interstitial to alveolar soft tissue opacity is seen in the dorsal mid-right lung field. The gastric axis is normal. No rib fractures are evident. The 3rd thoracic vertebra is labeled (1) in 202c and 202d. There is misalignment of the ventral border of the spine at the T4/5 disk space, with T5 approximately 3 mm ventral to T4. The ventral cranial border of T5 overlaps with the T4/5 intervertebral disk space. Summary: mild/moderate pleural effusion (probably hemorrhage), mild pneumothorax, mild right-sided pulmonary opacity (likely contusions), and probable T5 compression fracture (202c, d).

ii. Because of the suspected T5 compression fracture, a more thorough neurologic evaluation is warranted. Although reluctance to stand or walk may relate to generalized pain from the trauma, evaluation for spinal pain and neurologic deficits is indicated. Based on the results of neurologic examination, additional imaging, such as myelography, CT, or MRI, may be needed to assess further the vertebra and spinal cord.

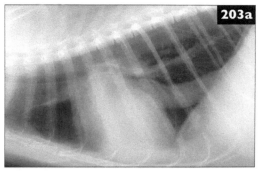

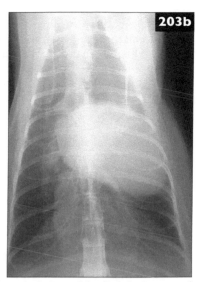

203 A 5-year-old spayed DSH cat becomes tired easily. She breathes heavily and her gums look slightly blue with moderate activity. Another veterinarian prescribed furosemide, suspecting hypertrophic cardiomyopathy (HCM), then referred the cat. She is alert but quiet. HR is 200 bpm; the rhythm is occasionally irregular. Respiratory rate is 30 breaths/min, with slightly increased effort. A soft systolic murmur is heard at the sternal border; lung sounds are normal. Mucous membrane color, capillary refill time, and femoral pulses appear normal. Lateral (203a) and DV (203b) thoracic radiographs are taken.

i. What is your radiographic interpretation?
ii. Do the radiographic findings support the presumptive diagnosis of HCM?
iii. What is your assessment of this case?
iv. Should furosemide be continued?

204 A 13-year-old male Miniature Schnauzer has episodic collapse with exercise and excitement. The dog will stagger and lie down abruptly or fall onto his side, then return to normal within 1–2 minutes. He appears alert and in good body condition. An irregular heart rhythm, but normal HR is heard. This ECG is recorded (204; leads I, II, and III at 25 mm/s, 1 cm = 1 mV).

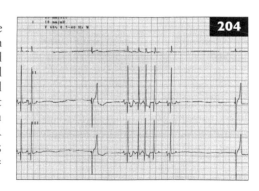

i. Describe the ECG abnormalities.
ii. What is the name of the syndrome associated with such abnormalities?
iii. How would you manage this case?

203 i. Generalized cardiomegaly (VHS of 9.4 v) and massive caudal vena cava (CaVC) enlargement are the most prominent findings. Normally the CaVC diameter is approximately that of the descending thoracic aorta. Persistent CaVC widening suggests increased systemic venous pressure, as with right ventricular failure, cardiac tamponade, pericardial constriction, or other obstruction to right heart inflow. Pulmonary parenchyma and vessels are unremarkable.

ii. Although there is generalized cardiomegaly, the marked CaVC enlargement without signs of congestive failure (usually pulmonary venous congestion with edema, or pleural effusion), is atypical for HCM.

iii. The history of cyanosis with activity suggests marked hypoxemia; polycythemia may be present. The normal pulmonary appearance along with the abnormal cardiovascular findings is consistent with a previously undiagnosed congenital cardiac malformation causing right-to-left shunting of blood. The murmur location suggests either a ventricular septal defect with pulmonary hypertension or a tetralogy of Fallot. An echocardiogram, ECG, and hematocrit measurement are recommended next. A large ventricular septal defect, marked pulmonary hypertension, and occasional ventricular premature beats were identified in this cat.

iv. No. Without evidence for pulmonary edema or pleural effusion, furosemide is unlikely to be helpful and can cause dehydration. This could further compromise tissue perfusion if the cat is polycythemic.

204 i. Two sinus complexes are followed by a long sinus pause or sinus arrest that is interrupted by a ventricular escape complex. A sinus complex then occurs, followed by a burst of three supraventricular premature complexes (P' waves not seen, but could be buried in the preceding T waves) and finally another sinus complex. Sinus arrest reoccurs, again interrupted by a ventricular escape complex.

ii. Periods of sinus arrest, often with intermittent tachycardia, are typical for sick sinus syndrome (sometimes called bradycardia–tachycardia syndrome). The diseased sinus node exhibits inappropriate periods of arrest. As sympathetic tone rises in response to the arrest, a burst of tachycardia can be stimulated. The tachycardia may cause overdrive suppression of the sick sinus node and additional sinus arrest.

iii. Some cases can be managed with oral anticholinergic, β-2 adrenergic, and/or methylxanthine bronchodilator drugs to minimize collapse episodes caused by the bradycardic periods (the most common cause of syncope); however, this may exacerbate tachycardias. Positive response to medical therapy, if it occurs, is often short-lived. Permanent pacemaker implantation is usually needed for advanced symptomatic sick sinus syndrome. Occasionally, paroxysmal tachycardia also causes syncopal episodes. Antiarrhythmic therapy for the tachyarrhythmia is warranted only after bradycardia is controlled by pacing.

205 A 5-year-old male English Bulldog developed progressive abdominal distension, weakness, and exercise intolerance. Physical findings include ascites, jugular venous distension with pulsation, and a loud left basilar systolic murmur. After other testing is done, the dog is anesthetized for cardiac catheterization. Simultaneous ECG and intracardiac pressures are recorded from the RA (205a) and a pullback from PA to RV (205b). Pressure reference range at left.

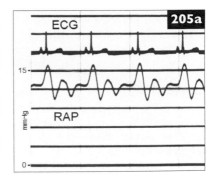

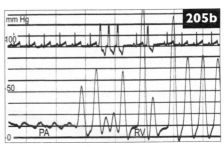

i. What information is evident from 205a?
ii. What is shown in 205b?
iii. What is the diagnosis?
iv. Is there any additional concern regarding the diagnosis given the breed of this dog?

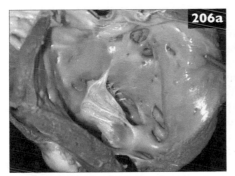

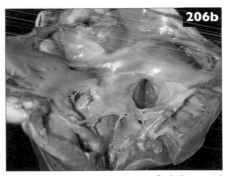

206 An 8-week-old Labrador Retriever puppy is presented because of abdominal distension (ascites), poor appetite, and stunted growth. Euthanasia and necropsy are requested by the breeder. The open RV, with pulmonary valve at top (206a), and the open RA, looking onto the tricuspid valve with RV below (206b), are shown.

i. Describe the abnormal findings
ii. What is the diagnosis?
iii. Does this explain the clinical findings?

205 i. RA pressure is elevated (estimated mean pressure ~12 mmHg) consistent with right-sided heart failure. The 'a' wave (from atrial contraction, 205c) is especially prominent, suggesting RV hypertrophy and increased stiffness.

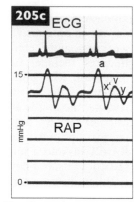

ii. PA pressures are normal (left side, 205b). As the catheter tip moves into the RV, a systolic pressure gradient becomes evident and premature ventricular contractions (VPCs) occur. Note the poor RV systolic pressure generated by the VPCs. After three VPCs, a sinus beat causes markedly increased RV systolic pressure ('post-extrasystolic potentiation'); this recurs after the following single VPC. RV systolic pressure then stabilizes, indicating a systolic PA to RV pressure gradient of about 60 mmHg. Doppler-estimated systolic pressure gradients in unanesthetized animals are usually 40–50% higher than those recorded during cardiac catheterization.

iii. Severe valvular pulmonic stenosis with congestive heart failure.

iv. Some English Bulldogs (and Boxers) have a single anomalous right coronary artery, from which a major left coronary branch courses around the PA and contributes to the stenosis. Balloon valvuloplasty and palliative surgical procedures are generally contraindicated because of the mortality risk from rupture of this vessel.

206 i. A malformed tricuspid valve apparatus is seen. The lateral leaflet inserts directly into a wide, abnormally-formed papillary muscle (206a). A large perforation of the leaflet, as well as abnormal chordal and papillary muscle formations of both leaflets, are also present (206b). Both RA and RV are dilated.

ii. Congenital tricuspid dysplasia. Malformations of the tricuspid valve and its support apparatus occur similarly to those of mitral valve dysplasia. Tricuspid dysplasia is diagnosed most frequently in large-breed dogs; heritability has been shown in Labrador Retrievers. Valve insufficiency most commonly results, but stenosis can also occur, as can abnormal ventral displacement of the valve (Ebstein-like anomaly). Supraventricular tachyarrhythmias are common. Tricuspid regurgitation leads to progressive RA and RV dilation.

iii. Yes. Severe tricuspid dysplasia leads to right-sided congestive heart failure. Initially, the animal may be asymptomatic; but fatigue, ascites, pleural effusion, anorexia, and cardiac cachexia often develop. Physical features include a tricuspid regurgitation murmur (not always audible) and jugular vein pulsation. Jugular distension, muffled heart and lung sounds, and ballotable abdominal fluid develop with congestive failure.

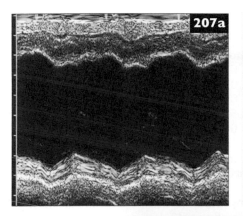

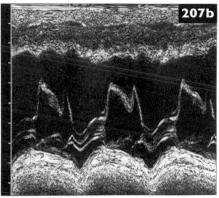

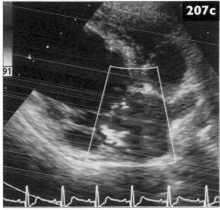

207 An 8-year-old 29 kg (64 lb) female Doberman Pinscher is presented for cardiac screening. The dog is in good condition. Other than two subcutaneous lipomatous masses on the thorax, physical examination is unremarkable. An echocardiogram is done; M-mode images at the ventricular (**207a**) and mitral valve (**207b**) levels and a right parasternal long axis systolic (**207c**) image are shown.

i. What are the echocardiographic findings?

ii. What is your diagnosis?

iii. How would you manage this case?

207 i. M-mode measurements are:

	Diastole (cm)	Systole (cm)
RV wall	0.4	0.9
RV chamber	0.2	0.2
IVS	0.9	1.2
LV chamber	5.7	4.5
LV wall	0.9	1.1

LV FS is 21%. Mitral E-point–septal separation (EPSS) is 1.2 cm (**207b**). Activation of LV wall and IVS is dyssynchronous. LV and LA dilation and mild mitral regurgitation (**207c**) are evident.

ii. Occult (preclinical) dilated cardiomyopathy (DCM), based on: diastolic LV dimension >4.6 cm (in Doberman Pinschers ≤42 kg), systolic LV dimension >3.8 cm, FS <25%, and EPSS >8 mm. Ventricular tachyarrhythmias also are common during occult DCM in Doberman Pinschers. Arrhythmia frequency increases as LV function deteriorates. A 24-hour ambulatory ECG recording is another screening tool for Doberman Pinscher (and Boxer) cardiomyopathy. Doberman Pinschers with >50 ventricular premature complexes (VPCs)/24 hours or any couplets or triplets are likely to develop DCM. Variability in VPC number between repeated Holter recordings in individual dogs can be extensive.

iii. Therapy with an angiotensin-converting enzyme inhibitor and sometimes pimobendan is initiated as LV function deteriorates during the occult phase. Chronic low-dose beta blocker therapy (e.g. carvedilol, metoprolol) is probably beneficial, if tolerated. Oral L-carnitine supplementation (e.g. 3–6 month trial) may help a few Doberman Pinschers.

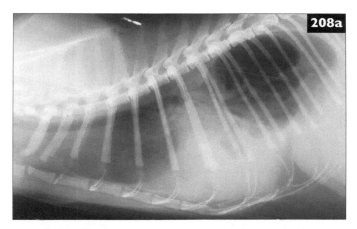

208 A 5-year-old spayed female DSH cat is brought in for re-evaluation because of increasing respiratory effort over the past few weeks. Two years ago you diagnosed hypertrophic cardiomyopathy (HCM) with congestive heart failure (pulmonary edema). The cat responded well to therapy with furosemide, benazepril, and low-dose aspirin. However, the cat was not returned for follow-up over the past year. The cat is alert and has a respiratory rate of 40 breaths/min, with increased effort in both inspiration and expiration. Mucous membranes are pink, pulses are normal bilaterally, HR is 200 bpm and regular. There is mild jugular distension. A soft systolic murmur is heard at the left sternal border; lung sounds are not heard. Lateral (208a) and DV (208b) radiographs are obtained.
i. Describe the radiographic findings.
ii. What would you do next?
iii. How would you change this cat's therapy?

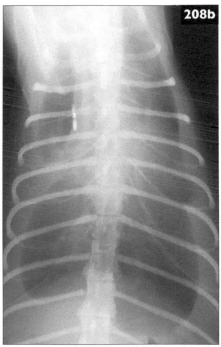

208 i. Large-volume pleural effusion is present, with rounded lung lobe borders suggesting chronicity. The cardiac borders are effaced, but tracheal elevation suggests cardiomegaly. Pulmonary vessels are not clear. A microchip is in the dorsal subcutis. Progressive cardiac disease with biventricular failure is likely in this cat. With lung lobes extending well into the cranial thorax, a mediastinal mass is unlikely.

ii. Thoracocentesis is indicated to improve lung expansion and obtain samples for fluid analysis. A modified transudate is expected with congestive heart failure, but chylous effusion is common in cats with advanced failure. Echocardiography can further characterize cardiac disease. A restrictive form of cardiomyopathy (RCM), can (and did here) develop as the end stage of myocardial failure and infarction from HCM. RCM is characterized by increasingly abnormal ventricular stiffness, restricted filling, and marked LA enlargement; right heart dilation and failure, arrhythmias, intracardiac thrombus, and reduced contractility often develop as well. CBC, serum biochemistries, BP measurement, and ECG would complete the initial database.

iii. Recommendations for intensified therapy in feline advanced biventricular heart failure include increasing furosemide dose and frequency, adding pimobendan and spironolactone, increasing to q12h benazepril, continuing aspirin or clopidogrel, and repeating thoracocentesis as needed. Carefully monitor renal function and electrolytes.

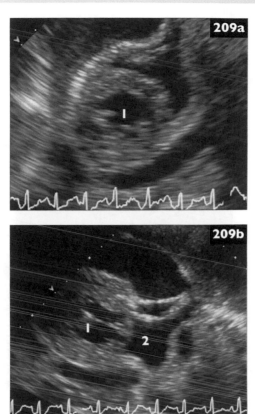

209 A 10-year-old male Golden Retriever is presented for signs of recurrent cardiac tamponade. Signs initially occurred 6 months ago (see case **144**). No evidence of neoplasia could be detected at that time or 2 months later when tamponade recurred. At the latter visit, balloon pericardiotomy was performed, allowing complete drainage of the pericardial effusion. The dog had been asymptomatic until recently. Chest radiographs now show pleural effusion. CBC and serum chemistries are unremarkable, except for mildly increased liver enzyme activities, attributed to hepatic congestion. Another echocardiogram is done; right parasternal short axis (**209a**) and long axis (**209b**) views are shown. 1 – LV, 2 – LA.

i. What is your echocardiographic interpretation?

ii. How could this happen?

iii. How would you proceed with this case?

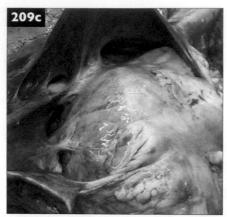

209 i. Recurrent pericardial effusion and tamponade is evidenced by RV and RA collapse (209b). The RV wall is adhered to the pericardium, deforming the RV chamber (209a). A discrete mass lesion could not be identified.

ii. Malignant mesothelioma with pericardial inflammation and scarring is the most likely cause in this older dog. Exaggerated inflammatory response to epicardial abrasion during pericardiotomy, with pericardial adherence, might be another possibility.

iii. Pericardiocentesis may relieve tamponade, but recurrence is likely. Surgical or thoracoscopic pericardectomy may prevent tamponade and allow biopsy, but continued pleural effusion is expected with mesothelioma. This dog developed acute respiratory distress and died before surgery could be pursued. Postmortem examination revealed mesothelioma (with local scar tissue reaction) involving the pericardium (209c) and pleura and a large pulmonary thromboembolus.

Mesothelioma can be difficult to diagnose. Tumor cells often grow diffusely along membrane surfaces, without a discrete mass. Reactive mesothelial cells appear cytologically similar to tumor cells. Even with biopsy, immunohistochemical stains may be required for definitive diagnosis. Prognosis is poor; doxorubicin and intracavitary cisplatin may prolong survival.

210 An adult male dog living in the central USA has recent onset of weakness, abdominal distension, rapid breathing, and inappetence. His mucous membranes are pale; femoral pulses are weak. Jugular distension with pulsation is evident. A regular HR at 180 bpm and a systolic murmur loudest at the right apex are heard. Respirations are rapid, with prominent breath sounds. An echocardiogram is done. A 2-D, right parasternal short axis view at the ventricular level in diastole is shown (210). 1 – RV, 2 – LV

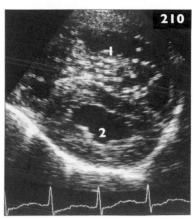

i. Describe the echo findings.
ii. What treatment do you recommend?
iii. What are your follow up recommendations?

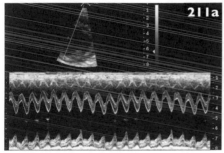

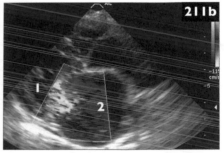

211 An 8-year-old male Cavalier King Charles Spaniel is receiving furosemide, benazepril, pimobendan, and spironolactone for congestive heart failure, initially diagnosed a year ago. Clinical signs of congestion are controlled and no coughing has been noticed. Recently, several collapse episodes have occurred with exertion or excitement.

The dog is alert and responsive. Respiratory rate (25 breaths/min) and pattern are normal. A grade 3/6 systolic heart murmur is loudest over the left apex region, but also heard at the right apex. Systolic BP is 130 mmHg. Echocardiographic images (from right parasternal position) are shown: M-mode at the ventricular level (211a) and 2-D color flow systolic frame from a long axis view (211b). Spectral Doppler interrogation of tricuspid valve regurgitation (TR) yields a peak velocity of 4.6 m/s. 1 – LV, 2 – LA.

i. What are the major echocardiographic abnormalities shown?
ii. How would you interpret the findings on the spectral Doppler study?
iii. What are some likely causes of episodic collapse in this dog?

210 i. Interventricular septal flattening indicates higher diastolic pressure in the RV compared to the LV. The RV wall is almost as thick as the left, consistent with chronic RV systolic pressure overload. Multiple, bright parallel echoes are seen within the RV; these are heartworms entangled in the tricuspid valve apparatus. This dog has caval syndrome, which develops when a mass of heartworms obstructs venous inflow to the heart.

ii. Heartworms must be removed from the heart quickly. Alligator forceps, an endoscopic basket retrieval instrument, or other device can be used to grasp and withdraw the worms via a right jugular venotomy, using local anesthesia and light sedation. The instrument is gently passed down the vein into the RA with fluoroscopic guidance, if available, to retrieve as many worms as possible. Unless treated, most dogs die within 1–3 days from cardiogenic shock complicated by metabolic acidosis, disseminated intravascular coagulation, anemia, and multi-organ failure. Supportive care includes IV fluid and other treatment depending on individual patient needs.

iii. Survivors of acute caval syndrome are given monthly heartworm preventive after being stabilized; adulticide treatment to eliminate the remaining worms can proceed a few weeks later.

211 i. LV motion appears hyperdynamic (FS = 46%; **211a**), as is typical with advanced mitral regurgitation (MR) and well preserved systolic function (increased LV preload with reduced afterload). Marked MR (**211b**) is present; the LA and LV are dilated consistent with chronic MR. Mitral thickening typical for degenerative (myxomatous) mitral valve disease was seen on 2-D views.

ii. The peak TR velocity (4.6 m/s) indicates a systolic pressure gradient of 84.6 mmHg across the tripcuspid valve, according to the Bernoulli relationship ($P = 4 \times v^2$). This suggests a RV systolic pressure of 89.6 mmHg, if RA pressure is normal (~5 mmHg). Because this also represents the estimated PA systolic pressure (if there is no RV outflow obstruction), this indicates concurrent severe pulmonary hypertension (normal PA systolic pressure <25 mmHg). Chronic MR and pulmonary venous hypertension often promote secondary PA hypertension, although usually to a lesser degree than seen here.

iii. Pulmonary hypertension can cause exercise intolerance and collapse by impairing pulmonary blood flow. Collapse could also stem from paroxysmal tachyarrhythmias (usually atrial) or inappropriate bradycardia from neuro-cardiogenic reflexes (e.g. vasovagal syncope).

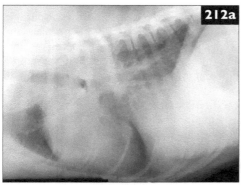

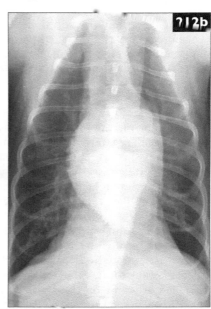

212 A 6-year-old spayed female Lhasa Apso is presented for coughing, which is worse at night. On physical examination there is mild respiratory distress, an occasional cough, and normal thoracic auscultatory findings. Right lateral (212a) and DV (212b) thoracic radiographs are taken.

i. What is the specific location of the major abnormality?
ii. What are the differentials for the lesion?

213 An 8-year-old spayed female DSH cat is presented for anorexia of 1-week duration. Thoracic radiographs reveal a mediastinal mass. After CT-guided biopsy yields a diagnosis of thymoma, a median sternotomy is performed for surgical excision. An intra-operative photograph is shown (213); the cranial aspect of the thorax is to the lower left.

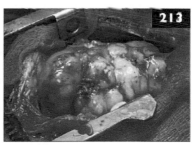

i. What would be the primary differential diagnosis for this mass (prior to confirmation of the diagnosis of thymoma)?
ii. What are the common presenting clinical signs for thymoma in cats?
iii. What paraneoplastic syndromes are possible with thymoma?
iv. What is the most consistent prognostic factor for long-term survival in cats and dogs that have surgical excision of thymoma?
v. What treatment modality can be used for non-resectable thymomas in cats and dogs and provide a reasonable chance of achieving 1–2-year survival?

212 i. There is uniform soft tissue opacity between the heart and the diaphragm. The border effaces the caudal vena cava, the mid-caudal border of the heart, and the central portion of the diaphragm. This suggests a lesion in the accessory lung lobe, a lesion arising from the diaphragm, or plica vena cava of the caudal mediastinum. There is also moderate widening of the mainstem bronchi, best seen in the DV view.

ii. The radiographic findings are non-specific. The general differentials of infection (bacterial or mycotic) and neoplasia are equally likely, both of which could also cause secondary tracheobronchial lymph node enlargement. Because of the normal location of the liver and gastric shadows, diaphragmatic hernia is considered unlikely. Further assessment by ultrasound and CT imaging may aid in defining the origin of the lesion and possibly identify a route for non-surgical biopsy. Surgical biopsy in this patient provided a diagnosis of undifferentiated sarcoma.

213 i. The primary differential diagnosis for mediastinal thymoma in cats is lymphosarcoma. Differentiating between these two tumors by minimally invasive means is important because of the divergent treatment recommendations; chemotherapy for lymphosarcoma versus surgical excision for thymoma.

ii. The most common clinical sign in cats with thymoma is dyspnea. Coughing, anorexia, lethargy, vomiting, and regurgitation are other reported signs.

iii. Paraneoplastic syndromes associated with thymoma, reported in both animals and people, include myasthenia gravis, megaesophagus, hypercalcemia, polymyositis, exfoliative dermatitis, cranial vena cava (cranial caval) syndrome, non-thymic neoplasia, cytopenias, glomerulonephritis, systemic lupus erythematosis, rheumatoid arthritis, thryoiditis, and cardiac arrhythmias.

iv. The percentage lymphocyte composition of the mass is the most consistent prognostic indicator in these cases. Cats and dogs with lymphocyte-rich thymomas live longer than animals with thymomas containing a low lymphocyte percentage. Tumor invasiveness is another factor related to prognosis. Cats and dogs with invasive thymomas have a high rate of immediately postoperative mortality. However, if the animal survives surgery, the chance for 1–2-year survival is good.

v. When a thymoma is determined to be non-resectable, external beam radiation therapy may be employed. While complete responses are rare with radiation therapy of feline and canine thymomas, long-term survival can be achieved.

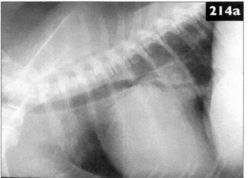

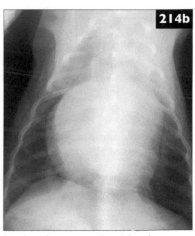

214 An older spayed female Terrier mix is presented for recurrence of a cough. Several months previously she presented for coughing and was diagnosed with chronic mitral valve disease and mild pulmonary edema. Furosemide, enalapril, and pimobendan were prescribed and her cough resolved. She has been doing well until recently. Lateral (214a) and DV (214b) chest radiographs are obtained.

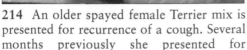

i. What additional historical or physical examination information would be helpful in this case?

ii. What is your radiographic interpretation?

iii. How would you manage this case?

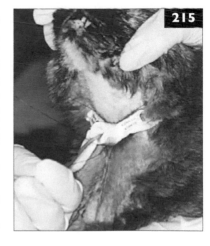

215 A 6-year-old spayed female DSH cat is evaluated for a pharyngeal mass, weight loss, and suspected tongue paresis. Temporary tube tracheostomy is performed when the cat is anesthetized for complete oral examination and biopsy of the mass (later identified as squamous cell carcinoma). The owners declined surgical excision with radiation and chemotherapy, and opted to maintain the tube at home for a time prior to euthanasia.

i. What is the principal indication for tracheostomy tube placement?

ii. List some situations where temporary tube tracheostomy is indicated.

iii. What are the key steps for tracheostomy tube placement?

iv. What two concerns are most important when a tracheostomy tube is in place?

214 i. Is the cough from recurrent pulmonary edema or another cause (e.g. airway collapse or compression, inflammatory small airway disease, parenchymal disease)? Findings more likely associated with decompensating heart failure include reduced exercise tolerance, increased resting respiratory rate, increased HR with minimal to no sinus arrhythmia, soft productive (rather than dry, honking) cough, and reduced appetite. In this case, no change in resting respiratory rate, exercise tolerance, or appetite was observed and a dry cough was described.

ii. There is generalized cardiomegaly (VHS ~12 v) with marked LA enlargement (LAE; note double 'apex' shadow, **214b**) causing left main bronchus compression. No pulmonary edema is evident.

iii. No increase in diuretic dosage is presently indicated. The dog should be screened for hypertension, which can exacerbate mitral regurgitant flow and LAE. Management strategies include enalapril dosing (q12h), if tolerated, and/or cautiously adding amlodipine or hydralazine to further increase forward cardiac output. Monitor BP to avoid hypotension. A cough suppressant helps reduce excessive mechanical or irritative coughing. Continued monitoring for future heart failure decompensation is important. If concurrent small airway disease is suspected, confirmation by airway washing cytology and culture is preferred; if declined, trials of antibiotic, bronchodilator, and anti-inflammatory glucocorticoid therapy can be tried.

215 i. The principal indication for temporary tracheostomy tube placement is to relieve life-threatening upper airway obstruction.

ii. Temporary tracheostomy may be necessary for oropharyngeal/laryngeal trauma, foreign body or tumor, and for laryngeal paralysis. Tube tracheostomy can also be used to facilitate removal of lower airway secretions when the cough reflex is compromised, to allow manual or mechanical ventilation when orotracheal intubation is not practical, to reduce airway resistance in patients with increased intracranial pressure, and to permit inhalant anesthesia during certain intraoral surgical procedures.

iii. After general anesthesia with endotracheal intubation, key surgical steps are to make a short ventral mid-line cervical incision, separate the sternohyoideus muscles, make an interannular tracheal incision less than 50% of the tracheal circumference, place long knotted stay sutures around the tracheal rings cranial and caudal to the incision, remove the endotracheal tube as the tracheostomy tube is inserted, and secure the tube with umbilical tape tied at the back of the neck.

iv. The two major concerns are to avoid obstruction of the tube and infection. Constant monitoring, frequent suctioning, and periodic hydration of the tracheal lumen via saline instillation help to prevent obstruction. Sterile or sanitized supplies and examination gloves are employed during manipulations to decrease contamination.

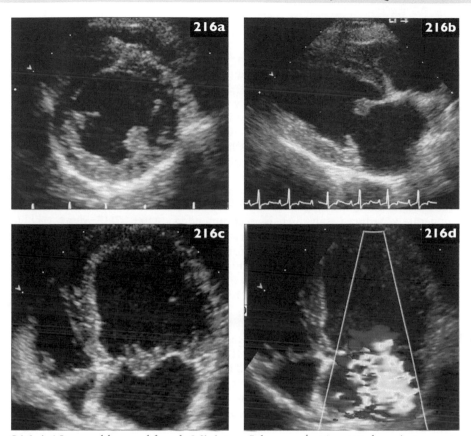

216 A 15-year-old spayed female Miniature Schnauzer has increased respiratory rate and effort, first noticed when sleeping. She also has a mild cough in the morning and is reluctant to go on walks. The dog's HR is 150 bpm; respirations are 50 breaths/min. A grade 4/6 systolic murmur is heard at the left apex. Increased breath sounds, but no crackles, are heard. The rest of the examination is unremarkable. Chest radiographs indicate moderate cardiomegaly with LA prominence and mild perihilar interstitial infiltrates. An echocardiogram is done; diastolic right parasternal short axis (216a) and long axis (216b) and systolic left apical (216c, d) frames are shown.

i. Describe the echo findings.

ii. What is your diagnosis?

iii. How would you manage this case?

217 What is amiodarone, and when is it indicated?

216 **i.** The images show LV and LA enlargement with knobby mitral valve thickening. Color flow Doppler shows marked mitral regurgitation (MR, **216d**). Right heart size appears normal, but the tricuspid valve is also thick.

ii. Advanced degenerative mitral valve disease, with left-sided congestive heart failure (CHF; stage C disease).

iii. Furosemide is used at doses necessary to control the CHF signs (e.g. 1–2 mg/kg q12h initially here). Pimobendan is also indicated now; its positive inotropic and vasodilatory effects should improve cardiac pump function. An angiotensin-converting enzyme inhibitor (ACEI) is also recommended; although conferring only modest diuretic and vasodilatory effects, ACEIs moderate excess neurohormonal responses. Enalapril and benazepril are the most commonly used ACEIs; benazepril's lesser dependence on renal elimination is advantageous with concurrent kidney disease. Exercise is not advised in decompensated CHF. A moderately reduced salt diet is recommended. After CHF signs resolve, furosemide is gradually titrated downward to the lowest effective dosage (and longest consistent dosing interval) for long-term therapy. At-home resting respiratory rate monitoring helps guide this process. Pimobendan and ACEI therapy are continued. Regular mild to moderate exercise can improve quality of life in chronic heart failure. Low-dose beta blocker therapy may be helpful long term.

217 Amiodarone HCl is a 'broad-spectrum' antiarrhythmic drug used for refractory tachyarrhythmias (both atrial and ventricular origin) in dogs. It is an iodinated compound that affects K^+ (and also Na^+ and Ca^{++}) channels and has non-competitive $alpha_1$- and beta-blocking properties. Classified as a class III antiarrhythmic drug, amiodarone prolongs action potential duration and refractoriness in both atrial and ventricular tissues. It may reduce risk of sudden death. Amiodarone's complex pharmacokinetics are characterized by delayed onset of action, prolonged time to steady state, and tissue accumulation of an active metabolite. Potential side-effects with long-term use are many and include depressed appetite, gastrointestinal upset, pneumonitis leading to pulmonary fibrosis, hepatopathy, thyroid dysfunction, and thrombocytopenia, among others. Occasional hypersensitivity reactions (with acute angioedema) or tremors occur, especially with IV use (which also can cause hypotension).

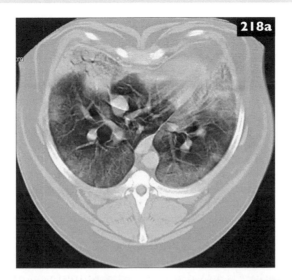

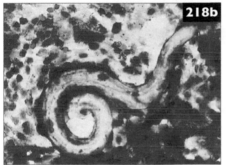

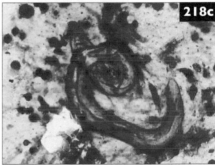

218 Additional testing is done on the dog described in **162**. A hemogram indicates mild anemia, mild neutrophilia, and monocytosis. Serum biochemistry tests are normal, but a coagulation profile shows moderately increased prothrombin and activated partial thromboplastin times. Thoracic CT imaging (**218a**, representative slice from caudal thorax, dog's back is at the bottom) and bronchoscopy are performed. Visual airway inspection reveals small areas of focal hemorrhage in larger airways and some mucus accumulation within the bronchi. BAL fluid cytology shows numerous inflammatory cells, especially macrophages containing hemosiderin pigment and neutrophils; there are also small numbers of eosinophils and parasitic larvae (**218b, c**).

i. What abnormalities can be observed on the CT image?

ii. What is your diagnosis?

iii. What are the available treatment options for this condition?

218 i. Areas of alveolar infiltrate peripherally and around dependant bronchi. This suggests a diffuse pneumonia, although the possible causes are numerous.

ii. The small larvae support a diagnosis of infection with *Angiostrongylus vasorum*, a nematode parasite that infects the PAs and RV of wild and domestic canids. Angiostrongylosis is common in western and northern Europe, but is also reported in several other regions worldwide. Verminous pneumonia and pulmonary vascular lesions are often observed, with thromboarteritis, intimal proliferation, and, in some cases, development of pulmonary hypertension, although this is less common than with heartworm disease (*Dicrofilaria immitis*). Coagulopathies and anemia are often present, as observed in this case.

A. vasorum larvae (L_1) are ~350 µm long and characterized by a kinked tail (**218b**) and dorsal spine (seen better in **218c**). Larvae may also be found on fecal examination (Baermann technique), as L_1 larvae migrate into small airways to be coughed up and swallowed. Multiple fecal samples may be needed for diagnosis because of intermittent shedding.

iii. Several anthelmintics can kill adult *A. vasorum* worms. Fenbendazole, imidacloprid/moxidectin, or milbemycin are commonly used (see case **154** for doses). Supportive care is provided as needed; post-treatment parasitic embolism, similar to heartworm disease, is possible.

219 A 9-year-old 40 kg (88 lb) male Laborador Retriever is referred for a 2-week history of exercise intolerance, non-productive cough, and ascites (modified transudate). Furosemide (40 mg q12h) and spironolactone (50 mg q12h) have been prescribed by another veterinarian. The dog is alert, well hydrated, overweight, and panting. Body temperature is 38.9°C (102°F); HR is 72 bpm. Mucous membranes and femoral pulses are normal. Jugular veins are mildly distended. No heart murmur is heard and lung sounds are normal. The abdomen is severely distended with ascites. Systolic BP is normal. Chest radiographs show minimal cardiac enlargment (VHS 11.6 v) with a moderate volume of pleural fluid. Laboratory tests reveal a stress leukogram, mild hyperglycemia, and mild hypoalbuminemia. Central venous pressure (CVP) is 16 mmHg (normal 0–5 mmHg). Echocardiography shows trivial AV valve insufficiency; right parasternal short axis (**219a**) and left apical 4-chamber (**219b**) images are shown.

i. Describe the echo findings.
ii. What is your assessment of this case?
iii. What are your recommendations?

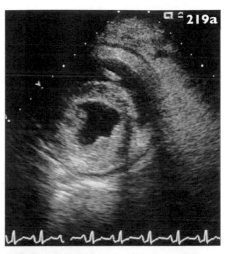

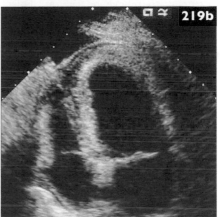

219 i. There is a tiny amount of pericardial effusion. Cardiac chamber proportions are unremarkable. A mass lesion is not evident. Some pleural effusion is seen near the cardiac apex (**219b**).

ii. Elevated CVP with bicavitary effusion occurs from diseases causing right-sided congestive heart failure, cardiac tamponade, restrictive pericardial disease, and other inflow obstruction. Evidence for primary right-sided heart disease, cardiac tamponade, or intracardiac obstruction is lacking here. Constrictive pericardial disease was diagnosed. This can develop subsequent to bouts of idiopathic pericardial effusion, but this dog has no history of this. Other causes include pericardial infection (e.g. actinomycosis, coccidioidomycosis), foreign body, and neoplasia (including mesothelioma), but the etiology often is unknown.

iii. Medical therapy (e.g. diuretic, vasodilator) is ineffective and further reduces cardiac output. Constrictive pericarditis requires surgical pericardiectomy to improve ventricular filling; pericardial window and balloon pericardiotomy procedures are generally inadequate. Pericardiectomy is more likely to succeed if parietal pericardium only is affected. Visceral pericardial involvement and adhesions require epicardial stripping to relieve restriction. This increases surgical difficulty and associated complications. Excised tissue should be biopsied (mesothelioma was diagnosed in this case). Complications can include myocardial bleeding, cardiac perforation, pulmonary thrombosis, disseminated intravascular coagulopathy, arrhythmias, and cardiac arrest.

Drugs used for cardiac and respiratory diseases

Drug	Dog doses	Cat doses
Acepromazine	0.02–0.1 mg/kg (up to 3 mg total) IV, IM, SC	Same
Albuterol	0.02–0.05 mg/kg PO q6–8h	Same
Amikacin	5–10 mg/kg IV, SC q8h	Same
Aminophylline	11 mg/kg PO, IM, IV q8h	5 mg/kg PO, IM, IV q12h
Amiodarone	10 mg/kg PO q12h for 7 days, then 8 mg/kg PO q24h (lower as well as higher doses have been used); 3(–5) mg/kg slowly (over 10–20 minutes) IV (can repeat, but do not exceed 10 mg/kg in 1 hour)	—
Amlodipine	0.05–0.3(–0.5) mg/kg PO q12–24h	0.625 (–1.25) mg/cat (or 0.1–0.5 mg/kg) PO q24(–12)h
Amoxicillin	22 mg/kg PO q8–12h	Same
Amoxicillin–clavulanate	20–25 mg/kg PO q8h	Same
Ampicillin	22 mg/kg PO, IV, SC q8h	Same
Azithromycin	5–10 mg/kg PO q24h for 3 days, then q48–72h	5–10 mg/kg PO q24h for 3 days, then q72h
Aspirin	0.5 mg/kg PO q12h	Low-dose, 5 mg/cat q72h (or 20–40 mg/cat [¼–½ baby aspirin] PO 2–3 times a week)
Atenolol	0.2–1.0 mg/kg PO q12–24h	6.25–12.5 mg/cat PO q(12–)24h
Atropine	0.02–0.04 mg/kg IV, IM, SC; 0.04 mg/kg PO q6–8h. Atropine response test: 0.04 mg/kg IV; record ECG 5–10 minutes after injection. If HR not increased by ≥150%, repeat ECG 15 (to 20) minutes after injection.	Same
Benazepril	0.25–0.5 mg/kg PO q(12–)24h	0.25–0.5 mg/kg PO q(12–)24h

Drugs used for cardiac and respiratory diseases

Drug	Dog doses	Cat doses
Buprenorphine	0.005–0.02 mg/kg IM, IV, SC q6–8h	0.005–0.02 mg/kg IM, IV, SC q6–8h
Butorphanol	0.2–0.4 mg/kg IM, IV, SC q2–4h; antitussive: 0.05–0.06 mg/kg SC q6–12h or 0.5 mg/kg PO	0.2–0.8 mg/kg IV, SC q2–6h; 1.5 mg/kg PO q4–8h
Captopril	0.5–2.0 mg/kg PO q8–12h	0.5–1.25 mg/kg PO q12–24h
Carvedilol	0.05 mg/kg q24h (initial dose, if cardiac disease), gradually titrate up to 0.2–0.4 mg/kg PO q12h as tolerated; possibly up to 1.5 mg/kg PO q12h PO if needed	—
Cefazolin	20–35 mg/kg IM, IV q8h	Same
Cephalexin	20–40 mg/kg q8h	Same
Chlorothiazide	10–40 mg/kg PO q12–48h (start low)	10–40 mg/kg PO q12–48h (start low)
Clindamycin	5.5–11(–20) mg/kg PO, SC, IM, IV q12(–24)h	5.5–11(–25) mg/kg PO, SC, IM, q12–24h
Clopidogrel	2–4 mg/kg PO q24h; oral loading dose, 10 mg/kg	¼ (–½?) of 75 mg tab/cat PO q24h
Codeine	0.1–0.3 mg/kg PO q4–6h (antitussive)	—
Dalteparin sodium	100–150 U/kg SC q12(–24)h	100 U/kg SC q12(–24)h
Dexamethasone	0.1–0.2 mg/kg IV, IM, PO q12–24h	Same
Dextro-methorphan	1–2 mg/kg q6–8h	—
Digoxin	PO: dogs <22 kg, 0.005–0.008 mg/kg q12h; dogs >22 kg, 0.22 mg/m^2 or 0.003–0.005 mg/kg q12h. Decrease by 10% for elixir. Maximum: 0.5 mg/day or 0.375 mg/day for Doberman Pinschers	0.007 mg/kg (or ¼ of 0.125 mgtab) PO q48h

Drugs used for cardiac and respiratory diseases

Drug	Dog doses	Cat doses
Diltiazem	Oral maintenance: initial dose 0.5 mg/kg (up to 2+ mg/kg) PO q8h; acute IV for supraventricular tachycardia: 0.15–0.25 mg/kg over 2–3 minutes IV, can repeat every 15 minutes until conversion or maximum 0.75 mg/kg; CRI: 5–15 mg/kg/hour; PO loading dose: 0.5 mg/kg PO followed by 0.25 mg/kg PO q1h to a total of 1.5(–2.0) mg/kg or conversion. Diltiazem (Dilacor) XR, 1.5–4 (–6) mg/kg PO q 12–24h	Same? For HCM: 1.5–2.5 mg/kg (or7.5–10 mg/cat) PO q8h; sustained-release preparations: Diltiazem (Dilacor) XR, 30 mg/cat/day (½ of a 60 mg controlled-release tablet within the 240 mg gelatin capsule), can increase to 60 mg/day in some cats if necessary; (45 mg/cat ~105 mg of Cardizem-CD, 10 mg/kg/day Cardizem-CD, or amount that fits into small end of a No. 4 gelatin capsule)
Diphenhydra-mine	1 mg/kg IM; 2–4 mg/kg PO q8h (or 25–50 mg/dog IV, IM, PO)	1 mg/kg IM, IV q6–8h; 2–4 mg/kg PO q6–8h
Dobutamine	1–20 mcg/kg/minute CRI; start low	1–5 mcg/kg/minute CRI; start low
Dopamine	1–10 mcg/kg/minute CRI; start low	1–5 mcg/kg/minute CRI; start low
Doxycycline	5–10 mg/kg PO, IV q12h	Same
Enalapril	0.5 mg/kg PO q12–24h	0.25–0.5 mg/kg PO q(12–)24h
Enalaprilat	0.2 mg/kg IV, repeated q1–2h as needed	—
Enoxaparin	0.8 mg/kg SC q6h	1–1.25 mg/kg SC q6–12h
Enrofloxacin	5–20 mg/kg PO, IM q24h	5 mg/kg PO q24h
Esmolol	0.1–0.5 mg/kg IV over 1 minute (loading dose), followed by infusion of 0.025–0.2 mg/kg/minute	Same
Fenbendazole	25–50 mg/kg PO q12h for 14 days (lungworms); 20–50 mg/kg for [5–] 21 days (*A. vasorum*)	Same (lungworms)
Flecainide	(?) 1–5 mg/kg PO q8–12h	—
Fosinopril	0.25–0.5 mg/kg PO q24h	—

Drugs used for cardiac and respiratory diseases

Drug	Dog doses	Cat doses
Furosemide	Acute: 2–5[–8] mg/kg IV or IM, q1–4h until respiratory rate decreases, then 1–4 mg/kg q6–12h, or 0.6–1 mg/kg/hour CRI. Long term: 1–3(or more) mg/kg PO q8–24h; use smallest effective dose	Acute: 1–2[–4] mg/kg IV or IM, q1–4h until respiratory rate decreases, then q6–12h. Long term: 1–2 mg/kg PO q8–12h; use smallest effective dose
Gentamicin	9–14 mg/kg IV. IM, SC q24h	5-8 mg/kg IV, IM, SC q24h
Glycopyrrolate	0.005–0.01 mg/kg IV or IM; 0.01–0.02 mg/kg SC as needed	Same
Heparin sodium	200–250 IU/kg IV, followed by 200–300 IU/kg SC q6–8h for 2–4 days or as needed	Same
Hydralazine	0.5–2 mg/kg PO q12h (to 1 mg/kg initial); for hypertensive crisis: 0.2 mg/kg IV or IM, repeated q2h as needed	2.5 (up to 10) mg/cat PO q12h
Hydro-chlorothiazide	0.5–4 mg/kg PO q12-48h (start low)	0.5–2 mg/kg PO q12–48h (start low)
Hydrocodone bitartrate	0.25 mg/kg PO q4–12h	Not recommended
Hydrocortisone sodium succinate	Shock: 50–150 mg/kg IV; anti-inflammatory: 5 mg/kg IV q12h	Same
Hyoscyamine	0.003–0.006 mg/kg PO q8h	—
Imidacloprid/ moxidectin	0.1 ml/kg (10[–25] mg/kg plus 2.5[–6.25] mg/kg) topical, single dose (*A. vasorum*)	—
Imidapril	0.25 mg/kg PO q24h	—
Isoproterenol	0.045–0.09 mcg/kg/minute CRI	Same
Isosorbide dinitrate	0.5–2 mg/kg PO q(8–)12h	—
Isosorbide mononitrate	0.25–2 mg/kg PO q12h	—
Ivermectin	Heartworm prevention: 6 mcg/kg PO q30days; endoparasites: 200–400 mcg/kg SC, PO weekly	Heartworm prevention: 24 mcg/kg PO q30days; endoparasites: same
l-Carnitine	1 g (for dogs <25 kg) to 2 g (for dogs 25–40 kg) q8h; mix with food	—

Drugs used for cardiac and respiratory diseases

Drug	Dog doses	Cat doses
Labetolol	0.25 mg/kg IV over 2 minutes, repeated up to a total dose of 3.75 mg/kg; follow with 25 mcg/kg/minute CRI	—
Lidocaine	Initial boluses of 2 mg/kg slowly IV, up to 8 mg/kg; or rapid IV infusion at 0.8 mg/kg/minute; if effective, then 25–80 mcg/kg/minute CRI; can also be used intratracheally for CPR	Initial bolus of 0.25–0.5 (or 1.0) mg/kg slowly IV; can repeat boluses of 0.15–0.25 mg/kg, up to total of 4 mg/kg; if effective, 10–40 mcg/kg/minute CRI
Lisinopril	0.25–0.5 mg/kg PO q(12–)24h	0.25–0.5 mg/kg PO q24h
Marbofloxacin	3–5.5 mg/kg PO q24h	Same
Melarsomine	2.5 mg/kg IM (see case 27 for instructions)	Not recommended
Metoprolol	Initial dose, 0.1–0.2 mg/kg PO q24(–12)h, up to 1 mg/kg q8(–12)h	—
Metronidazole	10 mg/kg PO q8h	10 mg/kg PO q12h
Mexiletine	4–10 mg/kg PO q8h	—
Milbemycin oxime	0.5–1.0 mg/kg PO q30days (heartworm prevention); 0.5 mg/kg PO once weekly for 4 weeks (*A. vasorum*)	2 mg/kg PO q30days (heartworm prevention)
Moxidectin	3 mcg/kg PO q30days (heartworm prevention)	—
Nitroglycerin 2% ointment	½–1½ inch percutaneously q4–6h	¼–½ inch percutaneously q4–6h
Nitroprusside	0.5–1 mcg/kg/minute CRI (initial) to 5–15 mcg/kg/minute CRI	Same
Oxtriphylline	14 mg/kg PO q8h	—
Phenoxy-benzamine	0.2–0.5 mg/kg PO q(8–)12h	0.2–0.5 mg/kg or 2.5 mg/cat PO q12h
Phentolamine	0.02–0.1 mg/kg IV bolus, followed by CRI to effect	Same
Phenytoin	10 mg/kg slowly IV; 30–50 mg/kg PO q8h	Do not use
Pimobendan	0.2–0.3 mg/kg PO q12h	As for dog, or 1.25 mg/cat PO q12h

Drugs used for cardiac and respiratory diseases

Drug	Dog doses	Cat doses
Praziquantel	23 mg/kg PO q8h for 3 days (for *Paragonimus*)	Same
Prazosin	0.05–0.2 mg/kg PO q8–12h	—
Prednisone	0.25–2 mg/kg PO q12h	Same
Prednisolone sodium succinate	Up to 10 mg/kg IV	Same
Procainamide	6 –10 (up to 20) mg/kg IV over 5–10 minutes; 10–50 mcg/kg/minute CRI; 6–20 (up to 30) mg/kg IM q4–6h; 10–25 mg/kg PO q6h (sustained release: q6–8h)	1.0–2.0 mg/kg slowly IV; 10–20 mcg/kg/minute CRI; 7.5–20 mg/kg IM or PO q(6–)8h
Propafenone	2–4 (up to 6) mg/kg PO q8h (start low)	—
Propantheline bromide	3.73–7.5 mg/dog PO q8–12h	—
Propranolol	0.02 mg/kg initial bolus slowly IV (up to maximum of 0.1 mg/kg); initial dose, 0.1–0.2 mg/kg PO q8h, up to 1 mg/kg q8h	Same IV instructions; 2.5 up to 10 mg/cat PO q8–12h
Quinidine	6–20 mg/kg IM q6h (loading dose, 14–20 mg/kg); 6–16 mg/kg PO q6h; sustained action preparations, 8–20 mg/kg PO q8h	6–16 mg/kg IM or PO q8h
Ramipril	0.125–0.25 mg/kg PO q24h	—
Selamectin	6–12 mg/kg, topical q30days (heartworm prevention)	Same
Sildenafil	0.5–2 (–3) mg/kg PO q8–12h	—
Sotalol	1–3.5 (–5) mg/kg PO q12h	10–20 mg/cat PO q12h (or 2–4 mg/kg PO q12h)
Spironolactone	0.5–2 mg/kg PO q(12–)24h	0.5–1 mg/kg PO q(12–)24h
Taurine	0.5–1 g (for dogs <25 kg) to 1–2 g (for dogs 25 – 40 kg) PO q(8–)12h	0.25 (–0.5) g PO q12(–24)h (myocardial failure)
Terbutaline	1.25–5 mg/dog PO q8–12h	$^{1}/_{8}$–$^{1}/_{4}$ of 2.5 mg tablet/cat q12h PO initially, up to ½ tablet q12h; 0.01 mg/kg SC, can repeat once in 5–10 minutes if needed
Tetracycline	22 mg/kg PO q8h	Same

Drugs used for cardiac and respiratory diseases

Drug	Dog doses	Cat doses
Theophylline base (immediate release)	9 mg/kg PO q8h	4 mg/kg PO q12h
Theophylline (long acting)	10 mg/kg PO q12h	15 mg/kg PO q24h (in evening)
Trimethoprim-sulfadiazine	15–30 mg/kg PO q12h	Same
Vitamin K_1	2–5 mg/kg PO, SC q24h	Same
Verapamil	Initial dose, 0.02–0.05 mg/kg slowly IV, can repeat q5minutes to total of 0.15(–0.2) mg/kg; 0.5–2 mg/kg PO q8h (**Note:** diltiazem preferred)	Initial dose, 0.025 mg/kg slowly IV, can repeat q5minutes to total of 0.15 (–0.2) mg/kg; 0.5–1 mg/kg PO q8h. (**Note:** diltiazem preferred)
Warfarin	0.1–0.2 mg/kg PO q24h	0.5 mg/cat PO q24h

HCM, hypertrophic cardiomyopathy; CRI, constant rate infusion; CPR, cardiopulmonary resuscitation; IM, intramuscularly; IV, intravenously; PO, orally; SC, subcutaneously; —, effective dosage not known.

Further reading

CARDIOPULMONARY SIGNS
Arterial pulses
Tidholm A (2010) Pulse alterations. In *Textbook of Veterinary Internal Medicine*, 7th edn. (eds SJ Ettinger, EC Feldman) Saunders Elsevier, St. Louis, pp. 264–265.

Ware WA (2011) The cardiovascular examination. In *Cardiovascular Disease in Small Animal Medicine*. (ed WA Ware) Manson Publishing, London, pp. 26–33.

Cardiac auscultation abnormalities
Prosek R (2010) Abnormal heart sounds and heart murmurs. In *Textbook of Veterinary Internal Medicine*, 7th edn. (eds SJ Ettinger, EC Feldman) Saunders Elsevier, St. Louis, pp. 259–263.

Ware WA (2011) The normal cardiovascular system; The cardiovascular examination; and Murmurs and abnormal heart sounds. In *Cardiovascular Disease in Small Animal Medicine*. (ed WA Ware) Manson Publishing, London, pp. 10–25, 26–33, and 92–97.

Cyanosis
Allen J (2010) Cyanosis. In *Textbook of Veterinary Internal Medicine*, 7th edn. (eds SJ Ettinger, EC Feldman) Saunders Elsevier, St. Louis, pp. 283–286.

Forrester SD, Moon ML, Jacobson JD (2001) Diagnostic evaluation of dogs and cats with respiratory distress. *Compend Contin Educ Pract Vet* 23:56–68.

Lee JA, Drobatz KJ (2004) Respiratory distress and cyanosis in dogs. In *Textbook of Respiratory Disease in Dogs and Cats*. (ed LG King) Elsevier Saunders, St. Louis, pp. 1–12.

Jugular vein distension or pulsation
Riel DL (2010) Jugular catheterization and central venous pressure. In *Textbook of Veterinary Internal Medicine*, 7th edn. (eds SJ Ettinger, EC Feldman) Saunders Elsevier, St. Louis, pp. 317–318.

Ware WA (2011) Jugular vein distension or pulsations. In *Cardiovascular Disease in Small Animal Medicine*. (ed WA Ware) Manson Publishing, London, pp. 117–120.

Respiratory distress and hypoxemia
Hackett TB (2009) Tachypnea and hypoxemia. In *Small Animal Critical Care Medicine*. (eds DC Silverstein, K Hopper) Elsevier, St. Louis, pp. 37–40.

Haskins SC (2004) Interpretation of blood gas measurements. In *Textbook of Respiratory Disease in Dogs and Cats*. (ed LG King) Elsevier Saunders, St. Louis, pp. 181–193.

Hawkins EC (2009) Diagnostic tests for the lower respiratory tract. In *Small Animal Internal Medicine*, 4th edn. (eds RW Nelson, CG Couto) Mosby, St. Louis, pp. 252–284.

Koch DA, Arnold S, Hubler M *et al.* (2003) Brachycephalic syndrome in dogs. *Compend Cont Educ Pract Vet* 25:48–54.

Lee JA, Drobatz KJ (2004) Respiratory distress and cyanosis in dogs. In *Textbook of Respiratory Disease in Dogs and Cats*. (ed LG King) Elsevier Saunders, St. Louis, pp. 1–12.

Miller CJ (2007) Approach to the respiratory patient. *Vet Clin Small Anim* 37:861–878.

Syncope
Ware WA (2011) Syncope or intermittent collapse. In *Cardiovascular Disease in Small Animal Medicine*. (ed WA Ware) Manson Publishing, London, pp. 139–144.

Yee K (2010) Syncope. In *Textbook of Veterinary Internal Medicine*, 7th edn. (eds SJ Ettinger, EC Feldman) Saunders Elsevier, St. Louis, pp. 275–277.

CARDIOPULMONARY TESTS
Biomarkers
Boswood A (2009) Biomarkers in cardiovascular disease: beyond natriuretic peptides. *J Vet Cardiol* 11:S23–S32.

Connolly DJ, Soares Magalhaes RJ, Syme HM *et al.* (2008) Circulating natriuretic peptides in cats with heart disease. *J Vet Intern Med* 22:96–105.

Herndon WE, Rishniw M, Schrope D *et al.* (2008) Assessment of plasma cardiac troponin I concentration as a means to differentiate cardiac and noncardiac causes of dyspnea in cats. *J Am Med Assoc* 232:1261–1264.

Ljungvall I, Hoglund K, Tidholm A *et al.*

(2010) Cardiac troponin I is associated with severity of myxomatous mitral valve disease, age, and C-reactive protein in dogs. *J Vet Intern Med* **24**:153–159.

MacDonald KA, Kittleson MD, Munro C *et al.* (2003) Brain natriuretic peptide concentration in dogs with heart disease and congestive heart failure. *J Vet Intern Med* **17**:172–177.

Oyama MA, Sisson DD (2004) Cardiac troponin-I concentration in dogs with cardiac disease. *J Vet Intern Med* **18**:831–839.

Oyama MA, Rush JE, Rozanski EA *et al.* (2009) Assessment of serum N-terminal pro-B-type natriuretic peptide concentration for differentiation of congestive heart failure from primary respiratory tract disease as the cause of respiratory signs in dogs. *J Am Med Assoc* **235**:1319–1325.

Prosek R, Ettinger SJ. (2010) Biomarkers of cardiovascular disease. In *Textbook of Veterinary Internal Medicine*, 7th edn. (eds SJ Ettinger, EC Feldman) Saunders Elsevier, St. Louis, pp. 1187–1196.

Serres F, Pouchelon JL, Poujol L *et al.* (2009) Plasma N-terminal pro-B-type natriuretic peptide concentration helps to predict survival in dogs with symptomatic degenerative mitral valve disease regardless of and in combination with the initial clinical status at admission. *J Vet Cardiol* **11**:103–121.

Spratt DP, Mellanby RJ, Drury N *et al.* (2005) Cardiac troponin I: evaluation of a biomarker for the diagnosis of heart disease in the dog. *J Small Anim Pract* **46**:139–145.

Wess G, Simak J, Mahling M *et al.* (2010) Cardiac troponin I in Doberman Pinschers with cardiomyopathy. *J Vet Intern Med* **24**:843–849.

Zimmering TM, Meneses F, Nolte IJ *et al.* (2009) Measurement of N-terminal proatrial natriuretic peptide in plasma of cats with and without cardiomyopathy *Am J Vet Res* **70**:216–222.

Echocardiography

Belanger MC (2010) Echocardiography. In *Textbook of Veterinary Internal Medicine*, 7th edn. (eds SJ Ettinger, EC Feldman) Saunders Elsevier, St. Louis, pp. 415–431.

Bonagura JD, Miller MW, Darke PG (1998) Doppler echocardiography I. Pulsed-wave and continuous wave examinations. *Vet Clin North Am Small Anim Pract* **28**:1325–1359.

Campbell FE, Kittleson MD (2007) The effect of hydration status on the echocardiographic measurements of normal cats *J Vet Intern Med* **21**:1008–1015.

Cornell CC, Kittleson MD, Torre PD *et al.* (2004) Allometric scaling of M-Mode cardiac measurements in normal adult dogs. *J Vet Intern Med* **18**:311.

Koffas H, Dukes-McEwan J, Corcoran BM *et al.* (2006) Pulsed tissue Doppler imaging in normal cats and cats with hypertrophic cardiomyopathy. *J Vet Intern Med* **20**:65–77.

Schober KE, Hart TM, Stern JA *et al.* (2010) Detection of congestive heart failure in dogs by Doppler echocardiography. *J Vet Intern Med* **20**:1358–1368.

Ware WA (2011) Overview of echocardiography. In *Cardiovascular Disease in Small Animal Medicine*. (ed WA Ware) Manson Publishing, London, pp. 68–90.

Electrocardiographic interpretation and abnormalities (see Cardiac arrhythmias for rhythm disturbances)

Bonagura JD (1981) Electrical alternans associated with pericardial effusion in the dog. *J Am Vet Med Assoc* **178**:574–579.

MacKie BA, Stepien RL, Kellihan HB (2010) Retrospective analysis of an implantable loop recorder for evaluation of syncope, collapse, or intermittent weakness in 23 dogs (2004–2008). *J Vet Cardiol* **12**:25–33.

Miller M, Tilley LP, Smith FWK *et al.* (1999) Electrocardiography. In *Textbook of Canine and Feline Cardiology*, 2nd edn. (eds PR Fox, D Sisson, NS Moise) WB Saunders, Philadelphia, pp. 67–105.

Rishniw M, Bruskiewicz K (1996) ECG of the month. Respiratory sinus arrhythmia and wandering pacemaker in a cat. *J Am Vet Med Assoc* **208**:1811–1812.

Stafford Johnson M, Martin M, Binns S *et al.* (2004) A retrospective study of clinical findings, treatment and outcome in 143 dogs with pericardial effusion. *J Small Anim Pract* **45**:546–552.

Tag TL, Day TK (2008) Electrocardiographic assessment of hyperkalemia in dogs and cats. *J Vet Emerg Crit Care* **18**:61–67.

Further reading

Tilley LP (1985) Artifacts. In *Essentials of Canine and Feline Electrocardiogpraphy*, 2nd edn. (ed LP Tilley) Lea & Febiger, Philadelphia, pp. 240–246.

Ware WA (2011) Overview of electrocardiography. In *Cardiovascular Disease in Small Animal Medicine*. (ed WA Ware) Manson Publishing, London, pp. 47–67.

Ware WA, Christensen WF (1999) Twenty-four-hour ambulatory electrocardiography in normal cats. *J Vet Intern Med* **13**:175–180.

Radiography

Berry CR, Graham JP, Thrall DE (2007) Interpretation paradigms for the small animal thorax. In *Textbook of Veterinary Diagnostic Radiology*, 5th edn. (ed DE Thrall) Saunders Elsevier, St. Louis, pp. 462–485.

Buchanan JW, Bücheler J (1995) Vertebral scale system to measure canine heart size in radiographs. *J Am Vet Med Assoc* **206**:194.

Buecker A, Wein BB, Neuerburg JM et al. (1997) Esophageal perforation: comparison of use of aqueous and barium-containing contrast media. *Radiology* **202**:683–686.

Coulson A, Lewis ND (2002) *An Atlas of Interpretive Radiographic Anatomy of the Dog and Cat*. Blackwell Science, Oxford.

Litster AL, Buchanan JW (2000) Vertebral scale system to measure heart size in radiographs of cats. *J Am Vet Med Assoc* **216**:210–214.

McAlister WH, Askin FB (1983) The effect of some contrast agents in the lung: an experimental study in the rat and dog. *Am J Roentgenol* **140**:245–251.

Moon ML, Keene BW, Lessard P et al. (1993) Age-related changes in the feline cardiac silhouette. *Vet Radiol Ultrasound* **34**:315–320.

Nawrocki MA, Mackin AJ, McLaughlin R et al. (2003) Fluoroscopic and endoscopic localization of an esophagobronchial fistula in a dog. *J Am Anim Hosp Assoc* **39**:257–261.

O'Brien RT (2001) *Thoracic Radiography for the Small Animal Practitioner*. Teton NewMedia, Jackson.

Reif JS, Rhodes WH (1966) The lungs of aged dogs: a radiographic–morphologic correlation. *J Am Vet Radiol Soc* **7**:5–11.

Sleeper MM, Buchanan JW (2001) Vertebral scale system to measure heart size in growing puppies. *J Am Vet Med Assoc* **219**:57–59.

Suter PF (1984) (ed) *Thoracic Radiography: A Text Atlas of Thoracic Diseases of the Dog and Cat*. Wettswil, Switzerland, pp. 533–537.

Ware WA (2011) Overview of cardiac radiography. In *Cardiovascular Disease in Small Animal Medicine*. (ed WA Ware) Manson Publishing, London, pp. 34–46.

CARDIAC THERAPY: ARRHYTHMIA MANAGEMENT

Bradyarrhythmias

Bulmer BJ, Sisson DD, Oyama MA et al. (2006) Physiologic VDD versus nonphysiologic VVI pacing in canine 3rd degree atrioventricular block. *J Vet Intern Med* **20**:257–271.

DeFrancesco TC, Hansen BD, Atkins CE et al. (2003) Noninvasive transthoracic temporary cardiac pacing in dogs. *J Vet Intern Med* **17**:663–667.

Estrada AH, Maisenbacher III HW, Prosek R et al. (2009) Evaluation of pacing site in dogs with naturally occurring complete heart block. *J Vet Cardiol* **11**:79–88.

Ferasin L, van de Stad M, Rudorf H et al. (2002) Syncope associated with paroxysmal atrioventricular block and atrial standstill in a cat. *J Small Anim Pract* **43**:124–128.

Fine DM, Tobias AH (2007) Cardiovascular device infections in dogs: report of 8 cases and review of the literature. *J Vet Intern Med* **21**:1265–1271.

Forterre S, Nürnberg J-H, Skrodzki M et al. (2001) Transvenous demand pacemaker treatment for intermittent complete heart block in a cat. *J Vet Cardiol* **3**:21–26.

Fox PR, Moise NS, Woodfield JA et al. (1991) Techniques and complications of pacemaker implantation in four cats. *J Am Vet Med Assoc* **199**:1742–1753.

Francois L, Chetboul V, Nicolle A et al. (2004) Pacemaker implantation in dogs: results of the last 30 years. *Schweiz Arch Tierheilkd* **146**:335–344.

Hildebrandt N, Stertmann WA, Wehner M et al. (2009) Dual chamber pacemaker implantation in dogs with atrioventricular block. *J Vet Intern Med* **23**:31–38.

Johnson MS, Martin MWS, Henley W (2007) Results of pacemaker implantation in 104 dogs. *J Small Anim Pract* 48:4–11.

Kaneshige T, Machida N, Itoh H *et al.* (2006) The anatomical basis of complete atrioventricular block in cats with hypertrophic cardiomyopathy. *J Comp Path* 135:25–31.

Kellum HB, Stepien RL (2006) Third-degree atrioventricular block in 21 cats (1997–2004). *J Vet Intern Med* 20:97–103.

MacAulay K (2002) Permanent transvenous pacemaker implantation in an Ibizan hound cross with persistent atrial standstill. *Can Vet J* 43:789–91.

Maisenbacher III HW, Estrada AH, Prosek R *et al.* (2009) Evaluation of the effects of transvenous pacing site on left ventricular function and synchrony in healthy anesthetized dogs. *Am J Vet Res* 70:455–463.

Oyama MA, Sisson DD (2009) Permanent cardiac pacing in dogs. In *Kirk's Current Veterinary Therapy XIV*. (eds JD Bonagura, DC Twedt) Saunders Elsevier, St. Louis, pp. 717–721.

Oyama MA, Sisson DD, Lehmkuhl LB (2001) Practices and outcome of artificial cardiac pacing in 154 dogs. *J Vet Intern Med* 15:229–239.

Penning VA, Connolly DJ, Gajanayake I *et al.* (2009) Seizure-like episodes in 3 cats with intermittent high-grade atrioventricular dysfunction. *J Vet Intern Med* 23:200–205.

Saunders A (2005) ECG of the month. Sick sinus syndrome. *J Am Vet Med Assoc* 227:51–52.

Van De Wiele CM, Hogan DF, Green III HW *et al.* (2008) Cranial vena caval syndrome secondary to transvenus pacemaker implantation in two dogs. *J Vet Cardiol* 10:155–161.

Ware WA (2011) Managment of arrhythmias. In *Cardiovascular Disease in Small Animal Medicine*. (ed WA Ware) Manson Publishing, London, pp. 194–226.

Wess G, Thomas WP, Berger DM *et al.* (2006) Applications, complications, and outcomes of transvenous pacemaker implantation in 105 dogs (1997–2002). *J Vet Intern Med* 20:877–884.

Zimmerman SA, Bright JM (2004) Secure pacemaker fixation critical for prevention of Twiddler's syndrome. *J Vet Cardiol* 6:40–44.

Tachyarrhythmias

Bright JM, Martin JM, Mama K (2005) A retrospective evaluation of transthoracic biphasic electrical cardioversion for atrial fibrillation in dogs. *J Vet Cardiol* 7:85–96.

Calvert CA, Brown J (2004) Influence of antiarrhythmia therapy on survival times of 19 clinically healthy Doberman Pinschers with dilated cardiomyopathy that experienced syncope, ventricular tachycardia, and sudden death (1985–1998). *J Am Anim Hosp Assoc* 40:24–28.

Calvert CA, Meurs KM (2009) Cardiomyopathy in Doberman Pinschers In *Kirk's Current Veterinary Therapy XIV*. (eds JD Bonagura, DC Twedt) Saunders Elsevier, St. Louis, pp. 800–803.

Cober RE, Schober KE, Hildebrandt N *et al.* (2009) Adverse effects of intravenous amiodarone in 5 dogs. *J Vet Intern Med* 23:657–661.

Cote E, Harpster NK, Laste NJ *et al.* (2004) Atrial fibrillation in cats: 50 cases (1979–2002). *J Am Vet Med Assoc* 225:256–260.

Gelzer ARM, Kraus MS (2004) Management of atrial fibrillation. *Vet Clin North Am Small Anim Pract* 34:1127–1144.

Gelzer ARM, Kraus MS, Rishniw M *et al.* (2009) Combination therapy with digoxin and diltiazem controls ventricular rate in chronic atrial fibrillation in dogs better than digoxin or diltiazem monotherapy: a randomized crossover study in 18 dogs. *J Vet Intern Med* 23:499–508.

Glaus TM, Hassig M, Keene BW (2003) Accuracy of heart rate obtained by auscultation in atrial fibrillation. *J Am Anim Hosp Assoc* 39:237–239.

Kraus MS, Thomason JD, Fallaw TL *et al.* (2009) Toxicity in Doberman Pinschers with ventricular arrhythmias treated with amiodarone (1996–2005). *Vet Intern Med* 23:1-6.

Menaut P, Belanger MC, Beauchamp G *et al.* (2005) Atrial fibrillation in dogs with and without structural or functional cardiac disease: a retrospective study of 109 cases. *J Vet Cardiol* 7:75–83.

Meurs KM, Spier AW (2009) Cardiomyopathy in Boxer Dogs. In *Kirk's Current Veterinary Therapy XIV*. (eds JD Bonagura, DC Twedt) Saunders Elsevier, St. Louis, pp. 797–799.

Meurs KM, Spier AW, Wright NA *et al.* (2002) Comparison of the effects of four antiarrhythmic treatments for familial ventricular arrhythmias in Boxers. *J Am Vet Med Assoc* **221**:522–527.

Miyamoto M, Nishijima Y, Nakayama T *et al.* (2001) Acute cardiovascular effects of diltiazem in anesthetized dogs with induced atrial fibrillation. *J Vet Intern Med* **15**:559–563.

Moise NS, Gelzer ARM, Kraus MS. Ventricular arrhythmias in dogs. (2009) In *Kirk's Current Veterinary Therapy XIV.* (eds JD Bonagura, DC Twedt) Saunders Elsevier, St. Louis, pp. 727–731.

Moise NS, Pariaut R, Gelzer ARM *et al.* (2005) Cardioversion with lidocaine of vagally associated atrial fibrillation in two dogs. *J Vet Cardiol* **7**:143–148.

Oyama MA, Prosek R (2006) Acute conversion of atrial fibrillation in two dogs by intravenous amiodarone administration. *J Vet Intern Med* **20**:1224–1227.

Santilli RA, Spadacini G, Moretti P *et al.* (2006) Radiofrequency catheter ablation of concealed accessory pathways in two dogs with symptomatic atrioventricular reciprocating tachycardia. *J Vet Cardiol* **8**:157–165.

Saunders AB, Miller MW, Gordon SG *et al.* (2006) Oral amiodarone therapy in dogs with atrial fibrillation. *J Vet Intern Med* **20**:921–926.

Smith CE, Freeman LM, Rush JE, *et al.* (2007) Omega-3 fatty acids in boxer dogs with arrhythmogenic right ventricular cardiomyopathy. *J Vet Intern Med* **21**:265–273.

Stafford Johnson M, Martin M, Smith P (2006) Cardioversion of supraventricular tachycardia using lidocaine in five dogs. *J Vet Intern Med* **20**:272–276.

Ware WA (2011) Managment of arrhythmias. In *Cardiovascular Disease in Small Animal Medicine.* (ed WA Ware) Manson Publishing, London, pp. 194–226.

Wright KN (2009) Assessment and treatment of supraventricular tachyarrhythmias. In *Kirk's Current Veterinary Therapy XIV.* (eds JD Bonagura, DC Twedt) Saunders Elsevier, St. Louis, pp. 731–739.

Wright KN, Knilans TK, Irvin HM (2006) When, why, and how to perform cardiac radiofrequency catheter ablation. *J Vet Cardiol* **8**:95–107.

CARDIAC THERAPY: HEART FAILURE MANAGEMENT

Abbott JA, Broadstone RV, Ward DL *et al.* (2005) Hemodynamic effects of orally administered carvedilol in healthy conscious dogs. *Am J Vet Res* **66**:637–641.

Adin DB, Hill RC, Scott KC (2003) Short-term compatibility of furosemide with crystalloid solutions. *J Vet Intern Med* **17**:724–726.

Adin DB, Taylor AW, Hill RC *et al.* (2003) Intermittent bolus injection versus continuous infusion of furosemide in normal adult greyhound dogs. *J Vet Intern Med* **17**:632–636.

Amberger C, Chetboul V, Bomassi E *et al.* (2004) Comparison of the effects of imidapril and enalapril in a prospective, multicentric randomized trial in dogs with naturally acquired heart failure. *J Vet Cardiol* **6**:9–16.

Arsenault WG, Boothe DM, Gordon SG *et al.* (2005) Pharmacokinetics of carvedilol after intravenous and oral administration in conscious healthy dogs. *Am J Vet Res* **66**:2172–2176.

Atkins C, Bonagura J, Ettinger S *et al.* (2009) Guidelines for the diagnosis and treatment of canine chronic valvular heart disease. ACVIM Consensus Statement. *J Vet Intern Med* **23**:1142–1150.

Atkins CE, Keene BW, Brown WA *et al.* (2007) Results of the veterinary enalapril trial to prove reduction in onset of heart failure in dogs chronically treated with enalapril alone for compensated, naturally occurring mitral valve insufficiency. *J Am Vet Med Assoc* **231**:1061–1069.

BENCH study group (1999) The effect of benazepril on survival times and clinical signs of dogs with congestive heart failure: results of a multicenter, prospective, randomized, double-blinded, placebo-controlled, long-term clinical trial. *J Vet Cardiol* **1**:7–18.

Bernay F, Bland JM, Haggstrom J *et al.* (2010) Efficacy of spironolactone on survival in dogs with naturally occurring mitral regurgitation caused by myxomatous mitral valve disease. *J Vet Intern Med* **24**:331–341.

Bonagura JB, Lehmkuhl LB, de Morais HA (2006) Fluid and diuretic therapy in heart failure. In *Fluid, Electrolyte, and Acid–Base Disorders in Small Animal Practice,* 3rd edn. (ed SP DiBartola) Elsevier Saunders, St. Louis, pp. 490–518.

Gordon SG, Arsenault WG, Longnecker M et al. (2006) Pharmacodynamics of carvedilol in conscious, healthy dogs. *J Vet Intern Med* 20:297–304.

Haggstrom J, Boswood A, O'Grady M et al. (2008) Effect of pimobendan or benazepril HCl on survival times in dogs with congestive heart failure caused by naturally occurring myxomatous mitral valve disease: the QUEST study. *J Vet Intern Med* 22:1124–1135.

Haggstrom J, Hansson K, Karlberg BE et al. (1996) Effects of long-term treatment with enalapril or hydralazine on the renin–angiotensin–aldosterone system and fluid balance in dogs with naturally acquired mitral valve regurgitation. *Am J Vet Res* 57:1645–1652.

Hood WB, Dans AL, Guyatt GH et al. (2004) Digitalis for treatment of congestive heart failure in patients in sinus rhythm: a systematic review and meta-analysis. *J Card Fail* 10:155–164.

Kvart C, Haggsrom J, Pedersen HD et al. (2002) Efficacy of enalapril for prevention of congestive heart failure in dogs with myxomatous valve disease and asymptomatic mitral regurgitation. *J Vet Intern Med* 16: 80–88.

Lefebvre HB, Brown SA, Chetbouls V et al. (2007) Angiotensin-converting enzyme inhibitors in veterinary medicine. *Curr Pharmaceut Design* 13:1347–1361.

Lefebvre HP, Jeunesse E, Laroute V et al. (2006) Pharmacokinetic and pharmacodynamic parameters of ramipril and ramiprilat in healthy dogs with reduced glomerular filtration rate. *J Vet Intern Med* 20:499–507.

Lombarde CW, Jöns O, Bussadori CM (2006) Clinical efficacy of pimobendan versus benazepril for the treatment of acquired atrioventricular valvular disease in dogs. *J Am Anim Hosp Assoc* 42:249–261.

Luis Fuentes V (2004) Use of pimobendan in the management of heart failure. *Vet Clin North Am Small Anim Pract* 34:1145–1155.

Luis Fuentes V, Corcoran B, French A et al. (2002) A double-blind, randomized, placebo-controlled study of pimobendan in dogs with cardiomyopathy. *J Vet Intern*

Med 16:255–261.

Marcondes Santos M, Tarasoutchi F, Mansur AP et al. (2007) Effects of carvedilol treatment in dogs with chronic mitral valvular disease. *J Vet Intern Med* 21:996–1001.

O'Grady MR, Minors SL, O'Sullivan ML et al. (2008) Efficacy of pimobendan on case fatality rate in Doberman Pinschers with congestive heart failure caused by dilated cardiomyopathy. *J Vet Intern Med* 22:897–904.

O'Grady MR, O'Sullivan ML, Minors SL et al. (2009) Efficacy of benazepril hydrochloride to delay the progression of occult dilated cardiomyopathy in Doberman Pinschers. *J Vet Intern Med* 23:977–983.

Oyama MA, Sisson DD, Prosek R et al. (2007) Carvedilol in dogs with dilated cardiomyopathy. *J Vet Intern Med* 21:1272–1279.

Pouchelon JL, King J, Martignoni L et al. (2004) Long-term tolerability of benazepril in dogs with congestive heart failure. *J Vet Cardiol* 6:7–13.

Rush JE, Freeman LM, Brown DJ et al. (2000) Clinical, echocardiographic, and neurohormonal effects of a sodium-restricted diet in dogs with heart failure. *J Vet Intern Med* 14:512–520.

Rush JE, Freeman LM, Hiler C et al. (2002) Use of metoprolol in dogs with acquired cardiac disease. *J Vet Cardiol* 4:23–28.

Sisson DD (2010) Pathophysiology of heart failure. In *Textbook of Veterinary Internal Medicine*, 7th edn. (eds SJ Ettinger, EC Feldman) Saunders Elsevier, St. Louis, pp. 1143–1158.

Smith PJ, French AT, Van Israël N et al. (2005) Efficacy and safety of pimobendan in canine heart failure caused by myxomatous mitral valve disease. *J Small Anim Pract* 46:121–130.

Uechi M, Sasaki T, Ueno K et al. (2002) Cardiovascular and renal effects of carvedilol in dogs with heart failure. *J Vet Med Sci* 64:469–475.

Ware WA. (2011) Management of heart failure. In *Cardiovascular Disease in Small Animal Medicine*. (ed WA Ware) Manson Publishing, London, pp. 164–193.

HEART DISEASES: CONGENITAL

Abdulla R, Blew GA, Holterman MJ (2004) Cardiovascular embryology. *Pediatr*

Cardiol **25**:191–200.

Oyama MA, Sisson DD, Thomas WP *et al.* (2010) Congenital heart disease. In *Textbook of Veterinary Internal Medicine*, 7th edn. (eds SJ Ettinger, EC Feldman) Saunders Elsevier, St. Louis, pp. 1250–1298.

Ware WA (2011) Congenital cardiovascular diseases. In *Cardiovascular Disease in Small Animal Medicine*. (ed WA Ware) Manson Publishing, London, pp. 228–262.

Shunts

Blossom JE, Bright JM, Griffiths LG (2010) Transvenous occlusion of patent ductus arteriosus in 56 consecutive dogs. *J Vet Cardiol* **12**:75–84.

Brockman DJ, Holt DE, Gaynor JW *et al.* (2007) Long-term palliation of tetralogy of Fallot in dogs by use of a modified Blalock–Taussig shunt. *J Am Vet Med Assoc* **231**:721–726.

Chetboul V, Charles V, Nicolle A *et al.* (2006) Retrospective study of 156 atrial septal defects in dogs and cats (2001–2005). *J Vet Med* **53**:179–184.

Cote E, Ettinger SJ (2001) Long-term clinical management of right-to-left ('reversed') patent ductus arteriosus in 3 dogs. *J Vet Intern Med* **15**:39–42.

Fujii Y, Fukuda T, Machida N *et al.* (2004) Transcatheter closure of congenital ventricular septal defects in 3 dogs with a detachable coil. *J Vet Intern Med* **18**:911–914.

Gordon SG, Miller MW, Roland RM *et al.* (2009) Transcatheter atrial septal defect closure with the Amplatzer atrial septal occlude in 13 dogs: short- and mid-term outcome. *J Vet Intern Med* **23**:995–1002.

Gordon SG, Saunders AB, Achen SE *et al.* (2010) Transarterial ductal occlusion using the Amplatz Canine Duct Occluder in 40 dogs. *J Vet Cardiol* **12**:85–92.

Miller MW, Gordan SG (2009) Patent ductus arteriosus. In *Kirk's Current Veterinary Therapy XIV.* (eds JD Bonagura, DC Twedt) Saunders Elsevier, St. Louis, pp. 744–747.

Miller MW, Gordon SG, Saunders AB *et al.* (2006) Angiographic classification of patent ductus arteriosus morphology in the dog. *J Vet Cardiol* **8**:109–114.

Miller SJ, Thomas WP (2009) Coil embolization of patent ductus arteriosus

via the carotid artery in seven dogs. *J Vet Cardiol* **11**:129–136.

Moore KW, Stepien RL (2001) Hydroxyurea for treatment of polycythemia secondary to right-to-left shunting patent ductus arteriosus in 4 dogs. *J Vet Intern Med* **15**:418–421.

Nguyenba TP, Tobias AH (2008) Minimally invasive per-catheter patent ductus arteriosus occlusion in dogs using prototype duct occluder. *J Vet Intern Med* **22**:129–134.

Oswald GP, Orton CE (1993) Patent ductus arteriosus and pulmonary hypertension in related Pembroke Welsh Corgis. *J Am Vet Med Assoc* **202**:761–764.

Saunders AB, Miller MW, Gordon SG *et al.* (2007) Echocardiographic and angiocardiographic comparison of ductal dimensions in dogs with patent ductus arteriosus. *J Vet Intern Med* **21**:68–75.

Schneider M, Hildebrandt N, Schweigl T *et al.* (2007) Transthoracic echocardiographic measurement of patent ductus arteriosus in dogs. *J Vet Intern Med* **21**:251–257.

Shimizu M, Tanaka R, Hirao H *et al.* (2005) Percutaneous transcatheter coil embolization of a ventricular septal defect in a dog. *J Am Vet Med Assoc* **226**:69–72.

Valve malformations

Buchanan JW (2001) Pathogenesis of single right coronary artery and pulmonic stenosis in English Bulldogs. *J Vet Intern Med* **15**:101–104.

Bussadori C, DeMadron E, Santilli RA *et al.* (2001) Balloon valvuloplasty in 30 dogs with pulmonic stenosis: effect of valve morphology and annular size on initial and 1-year outcome. *J Vet Intern Med* **15**:553–558.

Estrada A (2009) Pulmonic stenosis. In *Kirk's Current Veterinary Therapy XIV.* (eds JD Bonagura, DC Twedt) Saunders Elsevier, St. Louis, pp. 752–756.

Estrada A, Moise NS, Erb HN *et al.* (2006) Prospective evaluation of the balloon-to-annulus ratio for valvuloplasty in the treatment of pulmonic stenosis in the dog. *J Vet Intern Med* **20**:862–872.

Estrada A, Moise NS, Renaud-Farrell S (2005) When, how and why to perform a double ballooning technique for dogs with valvular pulmonic stenosis. *J Vet Cardiol* **7**:41–51.

Falk T, Jonsson L, Pedersen HD (2004) Intramyocardial arterial narrowing in dogs with subaortic stenosis. *J Small Anim Pract* 45:448–453.

Famula TR, Siemens LM, Davidson AP *et al.* (2002) Evaluation of the genetic basis of tricuspid valve dysplasia in Labrador Retrievers. *Am J Vet Res* 63:816–820.

French A, Luis Fuentes V, Dukes-McEwan J *et al.* (2000) Progression of aortic stenosis in the Boxer. *J Small Anim Pract* 41:451–456.

Fonfara S, Martinez Pereira Y, Swift S *et al.* (2010) Balloon valvuloplasty for treatment of pulmonic stenosis in English bulldogs with an aberrant coronary artery. *J Vet Intern Med* 24:354–359.

Hoffman G, Amberger CN, Seiler G *et al.* (2000) Tricuspid valve dysplasia in fifteen dogs. *Schweiz Arch Tierheilkd* 142:268–277.

Jenni S, Gardelle O, Zini E *et al.* (2009) Use of auscultation and Doppler echocardiography in Boxer puppies to predict development of subaortic or pulmonary stenosis. *J Vet Intern Med* 23:81–86.

Johnson MS, Martin M, Edwards D *et al.* (2004) Pulmonic stenosis in dogs: balloon dilation improves clinical outcome. *J Vet Intern Med* 18:656–662.

Kienle RD, Thomas WP, Pion PD (1994) The natural history of canine congenital subaortic stenosis. *J Vet Intern Med* 8:423–431.

Kunze CP, Abbott JA, Hamilton SM *et al.* (2002) Balloon valvuloplasty for palliative treatment of tricuspid stenosis with right-to-left atrial-level shunting in a dog. *J Am Vet Med Assoc* 220:491–496.

Lehmkuhl LB, Ware WA, Bonagura JD (1994) Mitral stenosis in 15 dogs. *J Vet Intern Med* 8:2–17.

Linde A, Koch J (2006) Screening for aortic stenosis in the Boxer: auscultatory, ECG, blood pressure and Doppler echocardiographic findings. *J Vet Cardiol* 8:79–86.

Meurs KM, Lehmkuhl LB, Bonagura JD (2005) Survival times in dogs with severe subvalvular aortic stenosis treated with balloon valvuloplasty or atenolol. *J Am Vet Med Assoc* 227:420–424.

Ristic JM, Marin C, Baines EA, Herrtage ME (2001) Congenital pulmonic stenosis. A retrospective study of 24 cases seen between 1990–1999. *J Vet Cardiol* 3:13–19.

Stafford Johnson M, Martin M, Edwards D *et al.* (2004) Pulmonic stenosis in dogs: balloon dilation improves clinical outcome. *J Vet Intern Med* 18:656–662.

Stamoulis ME, Fox PR (1993) Mitral valve stenosis in three cats. *J Small Anim Pract* 34:452–456.

Stepien RL, Bonagura JD (1991) Aortic stenosis: clinical findings in six cats. *J Small Anim Pract* 32:341–350.

Vascular and other malformations

Buchanan JW (2004) Tracheal signs and associated vascular anomalies in dogs with persistent right aortic arch. *J Vet Intern Med* 18:510–514.

delPalacio MJF, Bayon A, Agut A (1997) Dilated coronary sinus in a dog with persistent left cranial vena cava. *Vet Radiol Ultrasound* 38:376–379.

Fossum TW, Miller MW (1994) Cor triatriatum and caval anomalies. *Semin Vet Med Surg* 9:177–184.

Muldoon MM, Birchard SJ, Ellison GW (1997) Long-term results of surgical correction of persistent right aortic arch in dogs: 25 cases (1980–1995). *J Am Vet Med Assoc* 210:1761–1763.

Stafford Johnson M, Martin M, DeGiovanni JV *et al.* (2004) Management of cor triatriatum dexter by balloon dilatation in three dogs. *J Small Anim Pract* 45:16–20.

VanGundy T (1989) Vascular ring anomalies. *Compend Contin Educ Pract Vet* 11:36–48.

HEART DISEASES: MYOCARDIAL, CANINE

Boxer arrhythmogenic right ventricular cardiomyopathy

(also see Cardiac therapy: arrhythmia management)

Baumwart RD, Meurs KM, Atkins CE *et al.* (2005) Clinical, echocardiographic, and electrocardiographic abnormalities in Boxers with cardiomyopathy and left ventricular systolic dysfunction: 48 cases (1985–2003). *J Am Vet Med Assoc* 226:1102–1104.

Kraus MS, Moise NS, Rishniw M *et al.* (2002) Morphology of ventricular arrhythmias in the Boxer as measured by

12-lead electrocardiography with pace-mapping comparison. *J Vet Intern Med* **16**:153–158.

Meurs KM, Ederer MM, Stern JA (2007) Desmosomal gene evaluation in Boxers with arrhythmogenic right ventricular cardiomyopathy. *Am J Vet Res* **68**:1338–1341.

Meurs KM, Spier AW (2009) Cardiomyopathy in Boxer Dogs. In *Kirk's Current Veterinary Therapy XIV*. (eds JD Bonagura, DC Twedt) Saunders Elsevier, St. Louis, pp. 797–799.

Meurs KM, Spier AW, Wright NA *et al.* (2001) Comparison of in-hospital versus 24-hour ambulatory electrocardiography for detection of ventricular premature complexes in mature Boxers. *J Am Vet Med Assoc* **218**:222–224.

Oyama MA, Reiken S, Lehnart SE *et al.* (2008) Arrhythmogenic right ventricular cardiomyopathy in Boxer dogs is associated with calstabin2 deficiency. *J Vet Cardiol* **10**:1–10.

Smith CE, Freeman LM, Meurs KM *et al.* (2008) Plasma fatty acid concentrations in Boxers and Doberman Pinschers. *Am J Vet Res* **69**:195–198.

Spier AW, Meurs KM (2004) Evaluation of spontaneous variability in the frequency of ventricular arrhythmias in Boxers with arrhythmiogenic right ventricular cardiomyopathy. *J Am Vet Med Assoc* **24**:538–541.

Stern JA, Meurs KM, Spier AW *et al.* (2010) Ambulatory electrocardiographic evaluation of clinically normal adult Boxers. *J Am Vet Med Assoc* **236**:430–433.

Thomason JD, Kraus MS, Surdyk KK *et al.* (2008) Bradycardia-associated syncope in 7 Boxers with ventricular tachycardia (2002–2005). *J Vet Intern Med* **22**:931–936.

Dilated cardiomyopathy
(also see Cardiac therapy: heart failure management)

Backus RC, Cohen G, Pion PD *et al.* (2003) Taurine deficiency in Newfoundlands fed commercially available complete and balanced diets. *J Am Vet Med Assoc* **223**:1130–1136.

Borgarelli M, Santilli RA, Chiavegato D *et al.* (2006) Prognostic indicators for dogs with dilated cardiomyopathy. *J Vet Intern Med* **20**:104–110.

Calvert CA, Jacobs GJ, Smith DD (2000) Association between results of ambulatory electrocardiography and development of cardiomyopathy during long-term follow-up of Doberman Pinschers. *J Am Vet Med Assoc* **216**:34–39.

Calvert CA, Meurs KM (2009) Cardiomyopathy in Doberman Pinschers. In *Kirk's Current Veterinary Therapy XIV*. (eds JD Bonagura, DC Twedt) Saunders Elsevier, St. Louis, pp. 800–803.

Carroll MC, Cote E (2001) Carnitine: a review. *Compend Contin Educ Pract Vet* **23**:45–52.

Dukes-McEwan J, Borgarelli M, Tidholm A *et al.* (2003) Proposed guidelines for the diagnosis of canine idiopathic dilated cardiomyopathy. *J Vet Cardiol* **5**:7–19.

Everett RM, McGann J, Wimberly HC *et al.* (1999) Dilated cardiomyopathy of Doberman Pinschers: retrospective histomorphologic evaluation on hearts from 32 cases. *Vet Pathol* **36**:221–227.

Fascetti AJ, Reed JR, Rogers QR *et al.* (2003) Taurine deficiency in dogs with dilated cardiomyopathy:12 cases (1997–2001). *J Am Vet Med Assoc* **223**:1137–1141.

Freeman LM, Rush JE, Brown DJ *et al.* (2001) Relationship between circulating and dietary taurine concentration in dogs with dilated cardiomyopathy. *Vet Ther* **2**:370–378.

Kittleson MD, Keene B, Pion PD *et al.* (1997) Results of the multicenter spaniel trial (MUST): taurine- and carnitine-responsive dilated cardiomyopathy in American Cocker Spaniels with decreased plasma taurine concentration. *J Vet Intern Med* **11**:204–211.

Luis Fuentes, Corcoran B, French A *et al.* (2002) A double-blind, randomized, placebo-controlled study of pimobendan in dogs with dilated cardiomyopathy. *J Vet Intern Med* **16**:255–261.

Moneva–Jordan A, Lius Fuentes V, Corcoran B *et al.* (2002) Pulsus alternans in English Cocker Spaniels with dilated cardiomyopathy. *J Small Anim Pract* **43**:410.

Meurs KM, Fox PR, Norgard MM (2007) A prospective genetic evaluation of familial dilated cardiomyopathy in the Doberman Pinscher. *J Vet Intern Med* **21**:1016–1020.

Meurs KM, Hendrix KP, Norgard MM (2008) Molecular evaluation of five cardiac genes in Doberman Pinschers with dilated cardiomyopathy. *Am J Vet Res* **69**:1050–1053.

O'Grady MR, O'Sullivan ML, Minors SL *et al.* (2009) Efficacy of benazepril hydrochloride to delay the progression of occult dilated cardiomyopathy in Doberman Pinschers. *J Vet Intern Med* **23**:977–983.

O'Grady MR, O'Sullivan ML (2004) Dilated cardiomyopathy: an update. *Vet Clin North Am Small Anim Pract* **34**:1187–1207.

O'Sullivan ML, O'Grady MR, Minors SL (2007) Plasma big endothelin-1, atrial natriuretic peptide, aldosterone, and norepinephrine concentrations in normal Doberman Pinschers and Doberman Pinschers with dilated cardiomyopathy. *J Vet Intern Med* **21**:92–99.

Oyama MA, Chittur SV, Reynolds CA (2009) Decreased triadin and increased calstabin2 expression in Great Danes with dilated cardiomyopathy. *J Vet Intern Med* **23**:1014–1019.

Oyama MA, Fox PR, Rush JE *et al.* (2008) Clinical utility of serum N-terminal pro-B-type natriuretic peptide concentration for identifying cardiac disease in dogs and assessing disease severity. *J Am Vet Med Assoc* **232**:1496–1503.

Oyama MA, Sisson DD, Solter PF (2007) Prospective screening for occult cardiomyopathy in dogs by measurement of plasma atrial natriuretic peptide, B-type natriuretic peptide, and cardiac troponin-I concentrations. *Am J Vet Res* **68**:42–47.

Pion PD, Sanderson SL, Kittleson MD (1998) The effectiveness of taurine and levocarnitine in dogs with heart disease. *Vet Clin North Am Small Anim Pract* **28**:1495–1514.

Sanderson SL, Gross KL, Ogburn PH *et al.* (2001) Effects of dietary fat and L-carnitine on plasma and whole blood taurine concentrations and cardiac function in healthy dogs fed protein-restricted diets. *Am J Vet Res* **62**:1616–1623.

Vollmar AC, Fox PR, Meurs KM *et al.* (2003) Dilated cardiomyopathy in juvenile Doberman Pinscher dogs. *J Vet Cardiol* **5**:23–27.

Wess G, Schulze A, Geraghty N *et al.* (2010) Ability of a 5-minute electrocardiography (ECG) for predicting arrhythmias in Doberman Pinschers with cardiomyopathy in comparison with a 24-hour ambulatory ECG. *J Vet Intern Med* **24**:367–371.

Other myocardial disease/injury

Actis Dato GM, Arslanian A, DiMarzio P *et al.* (2003) Post-traumatic and iatrogenic foreign bodies in the heart: report of fourteen cases and review of the literature. *J Thoracic Cardiovasc Surg* **126**:408–414.

Breitschwerdt EB, Atkins CE, Brown TT *et al.* (1999) *Bartonella vinsonii* subsp. *berkhoffii* and related members of the alpha subdivision of the Proteobacteria in dogs with cardiac arrhythmias, endocarditis, or myocarditis. *J Clin Microbiol* **37**:3618–3626.

Falk T, Jonsson L (2000) Ischaemic heart disease in the dog: a review of 65 cases. *J Small Anim Pract* **41**:97–103.

Fritz CL, Kjemtrup AM (2003) Lyme borreliosis. *J Am Vet Med Assoc* **223**:1261–1270.

Hess RS, Kass PH, Van Winkle TJ (2003) Association between diabetes mellitus, hypothyroidism or hyperadrenocorticism and atherosclerosis in dogs. *J Vet Intern Med* **17**:489–494.

Kidd L, Stepien RL, Amrheiw DP (2000) Clinical findings and coronary artery disease in dogs and cats with acute and subacute myocardial necrosis: 28 cases. *J Am Anim Hosp Assoc* **36**:199–208.

Schmiedt C, Kellum H, Legendre AM *et al.* (2006) Cardiovascular involvement in 8 dogs with *Blastomyces dermatitidis* infection. *J Vet Intern Med* **20**:1351–1354.

Snyder PS, Cooke KL, Murphy ST *et al.* (2001) Electrocardiographic findings in dogs with motor vehicle-related trauma. *J Am Anim Hosp Assoc* **37**:55–63.

Ware WA (2011) Myocardial diseases of the dog. In *Cardiovascular Disease in Small Animal Medicine.* (ed WA Ware) Manson Publishing, London, pp. 280–299.

Heart diseases: myocardial, feline

Connolly DJ, Soares Magalhaes RJ, Syme HM *et al.* (2008) Circulating natriuretic peptides in cats with heart disease. *J Vet Intern Med* **22**:96–105.

Ferasin L (2009) Feline myocardial disease: classification, pathophysiology and clinical presentation. *J Feline Med Surg* **11**:3–13.

Ferasin L (2009) Feline myocardial disease:

diagnosis, prognosis, and clinical management. *J Feline Med Surg* **11**:183–194.

Ferasin L, Sturgess CP, Cannon MJ *et al.* (2003) Feline idiopathic cardiomyopathy: a retrospective study of 106 cats (1994–2001). *J Feline Med Surg* **5**:151–159.

Fox PR (2003) Hypertrophic cardiopathy. Clinical and pathologic correlates. *J Vet Cardiol* **5**:39–45.

Fox PR, Maron BJ, Basso C *et al.* (2000) Spontaneously occurring arrhythmogenic right ventricular cardiomyopathy in the domestic cat: a new animal model similar to the human disease. *Circulation* **102**:1863–1870.

Fries R, HeaneyAM, Meurs KM (2008) Prevalence of the myosin-binding protein C mutation in Maine coon cats. *J Vet Intern Med* **22**:893–896.

Harvey AM, Battersby IA, Faena M *et al.* (2005) Arrhythmogenic right ventricular cardiomyopathy in two cats. *J Small Anim Pract* **46**:151–156.

Koffas H, Dukes-McEwan J, Corcoran BM *et al.* (2006) Pulsed tissue Doppler imaging in normal cats and cats with hypertrophic cardiomyopathy. *J Vet Intern Med* **20**:65–77.

MacDonald KA, Kittleson MD, Kass PH *et al.* (2007) Tissue Doppler imaging in Maine Coon cats with a mutation of myosin binding protein C with or without hypertrophy. *J Vet Intern Med* **21**:232–237.

MacDonald KA, Kittleson MD, Kass PH (2008) Effect of spironolactone on diastolic function and left ventricular mass in Maine Coon cats with familial hypertrophic cardiomyopathy. *J Vet Intern Med* **22**:335–341.

MacDonald KA, Kittleson MD, Larson RF *et al.* (2006) The effect of ramipril on left ventricular mass, myocardial fibrosis, diastolic function, and plasma neurohormones in Maine Coon cats with familial hypertrophic cardiomyopathy without heart failure. *J Vet Intern Med* **20**:1093.

Meurs KM, Norgard MM, Kuan M *et al.* (2009) Analysis of 8 sarcomeric candidate genes for feline hypertrophic cardiomyopathy mutations in cats with hypertrophic cardiomyopathy. *J Vet Intern Med* **23**:840–843.

Meurs KM, Sanchez X, David RM *et al.* (2005) A cardiac myosin-binding protein C mutation in the Maine Coon cat with familial hypertrophic cardiomyopathy. *Hum Mol Genet* **14**:3587–3593.

Paige CF, Abbott JA, Elvinger F *et al.* (2009) Prevalence of cardiomyopathy in apparently healthy cats. *J Am Vet Med Assoc* **234**:1398–1403.

Rush JE, Freeman LM, Fenollosa NK *et al.* (2002) Population and survival characteristics of cats with hypertrophic cardiomyopathy: 260 cases (1990–1999). *J Am Vet Med Assoc* **220**:202–207.

Sampedrano CC, Chetboul V, Gouni V *et al.* (2006) Systolic and diastolic myocardial dysfunction in cats with hypertrophic cardiomyopathy or systemic hypertension. *J Vet Intern Med* **20**:1106–1115.

Sampedrano CC, Chetboul V, Mary J *et al.* (2009) Prospective echocardiographic and tissue Doppler imaging screening of a population of Maine coon cats tested for the A31P mutation in the myosin-binding protein C gene: a specific analysis of the heterozygous status. *J Vet Intern Med* **23**:91–99.

Schober KE, Maerz I (2006) Assessment of left atrial appendage flow velocity and its relation to spontaneous echocardiographic contrast in 89 cats with myocardial disease. *J Vet Intern Med* **20**:120–130.

Taillefer M, Di Fruscia R (2006) Benazepril and subclinical feline hypertrophic cardiomyopathy: a prospective, blinded, controlled study. *Can Vet J* **47**:437.

Ware WA. (2011) Myocardial diseases of the cat. In *Cardiovascular Disease in Small Animal Medicine*. (ed WA Ware) Manson Publishing, London, pp. 300–319.

Wess G, Schinner C, Weber K *et al.* (2010) Association of A31P and A74T polymorphisms in the myosin binding protein C3 gene and hypertrophic cardiomyopathy in Maine coon and other breed cats. *J Vet Intern Med* **20**:527–532.

Yang VK Freeman LM, Rush JE (2008) Comparisons of morphometric measurements and serum insulin-like growth factor concentration in healthy cats and cats with hypertrophic cardiomyopathy. *Am J Vet Res* **69**:1061–1066.

HEART DISEASES: NEOPLASTIC
(also see Acquired pericardial diseases and neoplasia)

Akkoc A, Ozyigit MO, Cangul IT (2007) Valvular cardiac myxoma in a dog. *J Vet Med A Physiol Pathol Clin Med* 54:356–358.

Aronsohn M (1985) Cardiac hemangiosarcoma in the dog: a review of 38 cases. *J Am Vet Med Assoc* 187:922–926.

Vicari ED, Brown DC, Holt DE et al. (2001) Survival times of and prognostic indicators for dogs with heart base masses: 25 cases (1986–1999). *J Am Vet Med Assoc* 219:485–487.

Ware WA, Hopper DL (1999) Cardiac tumors in dogs: 1982–1995. *J Vet Intern Med* 13:95–103.

Warman SM, McGregor R, Fews D et al. (2006) Congestive heart failure caused by intracardiac tumours in two dogs. *J Small Anim Pract* 47:480–483.

HEART DISEASES: PERICARDIAL
Acquired pericardial disease and neoplasia
Brisson BA, Reggeti F, Bienzle D (2006) Portal site metastasis of invasive mesothelioma after diagnostic thoracoscopy in a dog. *J Am Vet Med Assoc* 229:980–983.

Closa JM, Font A, Mascort J (1999) Pericardial mesothelioma in a dog: long-term survival after pericardiectomy in combination with chemotherapy. *J Small Anim Pract* 40:383–386.

Davidson BJ, Paling AC, Lahmers SL et al. (2008) Disease association and clinical assessment of feline pericardial effusion. *J Am Anim Hosp Assoc* 44:5–9.

Dunning D, Monnet E, Orton EC et al. (1998) Analysis of prognostic indicators for dogs with pericardial effusion: 46 cases (1985–1996). *J Am Vet Med Assoc* 212:1276–1280.

Hall DJ, Shofer F, Meier CK et al. (2007) Pericardial effusion in cats: a retrospective study of clinical findings and outcome in 146 cats. *J Vet Intern Med* 21:1002–1007.

Heinritz CK, Gilson SD, Soderstrom MJ et al. (2006) Subtotal pericardectomy and epicardial excision for treatment of coccidioidomycosis-induced effusive-constrictive pericarditis in dogs: 17 cases (1999–2003). *J Am Vet Med Assoc* 229:435–440.

Jackson J, Richter KP, Launer DP (1999) Thoracoscopic partial pericardiectomy in 13 dogs. *J Vet Intern Med* 13:529–533.

MacDonald KA, Cagney O, Magne ML (2009) Echocardiographic and clinicopathologic characterization of pericardial effusion in dogs: 107 cases (1985–2006). *J Am Vet Med Assoc* 235:1456–1461.

Machida N, Tanaka R, Takemura N et al. (2004) Development of pericardial mesothelioma in golden retrievers with a long-term history of idiopathic haemorrhagic pericardial effusion. *J Comp Path* 131:166–175.

McDonough SP, MacLachlan NJ, Tobias AH (1992) Canine pericardial mesothelioma. *Vet Path* 29:256–260.

Rush JE, Keene BW, Fox PR (1990) Pericardial disease in the cat: a retrospective evaluation of 66 cases. *J Am Anim Hosp Assoc* 26:39–46.

Stafford Johnson M, Martin M, Binns S et al. (2004) A retrospective study of clinical findings, treatment and outcome in 143 dogs with pericardial effusion. *J Small Anim Pract* 45:546–552.

Stepien RL, Whitley NT, Dubielzig RR (2000) Idiopathic or mesothelioma-related pericardial effusion: clinical findings and survival in 17 dogs studied retrospectively. *J Small Anim Pract* 41:342–347.

Thomas WP, Reed JR, Bauer TG et al. (1984) Constrictive pericardial disease in the dog. *J Am Vet Med Assoc* 184:546–553.

Tobias AH (2010) Pericardial diseases. In *Textbook of Veterinary Internal Medicine*, 7th edn. (eds SJ Ettinger, EC Feldman) Saunders Elsevier, St. Louis, pp. 1342–1352.

Ware WA (2011) Pericardial diseases and cardiac tumors. In *Cardiovascular Disease in Small Animal Medicine*. (ed WA Ware) Manson Publishing, London, pp. 320–339.

Congenital pericardial disease
Miller MW, Sisson D (2000) Pericardial disorders. In *Textbook of Veterinary Internal Medicine*, 5th edn. (eds SJ Ettinger, EC Feldman) WB Saunders, Philadelphia, pp. 923–936.

Reimer SB, Kyles AE, Filipowicz DE et al. (2004) Long-term outcome of cats treated conservatively or surgically for peritoneopericardial diaphragmatic hernia: 66 cases (1987–2002). *J Am Vet Med Assoc* **224**:728–732.

Evans SM, Biery DO (1980) Congenital peritoneopericardial diaphragmatic hernia in the dog and cat: a literature review and 17 additional case histories. *Vet Radiol* **21**:108–116.

Neiger R (1996) Peritoneopericardial diaphragmatic hernia in cats. *Compend Contin Educ Pract Vet* **18**:461–479.

Wallace J, Mullen HS, Lesser MB (1992) A technique for surgical correction of peritoneal pericardial diaphragmatic hernia in dogs and cats. *J Am Anim Hosp Assoc* **28**:503–510.

HEART DISEASES: VALVULAR
Chronic degenerative AV valve disease
(also see Cardiac therapy: heart failure management)

Atkins C, Bonagura J, Ettinger S *et al.* (2009) Guidelines for the diagnosis and treatment of canine chronic valvular heart disease. ACVIM Consensus Statement. *J Vet Intern Med* **23**:1142–1150.

Atkins CE, Keene BW, Brown WA *et al.* (2007) Results of the veterinary enalapril trial to prove reduction in onset of heart failure in dogs chronically treated with enalapril alone for compensated, naturally occurring mitral valve insufficiency. *J Am Vet Med Assoc* **231**:1061–1069.

Beardow AW, Buchanan JW (1993) Chronic mitral valve disease in Cavalier King Charles Spaniels: 95 cases (1987–1991). *J Am Vet Med Assoc* **203**:1023–1029.

Borgarelli M, Tarducci A, Zanatta R *et al.* (2007) Decreased systolic function and inadequate hypertrophy in large and small breed dogs with chronic mitral valve insufficiency. *J Vet Intern Med* **21**:61–67.

Corcoran BM, Black A, Anderson H *et al.* (2004) Identification of surface morphologic changes in the mitral valve leaflets and chordae tendineae of dogs with myxomatous degeneration. *Am J Vet Res* **65**:198–206.

Haggstrom J, Boswood A, O'Grady M *et al.* (2008) Effect of pimobendan or benazepril hydrochloride on survival times in dogs with congestive heart failure caused by naturally occurring myxomatous mitral valve disease: the QUEST study. *J Vet Intern Med* **22**:1124–1135.

Haggstrom J, Kvart C, Hansson K (1995) Heart sounds and murmurs: changes related to severity of chronic valvular disease in the Cavalier King Charles Spaniel. *J Vet Intern Med* **9**:75–85.

Kvart C, Haggstrom J, Pederson HD *et al.* (2002) Efficacy of enalapril for prevention of congestive heart failure in dogs with myxomatous valve disease and asymptomatic mitral regurgitation. *J Vet Intern Med* **16**:80–88.

Orton EC, Hackett TB, Mama K *et al.* (2005) Technique and outcome of mitral valve replacement in dogs. *J Am Vet Med Assoc* **226**:1508–1511.

Reineke EL, Burkett DE, Drobatz KJ (2008) Left atrial rupture in dogs: 14 cases (1990–2005) *J Vet Emerg Crit Care* **18**:158–164.

Ware WA (2011) Acquired valve diseases. In *Cardiovascular Disease in Small Animal Medicine*. (ed WA Ware) Manson Publishing, London, pp. 263–279.

Endocarditis

Breitschwerdt EB (2003) *Bartonella* species as emerging vector-transmitted pathogens. *Compend Contin Educ Pract Vet* **25(Suppl)**:12–15.

Dunn ME, Blond L, Letard D *et al.* (2007) Hypertrophic osteopathy associated with infective endocarditis in an adult boxer dog. *J Small Anim Pract* **48**:99–103.

MacDonald KA, Chomel BB, Kittleson MD *et al.* (2004) A prospective study of canine infective endocarditis in Northern California (1999–2001): emergence of *Bartonella* as a prevalent etiologic agent. *J Vet Intern Med* **18**:56–64.

Miller MW, Fox PR, Saunders AB (2004) Pathologic and clinical features of infectious endocarditis. *J Vet Cardiol* **6**:35–43.

Peddle G, Sleeper MM (2007) Canine bacterial endocarditis: a review. *J Am Anim Hosp Assoc* **43**:258–263.

Smith BE, Tompkins MB, Breitschwerdt EB (2004) Antinuclear antibodies can be detected in dog sera reactive to *Bartonella vinsonii* subsp. *berkhoffii*, *Ehrlichia canis* or *Leishmania infantum* antigens. *J Vet Intern Med* **18**:47–51.

Sykes JE, Kittleson MD, Chomel BB *et al.* (2006) Clinicopathologic findings and outcome in dogs with infective endocarditis: 71 cases (1992–2005). *J Am*

Vet Med Assoc **228**:1735–1747.

Tou SP, Adin DB, Castleman WL (2005) Mitral valve endocarditis after dental prophylaxis in a dog. *J Vet Intern Med* **19**:268–270.

Wall M, Calvert CA, Greene CE (2002) Infective endocarditis in dogs. *Compend Contin Educ Pract Vet* **24**:614–625.

HEARTWORM DISEASE AND ANGIOSTRONGYLOSIS

Canine angiostrongylosis (*Angiostrongylus vasorum*)

Boag AK, Lamb CR, Chapman PS *et al.* (2004) Radiographic findings in 16 dogs infected with *Angiostrongylus vasorum*. *Vet Rec* **154**:426–430.

Chapman PS, Boag AK, Guitian J *et al.* (2004) *Angiostrongylus vasorum* infection in 23 dogs (1999–2002). *J Small Anim Pract* **45**:435–440.

Helm JR, Morgan ER, Jackson MW *et al.* (2010) Canine angiostrongylosis: an emerging disease in Europe. *J Vet Emerg Crit Care* **20**:98–109.

Humm K, Adamantos S (2010) Is evaluation of a faecal smear a useful technique in the diagnosis of canine pulmonary angiostrongylosis? *J Small Anim Pract* **51**:200–203.

Kranjc A, Schnyder M, Dennler M *et al.* (2010) Pulmonary artery thrombosis in experimental *Angiostrongylus vasorum* infection does not result in pulmonary hypertension and echocardiographic right ventricular changes. *J Vet Intern Med* **24**:855–862.

Morgan ER, Shaw SE, Brennan SF *et al.* (2005) *Angiostrongylus vasorum*: a real heartbreaker. *Trends Parasitol* **21**:49–51.

Canine heartworm disease (*Dirofilaria immitis*)

American Heartworm Society (2010) Canine guidelines for the diagnosis, prevention, and management of heartworm (*Dirofilaria immitis*) infection in dogs. *American Heartworm Society Website* http://www.heartwormsociety.org/veterinary-resources/canine-guidelines.html

Atkins C (2010) Heartworm disease. In *Textbook of Veterinary Internal* Medicine, 7th edn. (eds SJ Ettinger, EC Feldman) Saunders Elsevier, St. Louis, pp. 1353–1380.

Atkins CE, Miller MW (2003) Is there a better way to administer heartworm adulticidal therapy? *Vet Med* **98**:310–317.

Bazzocchi C, Genchi C, Paltrinieri S *et al.* (2003) Immunological role of the endosymbionts of *Dirofilaria immitis*: the *Wolbachia* surface protein activates canine neutrophils with production of IL-8. *Vet Parasitol* **117**:73–83.

Bove CM, Gordon SG, Saunders AB *et al.* (2010) Outcome of minimally invasive surgical treatment of heartworm caval syndrome in dogs: 42 cases (1999–2007) *J Am Vet Med Assoc* **236**:187–192.

Hettlich BF, Ryan K, Bergman RL *et al.* (2003) Neurologic complications after melarsomine dihydrochloride treatment for *Dirofilaria immitis* in three dogs. *J Am Vet Med Assoc* **223**:1456–1461.

Litster A, Atkins C, Atwell R *et al.* (2005) Radiographic cardiac size in cats and dogs with heartworm disease compared with reference values using the vertebral heart scale method: 53 cases. *J Vet Cardiol* **7**:33–40.

McCall JW (2005) The safety-net story about macrocyclic lactone heartworm preventives: a review, an update, and recommendations. *Vet Parasitol* **133**:197–206.

Rawlings CA, Calvert CA, Glaus TM *et al.* (1994) Surgical removal of heartworms. *Semin Vet Med Surg* **9**:200–205.

Feline heartworm disease (*Dirofilaria immitis*)

Atkins C, DeFrancesco TC, Coats JR *et al.* (2000) Heartworm infection in cats: 50 cases (1985–1997). *J Am Vet Med Assoc* **217**:355–358.

Brawner WR, Dillon AR, Robertson-Plouch CK *et al.* (2000) Radiographic diagnosis of feline heartworm disease and correlation to other clinical criteria: results of a multicenter clinical case study. *Vet Therapeutics* **1**:81–87.

Browne LE, Carter TD, Levy JK *et al.* (2005) Pulmonary arterial disease in cats seropositive for *Dirofilaria immitis* but lacking adult heartworms in the heart and lungs. *Am J Vet Res* **66**:1544–1549.

DeFrancesco TC, Atkins CE, Miller MW *et al.* (2001) Use of echocardiography for the diagnosis of heartworm disease in cats: 43 cases (1985–1997). *J Am Vet Med Assoc* **218**:66–69.

Further reading

Dillon AR, Brawner WR, Robertson-Plouch CK et al (2000) Feline heartworm disease: correlations of clinical signs, serology, and other diagnostics: results of a multi-center study. *Vet Ther* 1:176–182.

Executive Board, American Heartworm Society (2007) 2007 guidelines for the diagnosis, prevention, and management of heartworm (*Dirofilaria immitis*) infection in cats. *American Heartworm Society* www.heartwormsociety.org

Kramer L, Genchi C (2002) Feline heartworm infection: serological survey of asymptomatic cats living in northern Italy. *Vet Parasitol* 104:43–50.

Hypertension: pulmonary

Atkinson KJ, Fine DM, Thombs LA et al. (2009) Evaluation of pimobendan and N-terminal probrain natriuretic peptide in the treatment of pulmonary hypertension secondary to degenerative mitral valve disease. *J Vet Intern Med* 23:1190–1196.

Bach JF, Rozanski EA, MacGregor J et al. (2006) Retrospective evaluation of sildenafil citrate as a therapy for pulmonary hypertension in dogs. *J Vet Intern Med* 20:1132–1135.

Brown AJ, Davison E, Sleeper MM (2010) Clinical efficacy of sildenafil in treatment of pulmonary arterial hypertension in dogs. *J Vet Intern Med* 24:850–854.

Henik RA. (2009) Pulmonary hypertension. In *Kirk's Current Veterinary Therapy XIV*. (eds JD Bonagura, DC Twedt) Saunders Elsevier, Philadelphia, pp. 697–702.

Kellum HB, Stepien RL (2007) Sildenafil citrate therapy in 22 dogs with pulmonary hypertension. *J Vet Intern Med* 21:1258–1264.

Schober KE, Baade H (2006) Doppler echocardiographic prediction of pulmonary hypertension in West Highland White Terriers with chronic pulmonary disease. *J Vet Intern Med* 20:912–920.

Serres F, Chetboul V, Tissier R et al. (2006) Doppler echocardiography-derived evidence of pulmonary arterial hypertension in dogs with degenerative mitral valve disease: 86 cases (2001–2005). *J Am Vet Med Assoc* 229:1772–1778.

Toyoshima Y, Kanemoto I, Arai S et al. (2007) Case of long-term sildenafil therapy in a young dog with pulmonary hypertension. *J Vet Med Sci* 69:1073–1075.

Ware WA (2011) Pulmonary hypertension. In *Cardiovascular Disease in Small Animal Medicine*. (ed WA Ware) Manson Publishing, London, pp. 340–350.

Hypertension: systemic

Brown S, Atkins C, Bagley R et al. (2007) Guidelines for the identification, evaluation, and management of systemic hypertension in dogs and cats. ACVIM Consensus Statement. *J Vet Intern Med* 21:542–558.

Chetboul V, Lefebvre HP, Pinhas C et al. (2003) Spontaneous feline hypertension: clinical and echocardiographic abnormalities, and survival rate. *J Vet Intern Med* 17:89–95.

Egner B (2003) Blood pressure measurement – basic principles and practical applications. In *Essential Facts of Blood Pressure in Dogs and Cats*. (eds B Egner, A Carr, S Brown) BE Vet Verlag, Germany, pp. 1–14.

Elliot J, Barber PJ, Syme HM et al. (2001) Feline hypertension: clinical findings and response to antihypertensive treatment in 30 cases. *J Small Anim Pract* 42:122–129.

Jepson RE, Elliot J, Brodbelt D et al. (2007) Effect of control of systolic blood pressure on survival in cats with systemic hypertension. *J Vet Intern Med* 21:402–409.

Kraft W, Egner B (2003) Causes and effects of hypertension. In *Essential Facts of Blood Pressure in Dogs and Cats*. (eds B Egner, A Carr, S Brown) BE Vet Verlag, Germany, pp. 61–86.

Nelson OL, Riedesel E, Ware WA et al. (2002) Echocardiographic and radiographic changes associated with systemic hypertension in cats. *J Vet Intern Med* 16:418–425.

Sansom J, Rogers K, Wood JLN (2004) Blood pressure assessment in healthy cats and cats with hypertensive retinopathy. *Am J Vet Res* 65:245–252.

Stepien RL (2003) The heart as a target organ. In *Essential Facts of Blood Pressure in Dogs and Cats*. (eds B Egner, A Carr, S Brown) BE Vet Verlag, Germany, pp. 103–111.

Syme HM, Barber PJ, Markwell PJ et al. (2002) Prevalence of systolic hypertension in cats with chronic renal failure at initial evaluation. *J Am Vet Med Assoc* 220:1799–1804.

Tissier R, Perrot S, Enriquez B (2005) Amlodipine: one of the main anti-hypertensive drugs in veterinary therapeutics. *J Vet Cardiol* 7:53–58.

RESPIRATORY DISEASES: AIRWAY
Laryngeal and upper airway disease
Flanders MM, Adams B (1999) Managing patients with a temporary tracheostomy tube. *Vet Technician* 20:605–613.

Guenther–Yenke C, Rozanski EA (2007) Tracheostomy in cats: 23 cases (1998–2006). *J Feline Med Surg* 9:451–457.

Hendricks JC, Kline LR, Kovalski RJ et al. (1987) The English bulldog: a natural model of sleep-disordered breathing. *J Appl Physiol* 63:1344–1350.

Jakubiak MJ, Siedlecki CT, Zenger E et al. (2005) Laryngeal, laryngotracheal, and tracheal masses in cats: 27 cases (1998–2003). *J Am Anim Hosp Assoc* 41:310–316.

Koch DA, Arnold S, Hubler M et al. (2003) Brachycephalic syndrome in dogs. *Compend Contin Educ Vet Pract* 25:48–55.

MacPhail CM, Monet E (2009) Laryngeal diseases. In *Kirk's Veterinary Therapy XIV*. (eds JD Bonagura, DC Twedt) Saunders Elsevier, St. Louis, pp. 627–629.

Schachter S, Norris, CR (2000) Laryngeal paralysis in cats: 16 cases (1990–1999). *J Am Vet Med Assoc* 216:1100–1103.

Ticehurst K, Zaki S, Hunt GB et al. (2008) Use of continuous positive airway pressure in the acute management of laryngeal paralysis in a cat. *Aust Vet J* 86:395–397.

Torrez CV, Hunt GB (2006) Results of surgical correction of abnormalities associated with brachycephalic airway obstruction syndrome in dogs in Australia. *J Small Anim Pract* 47:150–154.

Tracheal/large airway disease
Ayres SA, Holmberg DL (1999) Surgical treatment of tracheal collapse using pliable total ring prostheses: results in one experimental and 4 clinical cases. *Can Vet J* 40:787–791.

Buback JL, Boothe HW, Hobson HP (1996) Surgical treatment of tracheal collapse in dogs: 90 cases (1983–1993). *J Am Vet Med Assoc* 208:380–384.

Clarke DL, Holt DE, Macintire DK (2008) Tracheal collapse in dogs. *Standards of Care Emerg Crit Care Med* 10:1–6.

Coyne BE and Fingland RB (1992) Hypoplasia of the trachea in dogs: 103 cases (1974–1990) *J Am Vet Med Assoc* 201:768–772.

Hardie EM, Spodnick GJ, Gilson SD et al. (1999) Tracheal rupture in cats: 16 cases (1983–1998). *J Am Vet Med Assoc* 214:508–512.

Harvey CE and Fink EA (1982) Tracheal diameter: analysis of radiographic measurements in brachycephalic and nonbrachycephalic dogs. *J Am Anim Hosp Assoc* 18:570–576.

Hawkins EC, Clay LD, Bradley JM et al. (2010) Demographic and historical findings, including exposure to environmental tobacco smoke, in dogs with chronic cough. *J Vet Intern Med* 24:825–831.

Johnson L (2000) Tracheal collapse: diagnosis and medical and surgical treatment. *Vet Clin North Am Small Anim Pract* 30:1253–1266.

Johnson LR, Drazenovich TL (2007) Flexible bronchoscopy and bronchoalveolar lavage in 68 cats (2001–2006). *J Vet Intern Med* 21:219–225.

Johnson LR, Pollard RE (2010) Tracheal collapse and bronchomalacia in dogs: 58 cases (7/2001–1/2008). *J Vet Intern Med* 24:298–305.

Kaki A, Crosby ET, Lui AC (1997) Airway and respiratory management following non-lethal hanging. *Can J Anaesth* 44:445–450.

Lekeux P, Desmecht D (1993) Ventilatory failure and respiratory muscle fatigue. In *Pulmonary Function in Healthy Exercising and Diseased Animals*. Flemish Vet Journal Special Issue, pp. 331–350.

Macready DM, Johnson LR, Pollard RE (2007) Fluoroscopic and radiographic evaluation of tracheal collapse in dogs: 62 cases (2001–2006). *J Am Vet Med Assoc* 230:1870–1876.

Mitchell SL, McCarthy R, Rudloff E et al. (2000) Tracheal rupture associated with intubation in cats 20 cases (1996–1998). *J Am Vet Med Assoc* 216:1592–1595.

Queen EV, Vaughan MA, Johnson LR (2010) Bronchoscopic debulking of tracheal carcinoma in 3 cats using a wire snare. *J Vet Intern Med* 24:990–993.

Roach W, Krahwinkel DJ (2009) Obstructive

lesions and traumatic injuries of the canine and feline tracheas. *Compend Contin Ed Pract Vet* 31:86–93.

Robinson NE (2007) Overview of respiratory function: ventilation of the lung. In *Textbook of Veterinary Physiology*, 4th edn. (eds JG Cunningham, BG Klein) Saunders Elsevier, St. Louis, pp. 566–578.

Sura PA, Krahwinkel DJ (2008) Self-expanding nitinol stents for the treatment of tracheal collapse in dogs: 12 cases (2001–2004). *J Am Vet Med Assoc* 232:228–236.

Suter PF (1984) (ed) *Thoracic Radiography: A Text Atlas of Thoracic Diseases of the Dog and Cat*. Wettswil, Switzerland, pp. 533–537.

Tenwolde AC, Johnson LR, Hunt GB *et al.* (2010) The role of bronchoscopy in foreign body removal in dogs and cats: 37 cases (2000–2008). *J Vet Intern Med* 24:1063–1068.

Weisse CWC (2009) Intraluminal stenting for tracheal collapse. In *Kirk's Current Veterinary Therapy XIV*. (eds JD Bonagura, DC Twedt) Saunders Elsevier, St Louis, pp. 635–641.

Bronchitis/small airway disease

Gadbois J, d'Anjou MA, Dunn M *et al.* (2009) Radiographic abnormalities in cats with feline bronchial disease and intra- and interobserver variability in radiographic interpretation: 40 cases (1999–2006). *J Am Vet Med Assoc* 234:367–375.

Hawkins EC (2009) Disorders of the trachea and bronchi. In *Small Animal Internal Medicine*, 4th edn. (eds RW Nelson, CG Couto) Lea & Febiger, Philadelphia, pp. 285–301.

Hawkins EC (2009) Diagnostic tests for the lower respiratory tract. In *Small Animal Internal Medicine*, 4th edn. (eds RW Nelson, CG Couto) Lea & Febiger, Philadelphia, pp. 252–284.

Johnson LR (2005) Diseases of the small airways. In *Textbook of Veterinary Internal Medicine*. 6th edn. (eds SJ Ettinger, EC Feldman) Saunders Elsevier, St. Louis, pp. 1233–1238.

Suter PF (1984) (ed) *Thoracic Radiography: A Text Atlas of Thoracic Diseases of the Dog and Cat*. Wettswil, Switzerland, pp. 533–537.

RESPIRATORY DISEASES: LUNG

Cohn LA (2010) Pulmonary parenchymal diseases. In *Textbook of Veterinary Internal Medicine*, 7th edn. (eds SJ Ettinger, EC Feldman) Saunders Elsevier, St. Louis, pp. 1096–1118.

McNiel EA, Ogilvie GK, Powers BE *et al.* (1997) Evaluation of prognostic factors for dogs with primary lung tumors: 67 cases (1985–1992). *J Am Vet Med Assoc* 211:1422–1427.

Nemanic S, London CA, Wisner ER (2006) Comparison of thoracic radiographs and single breath-hold helical CT for detection of pulmonary nodules in dogs with metastatic neoplasia. *J Vet Intern Med* 20:508–515.

Paoloni MC, Adams WM, Dubielzig RR *et al.* (2006) Comparison of results of computed tomography and radiography with histopathologic findings in tracheobronchial lymph nodes in dogs with primary lung tumors: 14 cases (1999–2002). *J Am Vet Med Assoc* 228:1718–1722.

Acute respiratory distress syndrome and noncardiogenic pulmonary edema

DeClue AE, Cohn LA (2007) Acute respiratory distress syndrome in dogs and cats: a review of clinical findings and pathophysiology. *J Vet Emerg Crit Care* 17:340–347.

Dobratz KJ, Saunders HM *et al.* (1995) Noncardiogenic pulmonary edema in dogs and cats: 26 cases (1987–1993). *J Am Vet Med Assoc* 206:1732–1736.

Hsu YH, Cho LC, Wang LS *et al.* (2006) Acute respiratory distress syndrome associated with rabies: a case report. *Kaohsiung J Med Sci* 22:94–98.

Lemos LB, Baliga M, Guo M (2001) Acute respiratory distress syndrome and blastomycosis: presentation of nine cases and review of the literature. *Ann Diag Path* 5:1–9.

Meyer KC, McManus EJ, Maki DG (1993) Overwhelming pulmonary blastomycosis associated with the adult respiratory distress syndrome. *New Engl J Med* 329:1231–1236.

Parent C, King LG, Walker LM *et al.* (1996) Clinical and clinicopathologic findings in dogs with acute respiratory distress syndrome: 19 cases (1985–1993). *J Am Vet Med Assoc* 208:1419–1427.

Walker T, Tidwell AS, Rozanski EA et al. (2005) Imaging diagnosis: acute lung injury following massive bee envenomation in a dog. Vet Radiol Ultrasound 46:300–303.

Pneumonias

Forrester SD, Moon ML, Jacobson JD (2001) Diagnostic evaluation of dogs and cats with respiratory distress. Compend Contin Educ Pract Vet 23:56–69.

Greene CE (2006) (ed) Infectious Diseases of the Dog and Cat, 3rd edn. Elsevier Saunders, St. Louis.

Kogan DA, Johnson LR, Jandrey KE et al. (2008) Clinical, clinicopathologic, and radiographic findings in dogs with aspiration pneumonia: 88 cases (2004–2006). J Am Vet Med Assoc 233:1742–1747.

Kogan DA, Johnson LR, Sturges BK et al. (2008) Etiology and clinical outcome in dogs with aspiration pneumonia: 88 cases (2004–2006). J Am Vet Med Assoc 233:1748–1755.

Rochat MC, Cowell RL, Tyler RD et al. (1990) Paragonimiasis in dogs and cats. Compend Contin Educ Pract Vet 12:1093–1100.

Wray JD, Sparkes AH (2006) Use of radiographic measurements in distinguishing myasthenia gravis from other causes of canine megaesophagus. J Small Anim Pract 47:256–263.

Other pulmonary parenchymal disease

Berry CR, Graham JP, Thrall DE (2007) Interpretation paradigms for the small animal thorax. In Textbook of Veterinary Diagnostic Radiology, 5th edn. (ed DE Thrall) Saunders Elsevier, St Louis, pp. 462–485.

Brown AJ, Waddell LS (2009) Rodenticides. In Small Animal Critical Care Medicine. (eds DC Silverstein, K Hopper) Elsevier, St. Louis, Elsevier. pp. 346–350.

Clercx C, Peeters D (2007) Canine eosinophilic bronchopneumopathy. Vet Clin North Am Small Anim Pract 37:917–935.

Clercx C, Peeters D, German AJ et al. (2002) An immunologic investigation of canine eosinophilic bronchopneumopathy. J Vet Intern Med 16:229–237.

Clercx C, Peeters D, Snaps F et al. (2000) Eosinophilic bronchopneumopathy in dogs. J Vet Intern Med 14:282–291.

Drobatz DJ, Walker LM, Hendricks JC (1999) Smoke exposure in dogs: 27 cases (1986–1997) J Am Vet Med Assoc 215:1306–1311.

Drobatz DJ, Walker LM, Hendricks JC (1999) Smoke exposure in cats: 22 cases (1986–1997). J Am Vet Med Assoc 215:1312–1316.

Fitzgerald KT, Flood AA (2006) Smoke inhalation. Clin Tech Small Anim Pract 21:205–214.

Goldkamp CE, Schaer M (2008) Canine drowning. Compend Contin Educ Pract Vet 30:340–352.

Heffner GG, Rozanski EA, Beal MW et al. (2008) Evaluation of freshwater submersion in small animals: 28 cases (1996–2006). J Am Vet Med Assoc 232:244–248.

Johnson VS, Corcoran BM, Wotton PR et al. (2005) Thoracic high-resolution computed tomographic findings in dogs with canine idiopathic pulmonary fibrosis. J Small Anim Pract 46:381–388.

Norris AJ, Naydan DK, Wilson DW (2005) Interstitial lung disease in West Highland White Terriers. Vet Pathol 42:35–41.

Polton GA, Brearley MJ, Powell SM et al. (2008) Impact of primary tumour stage on survival in dogs with solitary lung tumours. J Small Anim Pract 49:66–71.

Rissetto KC, Lucas PW, Fan TM (2008) An update on diagnosing and treating primary lung tumors. Vet Med 103:154–169.

Ventilator therapy

Ethier MR, Mathews KA, Valverde A et al. (2008) Evaluation of the efficacy and safety for use of two sedation and analgesia protocols to facilitate assisted ventilation of healthy dogs. Am J Vet Res 69:1351–1359.

Hopper K, Haskins SC, Kass PH et al. (2007) Indications, management, and outcome of long-term positive-pressure ventilation in dogs and cats: 148 cases (1990–2001). J Am Vet Med Assoc 230:64–75.

Sereno RL (2006) Use of controlled ventilation in a clinical setting. J Am Anim Hosp Assoc 42:477–480.

RESPIRATORY DISEASES: PLEURAL SPACE

Pleural effusion

D'Anjou MA, Tidwell AS, Hecht S (2005) Radiographic diagnosis of lung lobe torsion. Vet Radiol Ultrasound 46:478–484.

Further reading

Boothe HW, Howe LM, Boothe DM *et al.*
(2010) Evaluation of outcomes in dogs
treated for pyothorax: 46 cases (1983–
2001). *J Am Vet Med Assoc* **236**:657–663.

Fossum TW, Forrester SD, Swenson CL *et al.*
(1991) Chylothorax in cats: 37 cases
(1969–1989). *J Am Vet Med Assoc*
198:672–678.

La Fond E, Weirich WE, Salisbury SK (2002)
Omentalization of the thorax for treatment
of idiopathic chylothorax with constrictive
pleuritis in a cat. *J Am Anim Hosp Assoc*
38:74–78.

Ludwig LL, Simpson AM, Han E (2010)
Pleural and extrapleural diseases. In
Textbook of Veterinary Internal Medicine,
7th edn. (eds SJ Ettinger, EC Feldman)
Saunders Elsevier, St. Louis, pp. 1125–
1137.

McGavin MD, Zachary JF (2007) (eds)
Pathologic Basis of Veterinary Disease, 4th
edn. Elsevier, St. Louis.

Moore AS, Kirk C, Cardona A (1991)
Intracavitary cisplatin chemotherapy
experience with six dogs. *J Vet Intern Med*
5:227–231.

Murphy KA, Brisson BA (2006) Evaluation
of lung lobe torsion in Pugs: 7 cases (1991–
2004). *J Am Vet Med Assoc* **228**:86–90.

Neath PJ, Brockman DJ, King LG (2000)
Lung lobe torsion in dogs: 22 cases (1981–
1999). *J Am Vet Med Assoc* **217**:1041–
1044.

Seiler G, Schwarz T, Rodriguez D (2008)
Computed tomographic features of lung
lobe torsion. *Vet Radiol Ultrasound*
49:504–508.

Spugnini EP, Crispi S, Scarabello A *et al.*
(2008) Piroxicam and intracavitary
platinum-based chemotherapy for the
treatment of advanced mesothelioma in
pets: preliminary observations. *J Exp Clin
Cancer Res* **27**:6–10.

Pneumothorax

Au JJ, Weisman DL, Stefanacci JD *et al.*
(2006) Use of computed tomography for
evaluation of lung lesions associated with
spontaneous pneumothorax in dogs: 12
cases (1999–2002). *J Am Vet Med Assoc*
228:733–737.

Lipscomb VJ, Hardie RJ, Dubielzig RR
(2003) Spontaneous pneumothorax caused
by pulmonary blebs and bullae in 12 dogs.
J Am Anim Hosp Assoc **39**:435–445.

Ludwig LL, Simpson AM, Han E (2010)
Pleural and extrapleural diseases. In
Textbook of Veterinary Internal Medicine,
7th edn. (eds SJ Ettinger, EC Feldman)
Saunders Elsevier, St. Louis, pp. 1125–
1137.

Maritato KC, Cokon KA, Kergosien DH
(2009) Pneumothorax. *Compend Contin
Educ Pract Vet* **31**:232–242.

Puerto DA, Brockman DJ, Lindquist C *et al.*
(2002) Surgical and nonsurgical
management of and selected risk factors
for spontaneous pneumothorax in dogs: 64
cases (1986–1999). *J Am Vet Med Assoc*
220:1670–1674.

THORACIC DISEASE AND OTHER ABNORMALITIES

Diaphragmatic disease

Bellenger CR, Milstein M, McDonell W
(1975) Herniation of gravid uterus into the
thorax of a dog. *Mod Vet Pract* **56**:553–
555.

Lin JL, Lee CS, Chen PW *et al.* (2007)
Complications during labour in a
Chihuahua due to diaphragmatic hernia.
Vet Rec **161**:103–104.

Tadmor A, Zuckerman E, Birnbaum SC
(1978) Diaphragmatic hernia in a pregnant
bitch. *J Am Vet Med Assoc* **172**:585–586.

Heinz body anemia

Court MH. Greenblatt DJ (2000) Molecular
genetic basis for deficient acetaminophen
glucuronidation by cats: UGT1A6 is a
pseudogene, and evidence for reduced
diversity of expressed hepatic UGT1A
isoforms. *Pharmacogenetics* **10**:355–369.

Hill AS, O'Neill S, Rogers QR *et al.* (2001)
Antioxidant prevention of Heinz body
formation and oxidative injury in cats. *Am
J Vet Res* **62**:370–374.

Robertson JE, Christopher MM, Rogers QR
(1998) Heinz body formation in cats fed
baby food containing onion powder. *J Am
Vet Med Assoc* **212**:1260–1266.

Villar D, Buck WB, Gonzales JM (1998)
Ibuprofen, aspirin and acetaminophen
toxicosis and treatment in dogs and cats.
Vet Hum Toxicol **40**:156–162.

Mediastinal disease

Biller DS, Larson MM (2010) Mediastinal
disease. In *Textbook of Veterinary Internal
Medicine*, 7th edn. (eds SJ Ettinger, EC

Feldman) Saunders Elsevier, St. Louis, pp. 1119–1124.

Fidel JL, Pargass IS, Dark MJ et al. (2008) Granulocytopenia associated with thymoma in a domestic shorthaired cat. *J Am Anim Hosp Assoc* **44**:210–217.

Palmer KG, King LG, Van Winkle TJ (1998) Clinical manifestations and associated disease syndromes in dogs with cranial vena cava thrombosis: 17 cases (1989–1996). *J Am Vet Med Assoc* **213**:220–224.

Rottenberg S, von Tscharner C, Roosje PJ (2004) Thymoma-associated exfoliative dermatitis in cats. *Vet Pathol* **41**:429–433.

Smith AN, Wright, JC, Brawner WR et al. (2001) Radiation therapy in the treatment of canine and feline thymomas: a retrospective study (1985–1999). *J Am Anim Hosp Assoc* **37**:489–496.

Stephens JA, Parnell NK, Clarke K et al. (2002) Subcutaneous emphysema, pneumomediastinum, and pulmonary emphysema in a young schipperke. *J Am Anim Hosp Assoc* **38**:121–124.

Yoon J, Feeney DA, Cronk KL (2004) Computed tomographic evaluation of canine and feline mediastinal masses in 14 patients. *Vet Radiol Ultrasound* **45**:542–546.

Zitz JC, Birchard SJ, Couto GC et al. (2008) Results of excision of thymoma in cats and dogs: 20 cases (1984–2005) *J Am Vet Med Assoc* **232**:1186–1192.

Pectus excavatum

Boudrieau R, Fossum T, Hartsfield S et al. (1990) Pectus excavatum in dogs and cats. *Compend Contin Educ Pract Vet* **12**:341–355.

Fossum TW (2007) Pectus excavatum. In *Small Animal Surgery*, 3rd edn. (ed TW Fossum) Mosby, St. Louis, pp. 889–894.

Fossum TW, Boudrieau RJ, Hobson HP (1989) Pectus excavatum in eight dogs and six cats. *J Am Anim Hosp Assoc* **25**:595–605.

Yoon H, Mann FA, Jeong S (2008) Surgical correction of pectus excavatum in two cats. *J Vet Sci* **9**:335–337.

Thoracic trauma

Holt DE, Griffin G (2000) Bite wounds in dogs and cats. *Vet Clin North Am Small Anim Pract* **30**:669–679.

Toxicity: coagulopathy

Brown AJ, Waddell LS (2009) Rodenticides. In *Small Animal Critical Care Medicine*. (eds DC Silverstein, K Hopper) Elsevier, St. Louis, pp. 346–350.

Dunn ME (2010) Acquired coagulopathies. In *Textbook of Veterinary Internal Medicine*, 7th edn. (eds SJ Ettinger, EC Feldman) Saunders Elsevier, St. Louis, pp. 797–800.

VASCULAR DISEASE

Pulmonary thromboembolism

Carr AP, Panciera DL, Kidd L (2002) Prognostic factors for mortality and thromboembolism in canine immune-mediated hemolytic anemia: a retrospective study of 72 dogs. *J Vet Intern Med* **16**:504–509.

Hackner SG (2009) Pulmonary thromboembolism. In *Kirk's Current Veterinary Therapy XIV*. (eds JD Bonagura, DC Twedt) Saunders Elsevier, St Louis, pp. 689–697.

Systemic arterial thromboembolism

Alwood AJ, Downend AB, Brooks MB et al. (2007) Anticoagulant effects of low-molecular-weight heparins in healthy cats. *J Vet Intern Med* **21**:378–387.

Boswood A, Lamb CR, White RN (2000) Aortic and iliac thrombosis in six dogs. *J Small Anim Pract* **41**:109–114.

Carr AP, Panciera DL, Kidd L (2002) Prognostic factors for mortality and thromboembolism in canine immune-mediated hemolytic anemia: a retrospective study of 72 dogs. *J Vet Intern Med* **16**:504–509.

Good LI, Manning AM (2003) Thromboembolic disease: physiology of hemostasis and pathophysiology of thrombosis. *Compend Contin Educ Pract Vet* **25**:650–658.

Good LI, Manning AM (2003) Thromboembolic disease: predispositions and clinical management. *Compend Contin Educ Pract Vet* **25**:660–674.

Hogan DF, Andrews DA, Green HW et al. (2004) Antiplatelet effects and pharmacodynamics of clopidogrel in cats. *J Am Vet Med Assoc* **225**:1406–1411.

Laste NJ, Harpster NK (1995) A retrospective study of 100 cases of feline distal aortic thromboembolism: 1977–1993. *J Am Anim Hosp Assoc* **31**:492–500.

Further reading

Moore KE, Morris N, Dhupa N *et al.* (2000) Retrospective study of streptokinase administration in 46 cats with arterial thromboembolism. *J Vet Emerg Crit Care* **10**:245–257.

Nelson OL, Andreasen C (2003) The utility of plasma D-dimer to identify thromboembolic disease in dogs. *J Vet Intern Med* **17**:830–834.

Rossmeisl JH (2003) Current principles and applications of D-dimer analysis in small animal practice. *Vet Med* **98**:224–234.

Smith CE, Rozanski EA, Freeman LM *et al.* (2004) Use of low molecular weight heparin in cats: 57 cases (1999–2003). *J Am Vet Med Assoc* **225**:1237–1241.

Smith SA, Tobias AH (2004) Feline arterial thromboembolism: an update. *Vet Clin North Am Small Anim Pract* **34**:1245–1271.

Smith SA, Tobias AH, Jacob KA *et al.* (2003) Arterial thromboembolism in cats: acute crisis in 127 cases (1992–2001) and long-term management with low-dose aspirin in 24 cases. *J Vet Intern Med* **17**:73–83.

Stokol T, Brooks M, Rush JE, *et al.* (2008) Hypercoagulability in cats with cardiomyopathy. *J Vet Intern Med* **22**:546–552.

Thompson MF, Scott-Moncrieff JC, Hogan DF (2001) Thrombolytic therapy in dogs and cats. *J Vet Emerg Crit Care* **11**:111–121.

Van De Wiele CM, Hogan DF, Green III HW *et al.* (2010) Antithrombotic effect of enoxaparin in clinically healthy cats: a venous stasis model. *J Vet Intern Med* **24**:185–191.

Van Winkle TJ, Hackner SG, Liu SM (1993) Clinical and pathological features of aortic thromboembolism in 36 dogs. *J Vet Emerg Crit Care* **3**:13–21.

Ware WA. (2011) Thromboembolic disease. In *Cardiovascular Disease in Small Animal Medicine*. (ed WA Ware) Manson Publishing, London, pp. 145–163.

Welch KM, Rozanski EA, Freeman LM *et al.* (2010) Prospective evaluation of tissue plasminogen activator in 11 cats with arterial thromboembolism. *J Feline Med Surg* **12**:122–128.

Index

Note: References are to case numbers

abdominal distension 44, 111, 120, 121, 205, 206
abdominal mass 183
acetaminophen toxicity 138
acidosis 102
activated partial thromboplastin time 97, 104
acute respiratory distress syndrome 105, 106, 197
Addison's disease 54
aerophagia 56, 105, 179, 191
air bronchogram 62, 65, 66, 89, 101, 166
airway collapse 15, 57, 58, 164, 195
airway obstruction 1
  bronchial foreign body 102, 103
  upper airway 9, 50, 57, 58, 116, 133
albuterol 96, 100
allergens 96, 99, 151
alveolar–arterial gradient 68
aminophylline 181
amiodarone 49, 87, 217
amlodipine 132, 201
amoxicillin–clavanulate 150, 166
anemia 82
angiography 45, 88, 110, 121, 163
angiostrongylosis 64, 154, 162, 218
angiotensin-converting enzyme inhibitors 95, 107, 110, 181, 187, 207, 216
anthelmintics 154, 199, 218
antiarrhythmic drugs 49, 91, 148, 217
antibiotic therapy
  bronchopneumonia 150, 177
  endocarditis 128
  infectious tracheo-bronchitis 166
antihypertensive therapy 132
aorta, dilation of ascending 132

aortic body tumor 158
aortic stenosis, *see* subaortic stenosis
aortic valve
  endocarditis 128
  insufficiency/regurgitation 85, 86, 88, 127, 171, 186
apical impulse, right 156
arrhythmias
  accelerated idioventricular rhythm 173
  atrial fibrillation 18, 67, 145, 149, 175, 188
  atrial standstill 53, 115
  atrial tachyarrhythmias 38, 80, 87, 181, 189, 217
  atrioventricular block 23, 37, 77, 113, 114, 143, 183
  bradyarrhythmias 23, 37, 102, 103, 114, 143
  re-entrant supraventricular tachycardia 130
  sinus 21, 54, 102, 103, 173
  sinus arrest 135, 143, 204
  supraventricular tachycardia 49, 87
  ventricular tachycardia 4, 36, 148, 172
arterial pulses (abnormal) 127, 146, 180, 188
arterial thromboembolism 97, 107, 180
  diagnosis 180
  diseases causing 180
  feline 34
  management 180
ascites 44, 111, 120, 121, 205, 206, 219
  categories 120
aspirin 35, 97, 107, 165, 208
asthma, feline 89, 99
atenolol 35
atrial fibrillation 18, 145, 149, 175, 188
  feline 67
  treatment 145
atrial premature complexes 38, 80, 181

atrial standstill 53, 115
  persistent 115
atrial tachyarrhythmias 38, 80, 87, 181, 189, 217
atrioventricular block 23, 37, 113, 114
  complete 183
  intermittent 23, 143
  symptomatic 77
atropine 143
atropine response test 37, 115
auscultation (cardiac)
  feline 41
  see also murmur

β2-adrenoreceptor agonists 96, 100
bacterial pneumonia 78, 150, 177
Balfour retractor 84
balloon valvuloplasty 45, 63
barium swallow 40
benazepril 35, 208, 216
beta blockers 32, 47, 49, 80, 132, 165, 207
  sotalol 91
biomarkers, cardiac 75, 95
bite wounds 178
blastomycosis 197
bloating, 'whole body' 182
blood gas analyses 68, 102
blood smears 138
bone, periosteal formation 142, 155
Bordetella spp. 166, 177
Boxer cardiomyopathy 36
brachycephalic breeds 158
bradyarrhythmias 23, 37, 114, 143
bradycardia, episodic 102, 103
bradycardia–tachycardia (sick sinus) syndrome 204
breathing, open mouth 21
breathing pattern 1, 133
bronchial collapse 15
bronchial pattern 16, 28, 72, 99, 176
bronchiectasis 72, 176
bronchitis
  allergic 96, 100, 151
  chronic 10, 72, 195

Index

bronchoalveolar carcinoma 17, 70, 168
bronchoalveolar lavage
  airway inflammation 96, 99
  angiostrongylosis 218
  bronchopneumonia 177
  chronic bronchitis 10, 72
  histoplasmosis 169
  tracheal thickening 82
bronchodilators 15, 96, 99, 100, 150, 204
bronchopneumonia 62, 150, 166, 177
bronchoscopy
  bronchial foreign body 103
  chronic bronchitis 195
  eosinophilic lung disease 153
  feline asthma 99
  pulmonary tumor 168
bronchus
  compression 214
  foreign body 103
bulla, pulmonary 134
Bulldogs 62
bullet wound 194

calcinosis cutis 126
calcium-channel blockers 201
cannon 'a' waves 23
cardiac catheterization 88, 163, 205
cardiac shift 98, 156, 193
cardiac silhouette
  horizontal orientation 132
  'valentine' shape 35
  vertical orientation 32
  see also cardiomegaly
cardiac size, assessment 20, 39
cardiac tamponade 44, 46, 69, 144
  recurrent 209
cardiac troponin I 75, 95
cardiomegaly 18, 32, 35, 46, 79, 107, 110, 114, 117, 132, 140, 149, 175, 189, 203
  assessment 20
  generalized 28, 46, 170, 171, 203, 214
  left heart 174, 175

cardiomyopathy
  arrhythmogenic RV ('Boxer') 26, 36
  dilated 4, 32, 95, 148, 170, 171, 207
  hypertrophic (HCM) 28, 35, 67, 90, 117
  hypertrophic obstructive 47
  restrictive 110, 165, 208
  thromboembolism 107
carnitine, plasma 171
carotid sinus massage 87
carvedilol 189
caval syndrome 55, 210
caval thrombosis 109
cavitary pulmonary lesions 108, 134, 153, 196
central venous pressure 29, 219
  measurement 29
cephalexin 150
chemodectoma 158
chemotherapy 123
chylothorax 25, 59, 60, 101
clopidogrel 35, 97, 107, 165
coagulopathies 65, 104
Cocker Spaniels 171
collapse 77, 102, 103, 112
  episodic 53, 130, 146, 172, 204, 211
  see also syncope
computed tomography 17, 108, 193, 196, 218
congenital disorders
  cor triatriatum dexter 120, 121
  laryngeal paralysis 5
  pectus excavatum 118, 119
  persistent left cranial vena cava 31
  persistent right aortic arch 139
  pulmonic valve stenosis 63
  subaortic stenosis 85, 86, 146
  tetralogy of Fallot 92, 125
  tracheal hypoplasia 62
  tricuspid dysplasia 87, 206
congestive heart failure 18, 32, 110, 117, 165, 170, 205
  biventricular 90, 208

congestive heart failure (continued)
  chronic patent ductus arteriosus 174, 175
  concurrent pulmonary hypertension 211
  decompensated 189, 216
  feline 26, 110, 208
  management 110, 171, 189, 214, 216
  re-evaluation 157
  stage D management 187
  staging 73
cor triatriatum dexter 120, 121
coronaviruses 61
corticosteroids 96, 99, 153, 184
cough
  causes in cats 137, 199
  chronic 1, 10, 176, 195, 199, 200
  with eating/drinking 40, 98
  with gagging 39, 40, 93, 200
  'honking' 164, 166
  intermittent/episodic 8, 9, 82, 164
  non-cardiac causes 39, 40, 102, 103
  persistent 38, 151, 162
  productive 151, 200
  recent onset 2, 8
  recurrent 2, 214
crackles, pulmonary 56, 66, 82, 90, 126, 162, 165, 191, 198
cranial caval syndrome 51, 52, 109
Curschmann's spiral 10
Cushing's disease 126
cyanosis 12, 50, 92, 102, 133, 194
  with activity 125, 203
  causes 12
  differential 131
cyclophosphamide 153
cyst, tracheal 9, 133
cytology 218

dalteparin sodium 97
dental procedures, history of 78
dexamethasone sodium phosphate 96

diaphragmatic hernia
  left-sided 98
  peritoneopericardial 140,
    188
  right-sided 3, 74
  traumatic 74, 84
digoxin 80, 181, 189
digoxin toxicity 143
diltiazem 49, 80, 87, 107,
  145, 149
diphenylhydantoin 143
dobutamine 95
drowning 66
dyspnea, see respiratory
  distress

echocardiogram 26
  cardiac tumor 76, 158
  cardiomyopathy 47, 90,
    165
  heartworm disease 185,
    210
  M-mode 47, 48, 90, 127,
    207
  mitral valve disease 149,
    188
  patent ductus arteriosus
    175
  penetrating cardiac wound
    194
  pericardial effusion 144
  peritoneopericardial
    diaphragmatic hernia
    188
  pulmonary hypertension
    129, 162
  pulmonic stenosis 63
  recurrent cardiac
    tamponade 209
  spontaneous contrast 107
  subaortic stenosis 146
  tetralogy of Fallot 125
  ventricular septal defect
    186
edema
  cranial subcutaneous 109
  pulmonary 81, 84, 105,
    106, 117, 170, 171
electrical alternans 44
electrocardiogram
  accelerated idioventricular
    rhythm 173
  artifacts 159, 183
  atrial fibrillation 67, 145,
    188

electrocardiogram
  (continued)
  atrial tachyarrhythmias
    80, 181
  atrioventricular block 183
  cardiac tumor 75
  digoxin toxicity 143
  electrical alternans 44
  Holter/ambulatory 36, 77,
    207
  hyperkalemia 33
  mean electrical axis 24
  mitral valve dysplasia 13
  right bundle branch block
    113, 152
  sick sinus syndrome 204
  sinus arrhythmias 54, 155
  ST segment elevation 75
  ventricular pre-excitation
    49, 130
  ventricular tachycardia 4,
    36, 148
emphysema, subcutaneous
  182
enalapril 38, 189, 214, 216
endocardiosis 48
endocarditis 85, 86, 127, 128
endotracheal tube trauma
  182
enoxaparin 97
enrofloxacin 166
eosinophilia 16, 96, 151, 153
erythrocytosis, primary 12,
  92
esmolol 87
esophageal reflux 200
esophagobronchial fistula
  39, 40
esophagram 39, 40, 139
esophagus
  abnormal thoracic 167
  distension/dilation 93,
    139, 191
  foreign body 179

feline infectious peritonitis 61
femoral pulses 23
fenbendazole 154, 199
fibrosarcoma 155
fire damage 56
fish oil 32
fluconazole 169
fluoroquinolones 166
foreign body
  bronchus 102, 103

foreign body (continued)
  esophagus 179
fractures
  ribs 147
  spinal compression 202
furosemide 38, 95, 110, 149,
  165, 170, 174, 189, 208,
  216
furosemide therapy 32

gagging 39, 40, 93
gallop sounds 32, 41, 117,
  132, 148, 165
gastroesophageal reflux 200
gentamicin 166
glycopyrrolate 143

heart failure
  acute 190
  chronic 174, 175, 181
  right-sided 69
  staging 73
  see also congestive heart
    failure
heartworm disease 136, 137,
  210
  diagnosis 136
  echocardiogram 185, 210
  feline 185
  severity grading 55
  treatment 27, 210
Heinz bodies 138
hemangiosarcoma 6, 75, 76
hematocrit 82, 92
hematoidin 6
hemoptysis 65, 108
hemorrhage 6, 65, 104, 147,
  162
hemosiderin 6
heparins 97, 107
hindlimb weakness 107,
  180
histoplasmosis 22, 169
Horner's syndrome 93
hydroxyurea 92
hyperadrenocorticism
  (Cushing's disease) 126
hyperkalemia 33, 53, 54
hypersensitivity response 16,
  96, 99, 151, 153
hypertension
  systemic 132
  see also pulmonary
    hypertension
hyperthyroidism 132

Index

hypoadrenocorticism
(Addison's disease) 54
hypotension 194
hypoventilation 42
hypoxemia 12, 42, 66, 68,
102, 103, 203
causes 102

imidacloprid 154
inflammation, airway 2, 82,
96, 99, 177
inhalation therapy 99, 100
insulin therapy 33
itraconazole 169

jugular veins,
pulsation/distension 23,
26, 51, 71, 111, 136,
210
jugular venotomy 210

kennel cough (infectious
tracheobronchitis) 166
ketoconazole 169

L-carnitine 32, 207
larynx
paralysis 5, 58
radiography 167
left atrial enlargement 4, 14,
15, 38, 81, 107, 110, 114,
115, 164, 165, 214, 216
left ventricle
enlargement 13, 86, 90,
95, 165, 186
fractional shortening
189, 207
hypertrophy 86, 90
wall motion 95
left ventricular outflow
obstruction 35, 47
lidocaine 49, 87, 143, 145
limb swelling 142
lipoma, abdominal 183
lung consolidation 191
lung lobe torsion 101
lung re-expansion edema
84
lung sounds (abnormal) 56,
66, 90, 116, 126, 153,
162, 165, 191, 198
classification 198
lymphadenopathy 22, 192
lymphoma 52, 94, 141, 192
diagnostic tests 141

mechanical ventilation 42, 43
mediastinal mass 51, 52, 93,
94, 109, 122, 213
megaesophagus 139, 191
causes 191
melarsomine
dihydrochloride 26
mesothelioma 71, 123, 209,
219
metallic projective injury 194
metastases, pulmonary 11,
168
metered dose inhaler 100
milbemycin oxime 154
mineralization, cutaneous
126
mitral regurgitation 7, 14,
48, 95, 164, 188, 189,
211, 214, 216
mitral valve
chronic degenerative
disease 38
dysplasia 13, 80, 149
moxidectin 154
murmur
aortic 127, 186
apical 20, 26, 38, 48
continuous (machinery)
79, 85, 139
diastolic 127, 128, 186
holosystolic 13, 14, 15,
114, 162, 186
important characteristics 7
mitral 7, 39, 47, 133, 149,
189
pectus excavatum 118
physiologic 7
pulmonic 45
systolic 4, 7, 12, 18, 24,
28, 29, 32, 35, 67, 141,
152, 186, 203
'to-and-fro' 85
muscular dystrophy, AV 115
myocardial disease, atrial 53
myocardial injury 173
myocardial tumor 172
myxoma, cardiac 111

N-acetylcysteine 138
nasal discharge 197
neoplasia
abdominal 183
cardiac 6, 69, 75, 76, 111,
158, 172
mesothelioma 71, 123, 209

neoplasia (continued)
pericardial effusion 6,
141, 144, 209
pulmonary 2, 17, 70, 82,
168
thoracic/mediastinal 51,
52, 93, 94, 109, 122,
142, 155, 212, 213
tracheal 116
nephropathy, protein-losing
19
nodules
airway 2, 8, 11, 108, 153
differentiation of benign
and malignant 11
NT-pro-BNP 95

octreotide 60
ocular pressure, bilateral 87
orthopnea 1, 104
Oslerus osleri 2
osteoma, pulmonary 11
osteopathy, hypertrophic 142
oxidative damage 138

pacemaker, artificial 113,
115, 135, 183
pancreatitis 105, 106
paragonimiasis 108, 199
paraneoplastic syndromes
213
parasympathetic tone 21
patent ductus arteriosus
79, 80, 139, 163, 174,
175
diagnostic tests 163
right-to-left shunting
(reversed) 131, 156
pectus excavatum 9, 118,
119
pericardial effusion 6, 44,
69, 144, 194
cardiac tamponade 46, 144
neoplastic 6, 141, 144,
209, 219
pericardial fluid samples 6,
71, 141, 161
pericardial space, soft tissue
188
pericardiectomy 69, 219
pericardiocentesis 6, 46,
160, 161
complications 161
equipment and technique
159

pericarditis, constrictive 219
periosteal new bone
    formation 142, 155
peritoneopericardial
    diaphragmatic hernia 140,
    188
persistent left cranial vena
    cava 31
persistent right aortic arch
    139
pharynx 167, 215
phlebotomy 92
phosphodiesterase-5
    inhibitors 83
physical deformities 9, 118,
    119
pimobendan 38, 95, 124,
    165, 181, 207, 216
    effects and indications 124
pleural effusion 29, 75, 101,
    208, 219
    chylous 25, 59, 60, 101
    differentiation from
        thoracic mass 155
    exudate 61
    modified transudate 26
    pseudochylous 25
    transudates 19, 155
    traumatic 194
pleural fluid samples 25, 59,
    61, 78
pleuritis 123
pneumomediastinum 30
pneumonia
    aspiration 191
    bacterial 150, 177
    embolic 78
    fungal 22, 169
    parasitic 108, 162, 199,
        218
    pyogranulomatous 89
pneumothorax 30
    recurrent 134
    spontaneous 193, 196
polycythemia rubra vera 12,
    92
positive end-expiratory
    pressure 43
praziquantel 199
precordial impulse 131, 156
prednisolone 96, 116
prednisone 153
pregnancy, diaphragmatic
    hernia 3
procainamide 49

propranolol 87
protein/creatinine ratio,
    urine 19
prothrombin time 104
pulmonary arteries,
    enlargement 137
pulmonary carcinoma
    bronchoalveolar 17, 168
    bronchogenic 70
pulmonary edema
    cardiogenic 117, 170,
        171, 214
    fluid analysis 106
    non-cardiogenic 81, 105,
        106
    re-expansion 84
pulmonary fibrosis,
    idiopathic 184
pulmonary granulomatosis,
    eosinophilic 153
pulmonary hypertension
    12, 129, 156, 162, 164,
    211
    echocardiography 129,
        162
    management 83
pulmonary infiltrates 162
pulmonary pattern
    alveolar 2, 56, 62, 66, 81,
        89, 101, 162, 191, 218
    alveolar–interstitial 65, 105
    bronchial 16, 28, 72, 99,
        176
    interstitial 2, 10, 22, 96,
        126, 137, 149, 162,
        168, 192, 197, 218
    nodular 11
    vascular 79, 117, 170,
        174, 185
pulmonary
    thromboembolism 27,
    185
pulmonary vessel dilation
    170, 174
pulmonic stenosis 45, 63,
    125, 205
purring
    discouraging during
        auscultation 41
    ECG artifact 159
pyothorax 78

radiography
    air bronchogram 62, 65,
        66, 89, 101, 166

radiography (continued)
    aspiration pneumonia
        191
    bronchiectasis 72, 176
    bronchitis 72
    cardiomegaly 20, 28, 32,
        35, 46, 170, 203
    cavitary pulmonary
        lesions 108, 196
    diaphragmatic hernia 3
    dilated cardiomyopathy
        170, 171
    esophagobronchial fistula
        39, 40
    feline asthma 89
    fire damage 56
    hypertrophic osteopathy
        142
    laryngeal/pharyngeal
        regions 167
    lymphadenopathy 22
    near drowning 66
    paragonimiasis 199
    patent ductus arteriosus
        79
    pleural effusion 60, 155,
        208
    pneumothorax 30, 193
    pulmonary edema 117,
        170
    pulmonary fibrosis 184
    pulmonary mass 17, 212
    pulmonary nodules 11
    strangulation 81
    thoracic mass 52, 93, 98,
        142, 155, 192
    thoracic trauma 74, 178,
        179, 202
    tracheal cyst 9
    tracheal hypoplasia 62
    tracheobronchitis 166
    upper airway 50
regurgitation (food) 139
renal disease 19
respiratory alkalosis 68
respiratory distress
    acetaminophen toxicity
        138
    acute respiratory distress
        syndrome 105, 106, 197
    airway obstruction 1, 5,
        9, 57, 58, 133
    asthma 99
    cardiac disease 28, 95,
        117, 149, 174

Index

respiratory distress
(*continued*)
  pulmonary bulla 134
  severe (orthopnea) 1, 104
  signs of in dog 1
  thoracic trauma 178
  tracheal tear 182
respiratory pattern 1, 133
retractor, Balfour 84
rhonchi 198
ribs
  fractures 147
  periosteal new bone
    formation 155
right atrial pressure 205
right bundle branch block
  113, 152
right ventricular enlargement
  162, 205
right ventricular pressure
  162
rodenticide toxicity 65, 104
rutin 60

saddle thrombus 34
sarcoma 142, 212
seizure activity 112
sick sinus syndrome 204
sildenafil 83, 184
sinus arrest 135, 143
soft palate, entrapment 50
sotalol 87, 91
spinal fracture 202
spironolactone 32, 38, 187
spleen, herniation 98
sputum histology,
  blastomycosis 197
sternotomy, median 134,
  213
sternum, luxation 178
strangulation 81
stridor 5, 50
subaortic stenosis 85, 86,
  146
subcutaneous emphysema
  182
subcutaneous hemorrhage
  104
synchronized intermittent
  mandatory ventilation 42
syncope 23, 36, 77, 112,
  113, 135, 204
  differentiation from
    seizure activity 112
  see also collapse

systemic inflammatory
  response 82

tachycardia
  AV reciprocating 49
  paroxysmal ventricular 4,
    148
  re-entrant
    supraventricular 130
  sinus 155, 181
  ventricular 36, 172
tachypnea 90, 138
taurine 171
terbutaline 96, 100
tetralogy of Fallot 92, 125
theophylline 38, 100
third eyelid, protrusion 93
thoracocentesis 25, 59, 60,
  61, 78, 123, 208
thoracoscopy 69, 123
thoracotomy 69
thromboembolism
  pulmonary 27, 185
  see also arterial
    thromboembolism
thymoma 122, 213
toxicities 104, 138, 143
trachea
  displacement 93, 122,
    140, 167, 179
  elevation 46, 117
  hypoplasia 62
  mass 9, 116, 133
  tear 182
  thickening 82
tracheal collapse 57, 58,
  164, 195
tracheal collapse complex
  15
tracheal diameter:thoracic
  inlet ratio 62
tracheal ring, prosthetic 58
tracheobronchitis, infectious
  166
tracheoscopy 58
tracheostomy tube
  placement 215
trauma
  bite wounds 178
  diaphragmatic hernia 74,
    84
  endotracheal tube
    placement 182
  penetrating cardiac
    wound 194

trauma (*continued*)
  post-traumatic arrhythmia
    173
  thoracic 74, 147, 178,
    202
tricuspid dysplasia 26, 87,
  206
tricuspid regurgitation 162

ultrasonography 34, 94
  survey 94
upper airway obstruction 1,
  9, 50, 57, 58, 116, 133
urethral obstruction 33
uterus, diaphragmatic
  herniation 3

vagal maneuvers 87
vascular ring anomaly 139
vehicle trauma 74, 84, 147,
  173
vena cava
  caudal enlargement 203
  cranial compression 52
  persistent left cranial 31
ventilation/perfusion (V/Q)
  mismatch 68, 102
ventilator therapy 42, 43
ventricular escape rhythm
  115
ventricular pre-excitation 49,
  130
ventricular premature
  complexes 4, 115, 143,
  205, 207
ventricular septal defect 13,
  88, 125, 186, 203
ventricular tachycardia 4,
  36, 148, 172
ventricular trigeminy 36
verapamil 49
vertebral heart score 20
vomiting 75, 140, 185, 188

water submersion 66
weight loss 109, 116
'Westie lung disease' 184
wheezes 66, 90, 116, 198
Wolff–Parkinson–White
  pre-excitation 130
Wright's stain 10

T - #0833 - 101024 - C288 - 210/148/13 - PB - 9781840761641 - Gloss Lamination